# Textbook of Neonatal Resuscitation, *6th Edition*

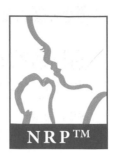

NRP™

**EDITOR**
John Kattwinkel, MD, FAAP

**ASSOCIATE EDITORS**
Jane E. McGowan, MD, FAAP
Jeanette Zaichkin, RN, MN, NNP-BC

**ASSISTANT EDITORS**
Khalid Aziz, MD, FRCPC
Christopher Colby, MD, FAAP
Marilyn Escobedo, MD, FAAP
Karen D. Fairchild, MD, FAAP
John Gallagher, RRT-NPS

Jay P. Goldsmith, MD, FAAP
Louis P. Halamek, MD, FAAP
Praveen Kumar, MD, FAAP
George A. Little, MD, FAAP
Barbara Nightengale, RN, MSN,
  NNP-BC

Jeffrey M. Perlman, MB, ChB,
  FAAP
Mildred Ramirez, MD, FACOG
Steven Ringer, MD, PhD, FAAP
Gary M. Weiner, MD, FAAP
Myra H. Wyckoff, MD, FAAP

**EDUCATIONAL DESIGN EDITOR**
Jerry Short, PhD

**MANAGING EDITORS**
Rachel Poulin, MPH
Wendy Marie Simon, MA, CAE

Based on original text by
Ronald S. Bloom, MD, FAAP
Catherine Cropley, RN, MN

*Textbook of Neonatal Resuscitation, 6th Edition, Interactive Multimedia DVD-ROM:*

**Editors**
Louis P. Halamek, MD, FAAP

Jeanette Zaichkin, RN, MN, NNP-BC

**Associate Editors**
JoDee Anderson, MD, MsEd, FAAP
Dana A. V. Braner, MD, FAAP

Susanna Lai, MPH
John Kattwinkel, MD, FAAP

**Assistant Editors**
Khalid Aziz, MD, FRCPC
Christopher Colby, MD, FAAP
Marilyn Escobedo, MD, FAAP
Karen D. Fairchild, MD, FAAP
John Gallagher, RRT-NPS
Jay P. Goldsmith, MD, FAAP

Louis P. Halamek, MD, FAAP
Praveen Kumar, MD, FAAP
Douglas T. Leonard, MD, FAAP
George A. Little, MD, FAAP
Barbara Nightengale, RN, MSN,
  NNP-BC

Jeffrey M. Perlman, MB, ChB,
  FAAP
Mildred Ramirez, MD, FACOG
Steven Ringer, MD, PhD, FAAP
Gary M. Weiner, MD, FAAP
Myra H. Wyckoff, MD, FAAP

**Contributors**
Julie Arafeh, RN, MSN
Kimberly D. Ernst, MD, MSMI,
  FAAP
Jay P. Goldsmith, MD, FAAP

Cheryl Major, RNC-NIC, BSN
Ptolemy Runkel
Scott Runkel
Bret Van Horn

**Animator**
Scott Eman

Sixth edition, 2011
Fifth edition, 2006
Fourth edition, 2000.
Third edition, 1994
Second edition, 1990
First edition, 1987

Library of Congress Catalog Card No. 2010907499

ISBN-13: 978-1-58110-498-1

NRP301

# Acknowledgments

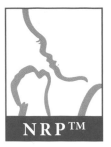

**NRP Steering Committee Members**
Louis P. Halamek, MD, FAAP, Co-chair, 2007-2011
Jane E. McGowan, MD, FAAP, Co-chair, 2009-2011
Christopher Colby, MD, FAAP
Marilyn Escobedo, MD, FAAP
Karen D. Fairchild, MD, FAAP
George A. Little, MD, FAAP
Steven Ringer, MD, PhD, FAAP
Gary M. Weiner, MD, FAAP
Myra H. Wyckoff, MD, FAAP

**Liaison Representatives**
Mildred Ramirez, MD, FACOG,
    American College of Obstetricians and Gynecologists
Barbara Nightengale, RN, MSN, NNP-BC,
    National Association of Neonatal Nurses
Praveen Kumar, MD, FAAP,
    AAP Committee on Fetus and Newborn
Khalid Aziz, MD, FRCPC,
    Canadian Paediatric Society
John Gallagher, RRT-NPS,
    American Association for Respiratory Care

**The committee would like to express thanks to the following reviewers and contributors to this textbook:**
American Academy of Pediatrics Committee on Fetus and Newborn
International Liaison Committee on Resuscitation, Neonatal Delegation
    Jeffrey M. Perlman, MB, ChB, FAAP, Co-chair
    Sam Richmond, MD, Co-chair
    Jonathan Wylie, MD
Francis Rushton, MD, FAAP, AAP Board-appointed Reviewer

**American Heart Association Emergency Cardiovascular Care Leadership**
Leon Chameides, MD, FAAP
Brian Eigel, PhD
Mary Fran Hazinski, RN, MSN
Robert Hickey, MD, FAAP
Vinay Nadkarni, MD, FAAP

**Associated Education Materials for the *Textbook of Neonatal Resuscitation, 6th Edition***

*Instructor Manual for Neonatal Resuscitation,* Jeanette Zaichkin, RN, MN, NNP-BC, Editor

*NRP Instructor DVD: An Interactive Tool for Facilitation of Simulation-based Learning,* Louis P. Halamek, MD, FAAP, and Jeanette Zaichkin, RN, MN, NNP-BC, Editors

*NRP Online Examination,* Steven Ringer, MD, PhD, FAAP, and Jerry Short, PhD, Editors

NRP Reference Chart, Code Cart Cards, and Pocket Cards, Karen D. Fairchild, MD, FAAP, Editor

NRP Simulation Poster, Louis P. Halamek, MD, FAAP, Editor

*Simply NRP*™, Gary Weiner, MD, FAAP, and Jeanette Zaichkin, RN, MN, NNP-BC, Editors

Neonatal Resuscitation Scenarios, Gary Weiner, MD, FAAP, and Jeanette Zaichkin, RN, MN, NNP-BC, Editors

## Hypix Media

Scott Runkel

Ptolemy Runkel

Bret Van Horn

## Photo Credits

Gigi O'Dea, RN, NICU at Sarasota Memorial Hospital

## AAP Life Support Staff

Wendy Marie Simon, MA, CAE

Rory K. Hand, EdM

Rachel Poulin, MPH

Kristy Crilly

Nancy Gardner

Melissa Marx

Bonnie Molnar

## NRP Education Workgroup Chair

Gary M. Weiner, MD, FAAP

## American Heart Association Emergency Cardiovascular Care Pediatric Subcommittee

Marc D. Berg, MD, FAAP, *Chair, 2009-2011*

Monica E. Kleinman, MD, FAAP,
*Immediate Past Chair, 2007-2009*

Dianne L. Atkins, MD, FAAP

Jeffrey M. Berman, MD

Kathleen Brown, MD, FAAP

Adam Cheng, MD

Laura Conley, BS, RRT, RCP, NPS

Allan R. de Caen, MD

Aaron Donoghue, MD, FAAP, MSCE

Melinda L. Fiedor Hamilton, MD, MSc

Ericka L. Fink, MD, FAAP

Eugene B. Freid, MD, FAAP

Cheryl K. Gooden, MD, FAAP

John Gosford, BS, EMT-P

Patricia Howard

Kelly Kadlec, MD, FAAP

Sharon E. Mace, MD, FAAP

Bradley S. Marino, MD, FAAP, MPP, MSCE

Reylon Meeks, RN, BSN, MS, MSN, EMT, PhD

Vinay Nadkarni, MD, FAAP

Jeffrey M. Perlman, MB, ChB, FAAP

Lester Proctor, MD, FAAP

Faiqa A. Qureshi, MD, FAAP

Kennith Hans Sartorelli, MD, FAAP

Wendy Simon, MA

Mark A. Terry, MPA, NREMT-P

Alexis Topjian, MD, FAAP

Elise W. van der Jagt, MD, FAAP, MPH

Arno Zaritsky, MD, FAAP

# Contents

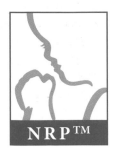

Appendix:

Evaluation Form

# Preface

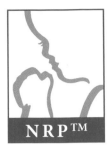

Birth is a beautiful, miraculous, and very personal event for all involved. It's an intimate and emotional time for a new mother and father when the baby they created together makes that initial cry and establishes first eye contact with the new parents. But it's also probably the single most dangerous event that most of us will ever encounter in our lifetimes. Our bodies are required to make more radical physiologic adjustments immediately following birth than they will ever have to do again. It's remarkable that more than 90% of babies make the transition from intrauterine to extrauterine life perfectly smoothly, with little to no assistance required, and it's important that we not disrupt that intimate and memorable moment for the 90% of families where an uncomplicated birth takes place smoothly. It's for the remaining few percent that the Neonatal Resuscitation Program™ (NRP™) was designed. While the proportion of newborns requiring assistance may be small, the real number of babies requiring help is substantial because of the large number of births taking place. The implications of not receiving that

help can be associated with problems that last a lifetime or even lead to death. The most gratifying aspect of providing skillful assistance to a compromised newborn is that your efforts are most likely to be successful, in contrast to the discouraging statistics associated with resuscitation attempts of adults or older children. The time that you devote to learning how to resuscitate newborns is time very well spent.

This textbook has a long history, with many pioneers from both the American Academy of Pediatrics (AAP) and the American Heart Association (AHA) responsible for its evolution. National guidelines for resuscitation of adults were initially recommended in 1966 by the National Academy of Sciences. In 1978, a Working Group on Pediatric Resuscitation was formed by the AHA Emergency Cardiac Care Committee. The group quickly concluded that resuscitation of newborns required a different emphasis than resuscitation of adults, with a focus on ventilation, rather than restitution of cardiac activity, being paramount. The formal specialty of neonatology was

evolving at about that time and, by 1985, the AAP and the AHA expressed a joint commitment to develop a training program aimed at teaching the principles of neonatal resuscitation. The pioneering leaders of this effort were George Peckham and Leon Chameides. A committee was convened to determine the appropriate format for the program, and the material written by Ron Bloom and Cathy Cropley was selected to serve as the model for the new NRP textbook. Some of the text contained in this book has been unchanged from the original textbook.

Pediatric leaders, such as Bill Keenan, Errol Alden, Ron Bloom, and John Raye, developed a strategy for disseminating the NRP. The strategy first involved training a national faculty consisting of at least one physician-nurse team from each state. The national faculty taught regional trainers who then trained hospital-based instructors. By the end of 2010, more than 2.9 million health care providers in the United States had been trained in the techniques of neonatal resuscitation—quite an accomplishment when one considers that the original goal was to strive to have at least one person trained in neonatal resuscitation in attendance in each of the approximately 5,000 delivery rooms in the United States. The NRP also has been used as a model for similar neonatal resuscitation programs in 92 other countries.

The science behind the program has also undergone significant evolution. While the ABCD (Airway, Breathing, Circulation, Drugs) principles of resuscitation have been standard for several decades, the details of how and when to accomplish each of the steps and what to do differently for newborns versus older children or adults have required constant evaluation and change. Also, while the recommendations traditionally have been based on opinions from experts in the field, recently there has been a concerted effort to base the recommendations on experimental or experiential evidence, collected from studies performed in the laboratory, randomized control studies conducted in hospitals, and observational series systematically collected from clinicians.

The AHA has addressed this evaluation process by facilitating periodic international Cardiopulmonary Resuscitation and Emergency Cardiac Care (CPR-ECC) conferences every 5 to 8 years to establish guidelines for resuscitation of all age groups and for all causes of cardiopulmonary arrest. The AAP formally joined that process in 1992 for development of the guidelines for resuscitation of children and newborns.

The most recent CPR-ECC activity took place over nearly 5 years and was conducted in 2 parts. First, starting in late 2006, a series of 32 questions identifying controversial issues regarding neonatal resuscitation were identified by the neonatology subgroup of the International Liaison Committee on Resuscitation (ILCOR), led by Jeff Perlman from the United States and Jonathan Wyllie from the United Kingdom. Individual ILCOR members were then assigned to develop worksheets for each question. Advances in computerized databases and search engines facilitated the literature review and permitted updating of the voluminous AHA detailed database of publications regarding resuscitation. The information from the worksheets was debated in a series of conferences, following which an international document titled Consensus on Cardiopulmonary Resuscitation (CPR) and Emergency Cardiovascular Care (ECC) Science With Treatment Recommendations (CoSTR) was published simultaneously in *Circulation* (2010;122[suppl 2]:S516-S538), *Resuscitation* (2010;81[suppl]:e260-287), and *Pediatrics* (2010;126;e1319-e1344). Second, each resuscitation council that makes up ILCOR was charged with developing resuscitation guidelines appropriate for the health care resources existing in (each of) its own region(s) of the world, but based on the scientific principles defined in CoSTR. The neonatal portion of the U. S. Treatment Guidelines was published in *Circulation* (2010;122:S909-S919), and *Pediatrics* (2010;126;e1400-e1413), and is reprinted in the back of this textbook. As a result of this process, each successive edition of NRP contains more recommendations that are based on evidence, rather than simply reflecting common practice. We encourage you to review the evidence and, more importantly, to conduct the future studies necessary to further define the optimum practices.

The past edition of NRP introduced 2 new chapters to address the unique challenges presented by stabilization and resuscitation of the baby born preterm (Lesson 8) and to discuss the important issues related to the ethics of neonatal resuscitation (Lesson 9). Those chapters have been retained and updated in the 6th edition. You will note a new algorithm ("flow diagram") in this edition, with the evaluation and action blocks changed to better reflect scientific format. There are a few important changes that will be recognized by the seasoned NRP student. First, the initial questions posed at the top of the flow diagram have been reduced from 4 to 3, with "clear amniotic fluid?" removed. While the guidelines for suctioning meconium from the airway have not changed, a careful review of the evidence failed to demonstrate a need to intervene with a baby born at term who is meconium stained but is breathing easily and exhibiting good muscle tone. This situation will occur in more than 10% of births and the Committee felt that such babies should not be taken from their mothers, as further assessment can be done with minimal disruption of her first moments with her new daughter or son.

Second, far more evidence has been published to strengthen our understanding that increasing the blood oxygen levels above those exhibited by healthy babies born at term provides no advantage, and that administering excessive oxygen can be injurious to tissues that have been previously compromised. Therefore, the new edition introduces new strategies for avoiding hyperoxemia. Also, several studies have demonstrated that cyanosis can be normal for the first few minutes following birth and that skin color can be a very poor indicator of oxygen saturation. Therefore, color has been removed from the list of primary clinical signs unless cyanosis is felt to be persistent, and color has been replaced by oximetry as the more reliable means of judging oxygen need. It was the consensus of the Committee that if resuscitation is anticipated or required, the goal should be to try to match the increase in blood oxygenation exhibited by the uncompromised healthy baby born at term. These observations and this recommendation will result in some changes in the equipment required and the actions indicated in the early stages of the flow diagram. Oximeters, a compressed air source, and oxygen/air blenders will need to be readily available in the birthing area and are now recommended for use whenever sustained supplemental oxygen is thought to be necessary or whenever the stage in the flow diagram is reached at which positive pressure, either as positive-pressure ventilation (PPV) or continuous positive airway pressure (CPAP), is instituted. A table has been added to designate the $SpO_2$ target goals, which have been defined by studying healthy term babies. Accommodating this change will present challenges to some small hospitals and birthing centers that may not have all of the supplies mentioned above as standard equipment.

Third, while new recommendations for resuscitation of older children and adults have shifted focus to the importance of chest compressions, with a reduced emphasis on ventilation ("C-A-B", rather than "A-B-C"), the evidence continues to support the primary importance of assuring adequate ventilation ("A-B-C") when resuscitating the newly born baby. When confronted with this difference, some learners have asked, "When is the appropriate age to switch from ABC to the new CAB?" While there is no definitive data from which to be guided for this conundrum, probably the simplest answer is to consider the likely etiology of the subject's compromise; in the case of the newly born baby, the answer will almost always be respiratory, rather than cardiac. A related observation is that some resuscitators of the newborn have appeared to be initiating chest compressions before adequate ventilation has been assured. Therefore, an additional step has been inserted in the flow diagram, involving a new pneumonic ("MR SOPA"), to ensure the provision of adequate ventilation.

There are innumerable smaller but important changes in this new edition that may be overlooked without a careful reading. Watch for a stronger emphasis in the later stages of the flow diagram on establishing vascular access, a further de-emphasis of endotracheal administration of epinephrine, and some changes in the endotracheal dose of epinephrine if it is used. Also, there are some new strategies suggested for keeping extremely low birth weight (ELBW) babies warm during the resuscitation or stabilization process, and a stronger endorsement for considering therapeutic hypothermia for the term baby who has experienced a significant hypoxic-ischemic event. There are other changes scattered throughout the program, so we encourage even veteran students to read the entire new program. Also, the Guidelines publication at the back of the textbook and the Instructor Manual summarize most of these new issues.

Production of the NRP was accomplished only through the efforts of a large number of people and several organizations. The collaborative relationships of the AHA, AAP, ILCOR, and the Pediatric Subcommittee of the AHA provided the infrastructure for developing recommendations that are more evidence-based and, therefore, internationally endorsed. The members of the NRP Steering Committee, listed in the front of this book, tirelessly debated the evidence and managed to reach consensus on a multitude of recommendations, while remaining sensitive to the practical implications of change. In particular, Gary Weiner is recognized for his innovative thinking, leading to re-formatting of the flow diagram and creating "MR SOPA." Jane McGowan and Jeanette Zaichkin are superb coeditors, with Jeanette constantly reminding us how the recommendations will be interpreted in the real world. Jill Rubino is thanked for her steadfast copyediting, as is Theresa Wiener for her production expertise and success in achieving the new multi-color capability. Staff members Sheila Lazier and her successor Rachel Poulin worked tirelessly to coordinate the tasks and keep us reasonably on schedule, despite the challenges involved with creating a complicated project with a mostly volunteer group of busy professionals.

While this textbook serves as the content foundation of NRP, the evolving structure of the Program's delivery strategy and the production of the supporting materials reflect an equal or perhaps even greater expenditure of time, innovation, and personal effort. Lou Halamek's innovativeness, knowledge, and creative thinking have been the driving force behind the new focus of NRP on coordinated resuscitation performance rather than simple knowledge acquisition, and his team of education and production specialists at the CAPE (Center for Advanced Pediatric and Perinatal Education Center at Stanford) deserve high praise for steering the NRP toward a goal of truly improving perinatal mortality and morbidity, rather than merely achieving the capability to do so.

Others that should be specifically recognized include Jeanette Zaichkin (Instructor Manual, Instructor DVD, *Simply NRP™*, and essentially every other aspect of the NRP); Jerry Short (educational design expertise throughout the entire program and more recently with the online examination); Steven Ringer, for his filming contributions for the DVD and leadership in transitioning to the online test; Cochairs Lou Halamek and Jane McGowan for their excellent leadership of the NRP Steering Committee; Jeff Perlman for his thorough knowledge of the literature and continuing advice about maintaining our adherence to the evidence; and Dana Braner, JoDee Anderson, Susanna Lai, and Scott Runkel and their teams at Oregon Health & Science University Media Lab and Hypix Media for their work on the textbook DVD. I should also mention our strategic alliance partner, Laerdal Medical, for its support in the development of new educational technologies and tools to help increase the effectiveness of skill training through *Simply NRP™* and SimNewB and its catalogue of learning scenarios. Most importantly, this program owes its success to the commitment of the AHA and the devotion of the AAP to improving and maintaining child health. However, everyone involved with the production of this complex and ambitious project will agree that one person is really responsible for making each component fall into place within budget and within the necessary time frame. She also deserves special recognition for her perceptivity in recognizing where NRP may *not* always be the most effective strategy and for advocating and facilitating development of new related initiatives such as *Helping Babies Breathe* for regions with resources less plentiful than exist in the developed World. Thank you, Wendy Simon, for all that you have done and continue to do to improve the prospects for a healthy life for newly born babies throughout the world.

*John Kattwinkel, MD, FAAP*

# Neonatal Resuscitation Program™ Provider Course Overview

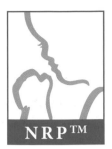

## Neonatal Resuscitation Scientific Guidelines

The Neonatal Resuscitation Program™ (NRP™) materials are based on the American Academy of Pediatrics (AAP) and American Heart Association (AHA) Guidelines for Cardiopulmonary Resuscitation and Emergency Cardiovascular Care of the Neonate (*Circulation.* 2010;122:S909-S919). A reprint of the Guidelines appears in the Appendix. Please refer to these pages if you have questions about the rationale for the current program recommendations. The Guidelines, originally published in October 2010, are based on the International Liaison Committee on Resuscitation (ILCOR) consensus on science statement. The evidence-based worksheets, prepared by members of ILCOR, which serve as the basis for both documents, can be viewed in the science area of the NRP Web site at www.aap.org/nrp.

## Level of Responsibility

The standard-length NRP Provider Course consists of 9 lessons; however, participants are eligible to receive a Course Completion Card by completing a minimum of Lessons 1 through 4 *and* Lesson 9. Resuscitation responsibilities vary from hospital to hospital, and you may be required to work through only the minimal course requirements and, perhaps, additional lessons appropriate to your level of responsibility. For example, in some institutions, nurses may be responsible for intubating the newborn, but in others, the physician or respiratory therapist may do so. The number of lessons you will need to complete depends on your personal level of responsibility and your hospital's policy for course completion requirements.

Before starting the course, you must have a clear idea of your exact responsibilities. If you have any questions about the level of your responsibilities during resuscitation, please consult your instructor or supervisor.

Special Note: Neonatal resuscitation is most effective when performed by a designated and coordinated team. It is important for you to know the neonatal resuscitation responsibilities of team members who are working with you. Periodic practice among team members will facilitate coordinated and effective care of the newborn.

## Lesson Completion

Successful completion of the online written examination is required *before* participants attend the classroom portion of the NRP course. Participants will be prompted to print a Certificate of Completion that they must bring to class and present to the instructor to be eligible for a Course Completion Card. Learners must attend the classroom portion of their NRP course within 30 days of completing the online examination. To successfully complete the course, participants must pass the required lessons of the online examination, demonstrate mastery of resuscitation skills in the Integrated Skills Station, and participate in simulated resuscitation scenarios, as determined by the course instructor(s).

Participants are encouraged to utilize *Simply NRP™* prior to attending an NRP course. *Simply NRP™* is a self-directed learning kit that provides video-based, hands-on instruction of the essential skills in the first four lessons of NRP. The kit allows learners to practice skills using the equipment required for neonatal resuscitation, including bag mask ventilation and chest compressions.

Upon successful completion of a minimum of Lessons 1 through 4 *and* Lesson 9, participants are eligible to receive a Course Completion Card. This verification of participation is not issued on the day of the course. Instructors will distribute Course Completion Cards after the Course Roster is received and processed by AAP Life Support staff. Course Completion Cards will not be distributed on the day of the course.

To learn more about online testing, please visit www.healthstream.com/hlc/aap or http://www.aap.org/nrp.

## Completion Does Not Imply Competence

The Neonatal Resuscitation Program is an educational program that introduces the concepts and basic skills of neonatal resuscitation. Completion of the program does not imply that an individual has the competence to perform neonatal resuscitation. Each hospital is responsible for determining the level of competence and qualifications required for someone to assume clinical responsibility for neonatal resuscitation.

## Standard Precautions

The US Centers for Disease Control and Prevention has recommended that standard precautions be taken whenever risk of exposure to blood or bodily fluids is high and the potential infectious status of the patient is unknown, as is certainly the case in neonatal resuscitation.

All fluid products from patients (blood, urine, stool, saliva, vomitus, etc) should be treated as potentially infectious. Gloves should be worn when resuscitating a newborn, and the rescuer should not use his or her mouth to apply suction via a suction device. Mouth-to-mouth resuscitation should be avoided by having a resuscitation bag and mask or T-piece resuscitator always available for use during resuscitation. Masks and protective eyewear or face shields should be worn during procedures that are likely to generate droplets of blood or other bodily fluids. Gowns or aprons should be worn during procedures that probably will generate splashes of blood or other bodily fluids. Delivery rooms must be equipped with resuscitation bags, masks, laryngoscopes, endotracheal tubes, mechanical suction devices, and the necessary protective shields.

### *Textbook of Neonatal Resuscitation, 6th Edition, Interactive Multimedia DVD-ROM*

The *Textbook of Neonatal Resuscitation, 6th Edition, Interactive Multimedia DVD-ROM* is located within this textbook. System requirements and content specifications are located on the inside front cover. In addition to all the content and illustrations contained in the textbook, the DVD-ROM contains footage of actual resuscitation events, laryngoscopic views of the airway, digitized animations, and several interactive video scenarios.

You may choose to learn the NRP content through reading the textbook, viewing the DVD-ROM, or a combination of the two. However, the NRP Steering Committee highly encourages learners to make use of all available resources. The DVD-ROM offers great learning value, as it shows real-time video footage of the NRP steps, and the interactive scenarios foster cognitive integration.

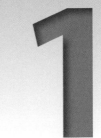

# Overview and Principles of Resuscitation

The Neonatal Resuscitation Program™ (NRP™) will help you learn to resuscitate newborns. By studying this book and practicing the skills, you will learn to be a valuable member of the resuscitation team.

Many concepts and skills are taught in the program. However, the following is the single most important concept emphasized throughout the program:

> **!** **Ventilation of the baby's lungs is the most important and effective action in neonatal resuscitation.**

## In Lesson 1 you will learn

- **The changes in physiology that occur when a baby is born**
- **The sequence of steps to follow during resuscitation**
- **The risk factors that can help predict which babies will require resuscitation**
- **The equipment and personnel needed to resuscitate a newborn**
- **The importance of communication and teamwork among team members during resuscitation**

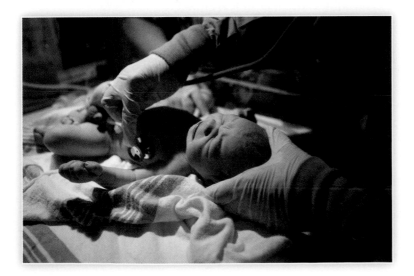

## Why learn neonatal resuscitation?

Birth asphyxia accounts for about 23% of the approximately 4 million neonatal deaths that occur each year worldwide (*Lancet.* 2010;375: 1969-1987). For many newborns, appropriate resuscitation is not readily available. Therefore, the outcomes of thousands of newborns per year can be improved by more widespread use of the resuscitation techniques taught in this program.

## Which babies require resuscitation?

Approximately 10% of newborns require some assistance to begin breathing at birth; fewer than 1% need extensive resuscitative measures to survive. In contrast, at least 90% of newly born babies make the transition from intrauterine to extrauterine life without difficulty. They require little to no assistance initiating spontaneous and regular respirations and completing the transition from the fetal to the neonatal blood-flow pattern. The presence of risk factors can help identify those who will need resuscitation, but you must always be prepared to resuscitate, as even some of those with no risk factors will require resuscitation.

> **ABCs of resuscitation:**
>
> - Airway (position and clear)
> - Breathing (stimulate to breathe)
> - Circulation (assess heart rate and oxygenation)

The "ABCs" of resuscitation are simple.* Ensure that the **A**irway is open and clear. Be sure that there is **B**reathing, whether spontaneous or assisted. Make certain that there is adequate **C**irculation of oxygenated blood. Newly born babies are wet following birth and heat loss is great. Therefore, it also is important to maintain the baby's body temperature in the normal range during resuscitation.

The diagram on the following page illustrates the relationship between resuscitation procedures and the number of newly born babies who need them. At the top are the procedures needed by all newborns. At the bottom are procedures needed by very few.

Every birth should be attended by someone who has been trained in initiating a neonatal resuscitation. Additional trained personnel are necessary when a full resuscitation is required.

---

*Note: The 2010 American Heart Association (AHA) Guidelines for CPR and ECC recommend, for adult resuscitation, that compressions be initiated before ventilations (ie, C-A-B, rather than A-B-C). However, since the etiology of newborn compromise is nearly always a breathing problem, newborn resuscitation should focus first on establishment of an airway and providing ventilation. Therefore, throughout this textbook, A-B-C will always be the recommended sequence.

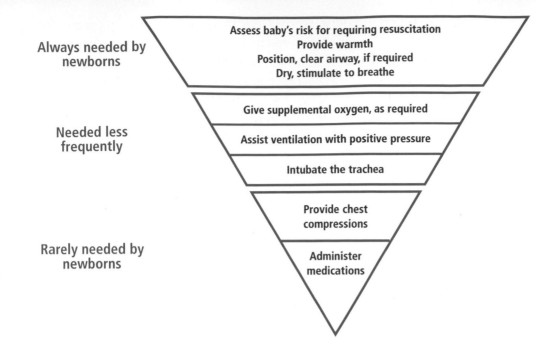

Always needed by
newborns

Assess baby's risk for requiring resuscitation
Provide warmth
Position, clear airway, if required
Dry, stimulate to breathe

Needed less
frequently

Give supplemental oxygen, as required

Assist ventilation with positive pressure

Intubate the trachea

Rarely needed by
newborns

Provide chest
compressions

Administer
medications

## Review

*(The answers are in the preceding section and at the end of the lesson.)*

1. About _____ % of newborns will require some assistance to begin regular breathing.

2. About _____ % of newborns will require extensive resuscitation to survive.

3. Careful identification of risk factors during pregnancy and labor can identify all babies who will require resuscitation. (True) (False).

4. Chest compressions and medications are (rarely) (frequently) needed when resuscitating newborns.

The Neonatal Resuscitation Program is organized in the following way:

Lesson 1: Overview and Principles of Resuscitation

Lesson 2: Initial Steps of Resuscitation

Lesson 3: Use of Resuscitation Devices for Positive-Pressure Ventilation

Lesson 4: Chest Compressions

Lesson 5: Endotracheal Intubation and Laryngeal Mask Airway Insertion

Lesson 6: Medications

Lesson 7: Special Considerations

Lesson 8: Resuscitation of Babies Born Preterm

Lesson 9: Ethics and Care at the End of Life

During your NRP course, you will have many opportunities to practice the steps involved in resuscitation and to use the appropriate resuscitation equipment. You also will work through simulated cases with other caregivers. You and the other members of the resuscitation team will gradually build proficiency and speed. In addition, you and your team will learn to evaluate a newborn together throughout the resuscitation process and make decisions about what actions to take next.

In the next section, you will learn the basic physiology involved in a baby's transition from intrauterine to extrauterine life. Understanding the physiology of breathing and circulation in the newborn will help you understand why prompt resuscitation is vital.

## How does a baby receive oxygen before birth?

Oxygen is essential for survival both before and after birth. Before birth, all the oxygen used by a fetus diffuses across the placental membrane from the mother's blood to the baby's blood.

Only a small fraction of fetal blood passes through the fetal lungs. The fetal lungs do not function as a route to transport oxygen into the blood or to excrete carbon dioxide. Therefore, blood flow to the lungs is not important to maintain normal fetal oxygenation and acid-base balance. The fetal lungs are expanded in utero, but the potential air sacs (alveoli) within the lungs are filled with fluid, rather than air. In addition, the arterioles that perfuse the fetal lungs are markedly constricted, partly due to the low partial pressure of oxygen ($Po_2$) in the fetus (Figure 1.1).

Before birth, most of the blood from the right side of the heart cannot enter the lungs because of the increased resistance to flow in the constricted blood vessels in the fetal lungs. Instead, most of this blood takes the lower resistance path through the ductus arteriosus into the aorta (Figure 1.2).

After birth, the newborn will no longer be connected to the placenta and will depend on the lungs as the only source of oxygen. Therefore, in a matter of seconds, the lung fluid must be absorbed from the alveoli, the lungs must fill with air that contains oxygen, and the blood vessels in the lungs must relax to increase blood flow to the alveoli so that oxygen can be absorbed and carried to the rest of the body.

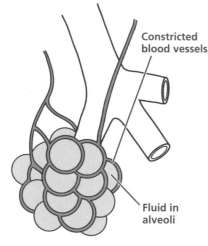

Constricted blood vessels

Fluid in alveoli

**Figure 1.1.** Fluid-filled alveoli and constricted blood vessels in the lung before birth

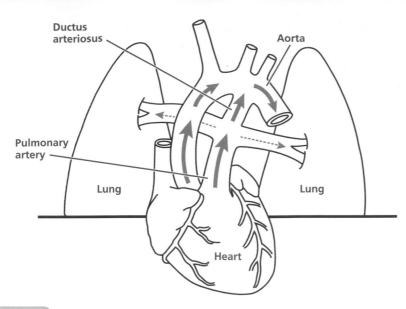

**Figure 1.2.** Shunting of blood through the ductus arteriosus and away from the lung before birth

## What normally happens at birth to allow a baby to get oxygen from the lungs?

Normally, 3 major changes begin immediately after birth.

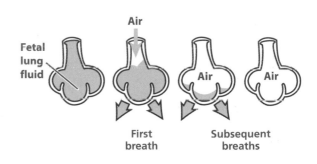

**Figure 1.3.** Fluid replaced by air in alveoli

1. The **fluid in the alveoli is absorbed** into pulmonary lymphatics and replaced by air (Figure 1.3). Because air contains 21% oxygen, filling the alveoli with air provides oxygen that can diffuse into the blood vessels that surround the alveoli.

2. The **umbilical arteries constrict and then the umbilical arteries and vein are closed when the umbilical cord is clamped.** This removes the low-resistance placental circuit and results in an increase in systemic blood pressure.

3. As a result of the distention of the alveoli with oxygen-containing gas and subsequent increased oxygen levels in the alveoli, the **blood vessels in the lung tissue relax, decreasing resistance to blood flow** (Figure 1.4).

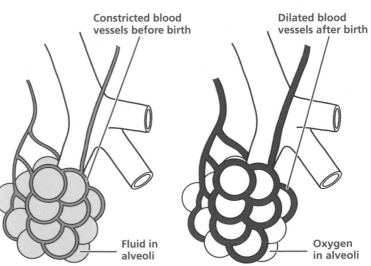

**Figure 1.4.** Dilation of pulmonary blood vessels at birth

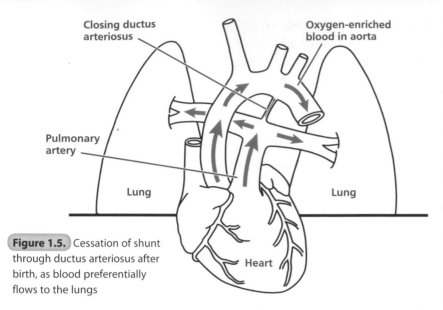

Closing ductus arteriosus

Oxygen-enriched blood in aorta

Pulmonary artery

Lung

Lung

Heart

**Figure 1.5.** Cessation of shunt through ductus arteriosus after birth, as blood preferentially flows to the lungs

This decreased resistance, together with the increased systemic blood pressure, leads to a dramatic increase in pulmonary blood flow and a decrease in flow through the ductus arteriosus. The oxygen from the alveoli is absorbed by the blood in the pulmonary vessels, and the oxygen-enriched blood returns to the left side of the heart, where it is pumped to the tissues of the newborn's body.

In most circumstances, air provides sufficient oxygen (21%) to initiate relaxation of the pulmonary blood vessels. As blood levels of oxygen increase and pulmonary blood vessels relax, the ductus arteriosus begins to constrict. Blood previously diverted through the ductus arteriosus now flows through the lungs, where it picks up more oxygen to transport to tissues throughout the body (Figure 1.5).

At the completion of this normal transition, the baby is breathing air and using his lungs to transport oxygen into his blood. His initial cries and deep breaths have been strong enough to help move the fluid from his airways. The oxygen and gaseous distention of the lungs are the main stimuli for the pulmonary blood vessels to relax. As adequate oxygen enters the blood, the baby's skin gradually turns from gray/blue to pink.

Although the initial steps in a normal transition occur within a few minutes of birth, the entire process may not be completed until hours or even several days after delivery. For example, studies have shown that, in normal newborns born at term, it may take up to 10 minutes to achieve an oxygen saturation of 90% or greater. Functional closure of the ductus arteriosus may not occur until 12 to 24 hours after birth, and complete relaxation of the lung vessels does not occur for several months.

## What can go wrong during transition?

A baby may encounter difficulty before labor, during labor, or after birth. If the difficulty begins in utero, either before or during labor, the problem usually reflects compromise in the uterine or placental blood flow. The first clinical sign can be a deceleration of the fetal heart rate, which may return to normal as steps are taken to improve placental oxygen transport, such as having the mother turn on her side, or giving the mother supplemental oxygen. Difficulties encountered after birth are more likely to reflect problems with the baby's airway and/or lungs. The following are some of the problems that may disrupt normal transition:

- *The lungs may not fill with air even when spontaneous respirations are present (inadequate ventilation).* The baby's initial breaths may not be strong enough to force fluid from the alveoli, or material such as meconium may block air from entering the alveoli. As a result, oxygen may not reach the blood circulating through the lungs.

- *The expected increase in blood pressure may not occur (systemic hypotension).* Excessive blood loss or neonatal hypoxia and ischemia may cause poor cardiac contractility or bradycardia (slow heart rate) and low blood pressure in the newborn.

- *The pulmonary arterioles may remain constricted after birth* because of complete or partial failure of gaseous distention of the lungs or lack of oxygen prior to or during delivery (persistent pulmonary hypertension of the newborn, frequently abbreviated as PPHN). As a result, blood flow to the lungs is decreased, reducing oxygen supply to body tissues. In some cases, the pulmonary arterioles may fail to relax even after the lungs are filled with air.

## How does a baby respond to an interruption in normal transition?

Normally, the newborn makes vigorous efforts immediately after birth to inhale air into the lungs. The increased pressure in the alveoli promotes absorption of fetal lung fluid. This also delivers oxygen to the pulmonary arterioles and causes the arterioles to relax. If this sequence is interrupted, the pulmonary arterioles can remain constricted, the alveoli remain filled with fluid instead of air, and the systemic arterial blood may not become oxygenated.

When the normal transition does not occur, oxygen supply to tissues is decreased, and the arterioles in the bowels, kidneys, muscles, and skin may constrict. A survival reflex maintains or increases blood flow to the heart and brain to try to keep oxygen delivery stable. This redistribution of blood flow helps preserve function of the vital organs. However, if oxygen deprivation continues, myocardial function and cardiac output ultimately deteriorate, blood pressure falls, and blood flow to all organs is reduced. The consequence of this lack of adequate blood perfusion and tissue oxygenation can be irreversible and may lead to brain damage, damage to other organs, or death.

The compromised baby may exhibit one or more of the following clinical findings:

- Depression of respiratory drive from insufficient oxygen delivery to the brain

- Poor muscle tone from insufficient oxygen delivery to the brain, muscles, and other organs

- Bradycardia from insufficient delivery of oxygen to the heart muscle or brain stem

- Tachypnea (rapid respirations) from failure to absorb fetal lung fluid

- Persistent cyanosis (blue color), or low saturation displayed on an oximeter, from insufficient oxygen in the blood

- Low blood pressure from insufficient oxygen to the heart muscle, blood loss, or insufficient blood return from the placenta before or during birth

Many of these same findings also may occur in other conditions, such as infection or hypoglycemia, or if the baby's respiratory efforts have been depressed by medications, such as narcotics or general anesthetic agents, given to the mother before birth.

## How can you tell if a newborn had in utero or perinatal compromise?

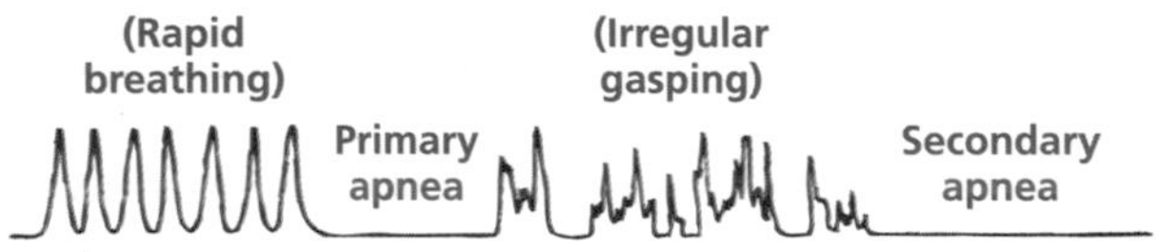

**Figure 1.6.** Primary and secondary apnea

> !
>
> **If a baby does not begin breathing immediately after being stimulated, he or she is likely in secondary apnea and will require positive-pressure ventilation. Continued stimulation will not help.**

Any problems that result in abnormal blood flow or oxygen supply in utero, during labor, and/or during delivery may compromise the status of the fetus and newborn. Laboratory studies have shown that cessation of respiratory efforts is the first sign that a newborn has had some perinatal compromise. Perinatal stress results in an initial period of rapid breathing followed by a period of *primary apnea* (no breathing or gasping) (Figure 1.6). During this period of primary apnea, stimulation, such as drying the newborn or slapping the feet, will cause a resumption of breathing.

However, if cardiorespiratory compromise continues during primary apnea, the baby will have an additional brief period of gasping breaths and then will enter a period of *secondary apnea* (Figure 1.6). During secondary apnea, stimulation will *not* restart the baby's breathing. Assisted ventilation must be provided to reverse the process.

Heart rate begins to fall at about the same time that the baby enters primary apnea. Blood pressure usually is maintained until the onset of secondary apnea unless blood loss has resulted in an earlier onset of hypotension (Figure 1.7).

Most of the time, the baby will be presented to you somewhere in the middle of the sequence described above. Often, the compromising event will have started before or during labor. Therefore, at the time of birth, it will be difficult to determine how long the baby's oxygenation and/or circulation have been compromised. Physical examination will not allow you to distinguish between primary and secondary apnea. However, the respiratory response to stimulation may help you estimate how recently the event began. If the baby begins breathing as soon as she is stimulated, she was in primary apnea; if she does not breathe right away, she is in secondary apnea and respiratory support must be initiated.

As a general rule, the longer a baby has been in secondary apnea, the longer it will take for spontaneous breathing to resume. However, the graph in Figure 1.8 demonstrates that, as soon as ventilation is established, most compromised newborns will show a very rapid improvement in heart rate.

If effective positive-pressure ventilation (PPV) does not result in a rapid increase in heart rate, the duration of the compromising event may have been such that myocardial function has deteriorated and blood pressure has fallen below a critical level. Under these circumstances, chest compressions and, possibly, medications will be required for resuscitation.

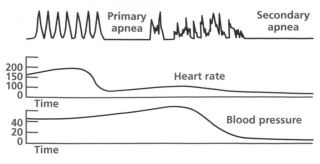

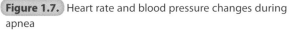

**Figure 1.7.** Heart rate and blood pressure changes during apnea

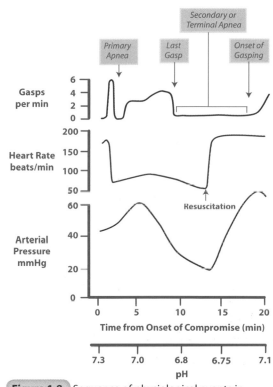

**Figure 1.8.** Sequence of physiological events in animal models from multiple species involving complete total asphyxia. Note the prompt increase in heart rate as soon as resuscitation is begun.

# Review

*(The answers are in the preceding section and at the end of the lesson.)*

5. Before birth, the alveoli in a baby's lungs are (collapsed) (expanded) and filled with (fluid) (air).

6. The air that fills the baby's alveoli during normal transition contains _____% oxygen.

7. The air in the baby's lungs causes the pulmonary arterioles to (relax) (constrict) so that the oxygen can be absorbed from the alveoli and distributed to all organs.

8. If a baby does not begin breathing in response to stimulation, you should assume she is in _____ apnea and you should provide _____.

9. If a baby enters the stage of secondary apnea, her heart rate will (rise) (fall) and her blood pressure will (rise) (fall).

10. Restoration of adequate ventilation usually will result in a (rapid) (gradual) (slow) improvement in heart rate.

## The resuscitation flow diagram

This flow diagram describes the steps necessary to determine the need for resuscitation and all the NRP resuscitation procedures. The diamonds indicate assessments and the rectangles show actions that may be required, depending on the result of the assessment. The diagram begins with the birth of the baby. Study the diagram as you read the description of each step and decision point. This diagram will be repeated in later lessons. Use it to help you remember the steps involved in a resuscitation.

*Initial Assessment Block.* At the time of birth, you should ask yourself 3 questions about the newborn: Was he born at term, is he breathing or crying, and does he have good tone (Figure 1.9)? If the answer to all 3 is "Yes," the baby should stay with the mother, where further stabilization and assessment can take place. If any answer is "No," you should continue to the initial steps of resuscitation.

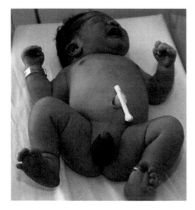

**Figure 1.9.** Normal newborn born at term. He is crying and has good tone.

**A** *Block A (Airway).* These are the initial steps you take to establish an Airway and begin resuscitating a newborn.

- Provide warmth, which can be accomplished by covering the baby with a towel and placing him skin-to-skin with mother, or, if the answer to any of the 3 questions is "No," placing him under a radiant warmer on a resuscitation table, where subsequent resuscitation can take place more easily.

- Position the head to open the airway. Clear the airway as necessary. Clearing the airway may involve suctioning the trachea to remove meconium; this procedure will be described in Lessons 2 and 5.

- Dry the skin, stimulate the baby to breathe, and reposition the head to maintain an open airway.

*Evaluation of the effect of Block A.* You evaluate the newborn during and immediately following these first interventions, which generally takes no more than 30 seconds to complete. You should simultaneously evaluate respirations and heart rate. If the newborn is not breathing (has apnea or is gasping) or has a heart rate below 100 beats per minute (bpm), you proceed immediately to Block B (left side). If the respirations appear labored or the baby appears persistently cyanotic, you proceed to Block B (right side).

Ⓑ *Block B (Breathing).* If the baby has apnea or has a heart rate below 100 bpm, you immediately begin to assist the baby's **B**reathing by providing PPV. If the baby is breathing but has persistent respiratory distress, many clinicians would administer continuous positive airway pressure (CPAP) with a mask, particularly if the baby was born preterm. If you initiate either PPV or CPAP, you should attach an oximeter to determine the need for supplemental oxygen. The technique of oximetry and interpretation of the oxygen saturation table shown in the resuscitation flow diagram will be discussed in Lesson 2.

*Evaluation of the effect of Block B.* After about 30 seconds of effective PPV, CPAP, and/or supplemental oxygen, you evaluate the newborn again to ensure that ventilation is adequate. It is critical to ensure that effective ventilation is being provided before moving to the next steps of resuscitation. In almost all cases, with appropriate ventilation technique, the heart rate will increase above 100 bpm. However, if the heart rate is below 60 bpm, you proceed to Block C.

Ⓒ *Block C (Circulation).* You support **C**irculation by starting chest compressions. Endotracheal intubation is strongly recommended at this point, if not already done, to facilitate and coordinate effective chest compressions and PPV.

*Evaluation of the effect of Block C.* After administering chest compressions and PPV, you evaluate the newborn again. If the heart rate is still below 60 bpm despite ventilation and chest compressions, you proceed to Block D.

Ⓓ *Block D (Drug).* You administer epinephrine as you continue PPV and chest compressions.

*Evaluation of the effect of Block D.* If the heart rate remains below 60 bpm, the actions in Blocks C and D are continued and repeated. This is indicated by the lower curved arrow.

When the heart rate improves and rises above 60 bpm, chest compressions are stopped. Positive-pressure ventilation is continued until the heart rate is above 100 bpm and the baby is breathing. Supplemental oxygen and/or CPAP can be administered, if necessary, based on oxygen saturation as measured by pulse oximetry ($Spo_2$). Care should be taken to avoid allowing the $Spo_2$ to exceed 95%. (See Lesson 2.)

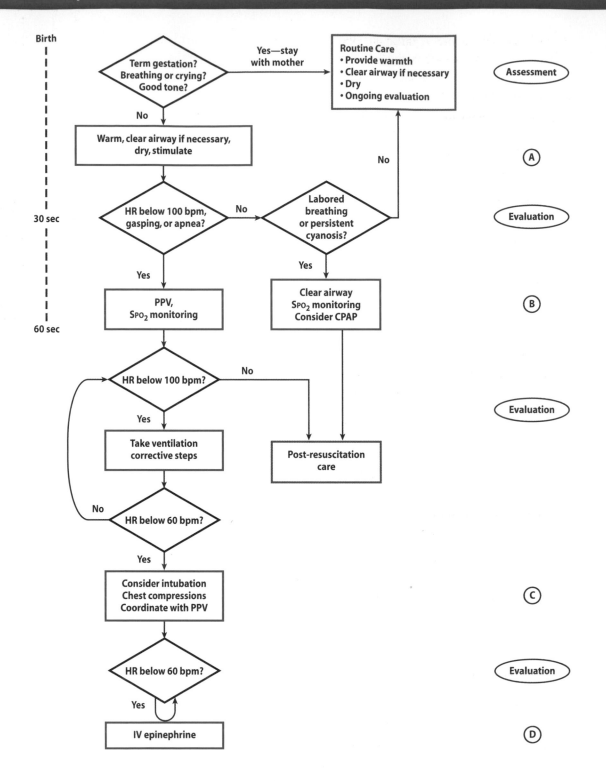

**Birth**

Term gestation?
Breathing or crying?
Good tone?

Yes—stay
with mother

**Routine Care**
• Provide warmth
• Clear airway if necessary
• Dry
• Ongoing evaluation

Assessment

No

Warm, clear airway if necessary,
dry, stimulate

Ⓐ

No

30 sec

HR below 100 bpm,
gasping, or apnea?

No

Labored
breathing
or persistent
cyanosis?

Evaluation

Yes

Yes

PPV,
SPO₂ monitoring

Clear airway
SPO₂ monitoring
Consider CPAP

Ⓑ

60 sec

HR below 100 bpm?

No

Evaluation

Yes

Take ventilation
corrective steps

Post-resuscitation
care

No

HR below 60 bpm?

Yes

Consider intubation
Chest compressions
Coordinate with PPV

Ⓒ

HR below 60 bpm?

Evaluation

Yes

IV epinephrine

Ⓓ

Evaluation occurs after initiation of each action and is based on
primarily the following 3 signs:

- Respirations

- Heart rate

- Assessment of oxygenation (color or, preferably, oximetry reading)

You will decide whether a particular step is effective by assessing each of these 3 signs. Although you will evaluate all 3 signs simultaneously, a low heart rate is most important for determining whether you should proceed to the next step. This process of evaluation, decision, and action is repeated frequently throughout resuscitation.

Note the following important points about the flow diagram:

- There are 2 heart rates to remember: 60 bpm and 100 bpm. In general, a heart rate below 60 bpm indicates that additional resuscitation steps are needed. A heart rate above 100 bpm usually indicates that resuscitation procedures beyond those in Block A can be stopped, unless the patient is apneic or has persistent low oxygen saturation levels.

- The asterisks (*) indicate points at which you should consider endotracheal intubation. The first point is for the special situation of removing meconium from the airway; intubation at the other points in resuscitation will optimize the most important step in neonatal resuscitation (ventilation) and/or maximize the efficacy of chest compressions.

- The primary actions in neonatal resuscitation are aimed at ventilating the baby's lungs (Blocks A and B). Once this has been accomplished, heart rate, blood pressure, and pulmonary blood flow usually will improve spontaneously, assuming there is continued *effective* ventilation. However, if blood and tissue oxygen levels are low, cardiac output may have to be assisted by chest compressions and epinephrine (Blocks C and D) for blood to reach the lungs to pick up oxygen. **Do not progress to chest compressions until you have assured adequate ventilation.**

- Although delivering oxygen to the heart and other tissues is important, excessive oxygen can also injure tissues. Therefore, from Block B forward it will be important to guide your use of supplemental oxygen by attaching an oximeter to the baby.

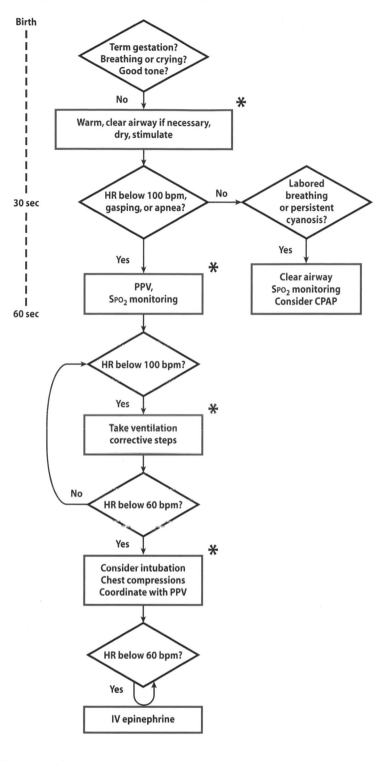

## How do you prioritize your actions?

It may take several hours for you to learn how to evaluate a baby's condition and how to perform each of the resuscitation steps. However, in the real world, you will need to implement them over seconds to minutes if you are to save a baby's life.

Think in terms of 30-second intervals as you progress through the flow diagram.

- As soon as a baby is born and handed to you and your team, you should be able to ask yourself the initial questions and perform the initial steps within approximately 30 seconds. Slightly more time may be required if special actions, such as suctioning of meconium, are required, as will be described in a later chapter.

- You should allow no more than another 30 seconds to go by to further stimulate the baby to breathe. Continuing to stimulate an apneic baby will be a waste of valuable time. The first 60 seconds after birth has been called "the Golden Minute®." If clearing the airway and stimulating the baby to breathe has not resulted in improvement after no more than 60 seconds from birth, you should begin PPV.

- The next 30 seconds should be spent evaluating respirations, heart rate, and oxygenation, and instituting respiratory support measures. Additional team members should be summoned at this point to assist with attaching an oximeter and to be available if more advanced resuscitation measures are required. If the heart rate has not improved, you should assure yourself that PPV is being performed effectively. If it is not, you should correct your technique and evaluate effectiveness again in 30 seconds. Do not proceed to the next step (Block C) until you assure yourself that PPV is being performed effectively. During this time, another member of the resuscitation team may start preparing an umbilical catheter to be used for administration of drugs, in case the next step should become necessary.

- Once you have started to administer chest compressions, you should evaluate the heart rate periodically to decide if chest compressions should be continued; however, frequent interruptions of chest compressions should be avoided as this will impair delivery of oxygenated blood to the heart.

- If the heart rate is still below 60 bpm, and PPV and chest compressions are being performed appropriately, you should move to the next step (Block D).

*Now take time to become familiar with the flow diagram, and learn the order of steps that will be presented in the following lessons. Also learn the heart rates you use to decide if the next step is needed.*

**Work as a team to accomplish each step.**

## Why is the Apgar score *not* used to guide resuscitation?

The Apgar score is an objective method of quantifying the newborn's condition and is useful for conveying information about the newborn's overall status and response to resuscitation. However, resuscitation must be initiated before the 1-minute score is assigned. Therefore, *the Apgar score is not used to determine the need for resuscitation, what resuscitation steps are necessary, or when to use them.* The 3 signs that you will use to decide how and when to resuscitate (respirations, heart rate, and color or oximetry assessment of oxygenation) do form part of the score. Two additional elements (muscle tone and reflex irritability) reflect neurologic status. It should be noted that the values of the individual elements of the score will be different if the baby is being resuscitated; therefore, the record should indicate what resuscitation measures, if any, are being taken each time the score is assigned. (See special form in the Appendix of this lesson.)

The Apgar score normally is assigned at 1 minute and again at 5 minutes of age. When the 5-minute score is less than 7, additional scores should be assigned every 5 minutes for up to 20 minutes. Although the Apgar score is not a good predictor of outcome, the change of score at sequential time points following birth can reflect how well the baby is responding to resuscitative efforts. The elements of the Apgar score are described in the Appendix at the end of this lesson.

## How do you prepare for a resuscitation?

At every birth, you should be prepared to resuscitate a newborn because the need for resuscitation can come as a complete surprise. For this reason, every birth should be attended by at least 1 person skilled in neonatal resuscitation whose only responsibility is management of the newborn. Additional personnel will be needed and should be immediately available in case resuscitation that is more complex is required. Those additional personnel should be at the delivery if the need for resuscitation is anticipated, as described in the next section.

With careful consideration of perinatal risk factors, more than half of all newborns who will need resuscitation can be identified prior to birth. If you anticipate the possible need for neonatal resuscitation, you should

- Recruit additional skilled personnel to be present at the delivery.

- Prepare all equipment that may be necessary.

# What risk factors may be associated with the need for neonatal resuscitation?

*Review this list of risk factors.*

*Consider having a copy readily available in the labor and delivery areas.*

## Antepartum Factors

| | |
|---|---|
| Maternal diabetes | Post-term gestation |
| Gestational hypertension or preeclampsia | Multiple gestation |
| Chronic hypertension | Size-dates discrepancy |
| Fetal anemia or isoimmunization | Drug therapy, such as magnesium |
| Previous fetal or neonatal death | Adrenergic agonists |
| Bleeding in second or third trimester | Maternal substance abuse |
| Maternal infection | Fetal malformation or anomalies |
| Maternal cardiac, renal, pulmonary, thyroid, or neurologic disease | Diminished fetal activity |
| Polyhydramnios | No prenatal care |
| Oligohydramnios | Mother older than 35 years |
| Premature rupture of membranes | |
| Fetal hydrops | |

## Intrapartum Factors

| | |
|---|---|
| Emergency cesarean section | Category 2 or 3 fetal heart rate patterns |
| Forceps or vacuum-assisted delivery | Use of general anesthesia |
| Breech or other abnormal presentation | Uterine tachysystole with fetal heart rate changes |
| Premature labor | Narcotics administered to mother within 4 hours of delivery |
| Precipitous labor | Meconium-stained amniotic fluid |
| Chorioamnionitis | Prolapsed cord |
| Prolonged rupture of membranes (>18 hours before delivery) | Abruptio placentae |
| Prolonged labor (>24 hours) | Placenta previa |
| Macrosomia | Significant intrapartum bleeding |

**!** **Always be prepared to resuscitate. Although identifying risk factors will be helpful to identify some at-risk babies, there still will be some with no risk factors who will need resuscitation.**

## Why are premature babies at higher risk?

Many of these risk factors may result in a baby being born before 37 completed weeks of gestation. Premature babies have anatomical and physiological characteristics that are quite different from babies born at term. These characteristics include

- Lungs deficient in surfactant, which may make ventilation difficult

- Immature brain development, which may decrease the drive to breathe

- Weak muscles, which may make spontaneous breathing more difficult

- Thin skin, large surface area, and decreased fat, which contribute to rapid heat loss

- Higher likelihood of being born with an infection

- Very fragile blood vessels in the brain, which may bleed during periods of stress

- Small blood volume, increasing susceptibility to the hypovolemic effects of blood loss

- Immature tissues, which may be more easily damaged by excessive oxygen

These and other aspects of prematurity should alert you to seek extra help when anticipating a preterm birth. The specific procedures and precautions associated with resuscitation of a premature baby will be presented in Lesson 8.

## What personnel should be present at delivery?

At every delivery, there should be at least 1 person in the delivery room who can be immediately available to the baby as his or her only responsibility and who is capable of initiating resuscitation, including administration of PPV and assisting with chest compressions. Either this person or someone else who is immediately available to the delivery area should have the necessary additional skills required to perform a complete resuscitation, including endotracheal intubation and administration of medications. It is not sufficient to have someone "on call" (either at home or in a remote area of the hospital) for newborn resuscitations in the delivery room. When resuscitation is needed, it must be initiated without delay.

If the delivery is anticipated to be high risk because of the presence of risk factors identified before birth, such as meconium staining of the amniotic fluid, more advanced neonatal resuscitation may be required. In these cases, at least 2 persons should be present solely to manage the baby—1 with complete resuscitation skills and 1 or more to assist. The goal is to provide a "resuscitation team," with a specified leader and an identified role for each member. (For multiple births, a separate complete team should be present in the delivery room for each baby.)

For example, if a delivery room nurse is present at an uncomplicated birth, this nurse might clear the airway if necessary, provide tactile stimulation, and evaluate the respirations and heart rate. If the newborn does not respond appropriately, the nurse would initiate PPV and call for assistance. A second person would help assess the efficacy of PPV. A physician or other health care professional with full resuscitation skills should be in the immediate vicinity and available to intubate the trachea and assist with coordinated chest compressions and ventilation, and to order medication.

In the case of an anticipated high-risk birth, 2, 3, or even 4 people with varying degrees of resuscitation skills may be needed at the delivery. One of them, with complete resuscitation skills, would serve as the leader of the team and would probably be the one to position the baby, open the airway, and intubate the trachea, if necessary. Two others would assist with positioning, suctioning, drying, and giving oxygen. They could administer PPV or chest compressions as directed by the leader. A fourth person would be helpful for administering medications and/or documenting the events.

## How can the team most effectively work together during a resuscitation?

Behavioral skills, such as teamwork, leadership, and efficient communication, are critical to successful resuscitation of the neonate. Even though individual team members may possess the knowledge and skills for a complete resuscitation, they will not be able to utilize these skills effectively if they are unable to communicate and coordinate with the other members of the team while working under the intense time pressure of a neonatal resuscitation. Because there may be several teams of caregivers (eg, obstetrics, anesthesia, and pediatrics/neonatology) in the delivery room, effective communication and coordination of interventions is critical. There is evidence that communication skills may be as important to the success of a neonatal resuscitation as performance of ventilation and chest compressions.

- Know your environment.
- Anticipate and plan.
- Assume the leadership role.
- Communicate effectively.
- Delegate workload optimally.
- Allocate attention wisely.
- Use all available information.
- Use all available resources.
- Call for help when needed.
- Maintain professional behavior.

(From the Center for Advanced Pediatric & Perinatal Education [CAPE], Lucile Packard Children's Hospital at Stanford University, http://www.cape.lpch.org.)

Thus, skills such as effective communication and assignment of tasks should be practiced regularly under conditions that are as realistic as possible, just as you practice bag-and-mask ventilation.

## What equipment should be available?

All the equipment necessary for a complete resuscitation must be in the delivery room and be fully operational. When a high-risk newborn is expected, appropriate equipment should be ready for immediate use. A complete list of neonatal resuscitation equipment is in the Appendix at the end of this lesson.

A baby in need of resuscitation should be moved quickly from the mother to a radiant warmer where caregivers can concentrate on evaluation and appropriate support.

All team members should know how to check for the presence and function of resuscitation equipment and supplies. It is not sufficient to simply look at what is on the radiant warmer. It is much more effective to establish an organized routine for checking equipment prior to every birth. In this way, you are checking for not only what is ready and available for resuscitation, you also will discover which pieces of equipment are missing. There are 2 equipment lists in the Appendix of this lesson. The "Neonatal Resuscitation Supplies and Equipment" lists all of the supplies needed to stock the resuscitation area. The "NRP Quick Pre-resuscitation Checklist" enables you to check your essential equipment and supplies in the same order as they are used according to the NRP flow diagram. Post the Pre-resuscitation Checklist and use it to check readiness of supplies and equipment prior to every birth.

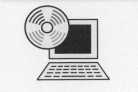

**You are encouraged to view this video on the DVD that accompanies this textbook:** *Equipment Check*

# What do you do after a resuscitation?

Babies who have required resuscitation are at risk even after their vital signs have returned to normal. You learned earlier in this lesson that the longer a baby has been compromised, the longer he or she will take to respond to resuscitation efforts. The NRP will refer to the following 2 levels of post-resuscitation care:

*Routine Care:* Nearly 90% of newborns are vigorous term babies with no risk factors. Similarly, babies who have prenatal or intrapartum risk factors, but have responded to the initial steps, will need close observation, but may not need to be separated from their mothers after birth to receive close monitoring and further stabilization. Thermoregulation can be provided by putting the baby directly on the mother's chest, drying the baby, and covering her with dry linen. Warmth is maintained by direct skin-to-skin contact with the mother. Clearing of the upper airway can be provided as necessary by wiping the baby's mouth and nose. It is recommended that suctioning following birth (including suctioning with a bulb syringe) should be reserved for babies who have obvious obstruction to spontaneous breathing or who require PPV. While the initial steps can be provided in modified form, ongoing observation of breathing, activity, and color must be carried out to determine any need for additional intervention.

*Post-resuscitation Care:* Babies who have depressed breathing or activity, and/or require supplemental oxygen to achieve target oximetry $Spo_2$ readings that match target levels will need closer assessment. These babies may still be at risk for developing problems associated with perinatal compromise and should be evaluated *frequently* during the immediate neonatal period. While some may be able to receive routine newborn care, many will require admission to a transitional area of the newborn nursery where cardiorespiratory monitoring is available and vital signs may be taken frequently. These babies often require ongoing support, such as mechanical ventilation, nasal CPAP, and/or administration of supplemental oxygen. They are at high risk for further episodes of altered cardiorespiratory status, and are also at risk for developing subsequent complications of an abnormal transition. Given these concerns, such babies generally should be managed in an environment where ongoing evaluation and monitoring are available. Transfer to an intensive care nursery may be necessary. Even in these cases, parents should be permitted and encouraged to see, touch, and, if possible, hold their baby, depending on the degree of stability.

Details of post-resuscitation care will be presented in Lesson 7.

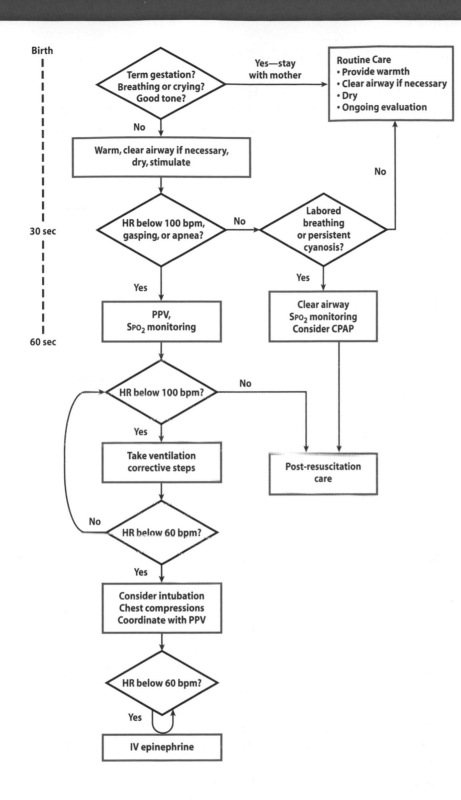

Birth

Term gestation?
Breathing or crying?
Good tone?

Yes—stay
with mother

Routine Care
• Provide warmth
• Clear airway if necessary
• Dry
• Ongoing evaluation

No

Warm, clear airway if necessary,
dry, stimulate

30 sec

HR below 100 bpm,
gasping, or apnea?

No

Labored
breathing
or persistent
cyanosis?

No

Yes

Yes

60 sec

PPV,
SpO₂ monitoring

Clear airway
SpO₂ monitoring
Consider CPAP

HR below 100 bpm?

No

Yes

Take ventilation
corrective steps

Post-resuscitation
care

No

HR below 60 bpm?

Yes

Consider intubation
Chest compressions
Coordinate with PPV

HR below 60 bpm?

Yes

IV epinephrine

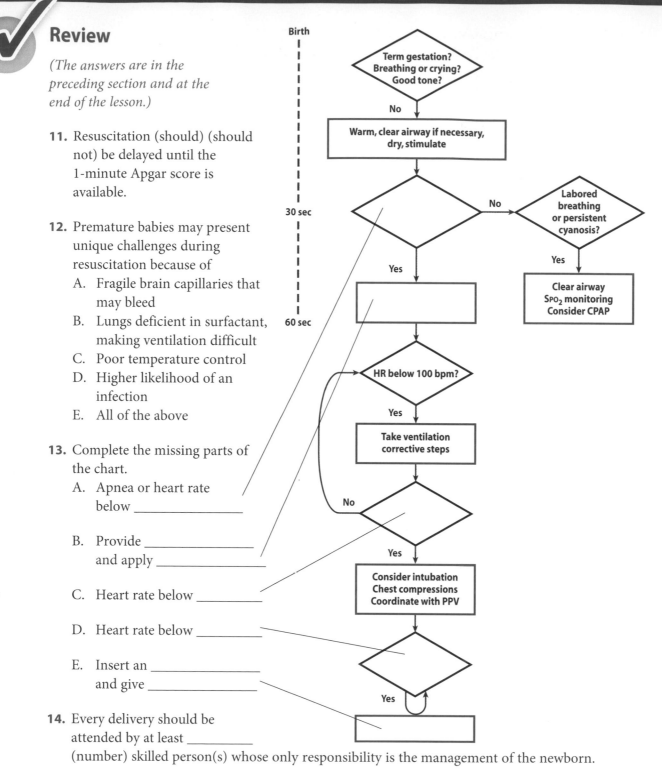

### Review

*(The answers are in the preceding section and at the end of the lesson.)*

**11.** Resuscitation (should) (should not) be delayed until the 1-minute Apgar score is available.

**12.** Premature babies may present unique challenges during resuscitation because of
  A. Fragile brain capillaries that may bleed
  B. Lungs deficient in surfactant, making ventilation difficult
  C. Poor temperature control
  D. Higher likelihood of an infection
  E. All of the above

**13.** Complete the missing parts of the chart.
  A. Apnea or heart rate below _____

  B. Provide _____ and apply _____

  C. Heart rate below _____

  D. Heart rate below _____

  E. Insert an _____ and give _____

**14.** Every delivery should be attended by at least _____ (number) skilled person(s) whose only responsibility is the management of the newborn.

**15.** If a high-risk delivery is anticipated, at least _____ (number) skilled person(s), whose only responsibility is resuscitation and the management of the baby, should be present at the delivery.

Flowchart labels:

Birth

Term gestation? Breathing or crying? Good tone? — No → Warm, clear airway if necessary, dry, stimulate

30 sec

(decision diamond) — No → Labored breathing or persistent cyanosis? — Yes → Clear airway SpO₂ monitoring Consider CPAP

Yes

60 sec

HR below 100 bpm? — Yes → Take ventilation corrective steps

No

Yes → Consider intubation Chest compressions Coordinate with PPV

Yes

16. When a depressed newborn is anticipated at a delivery, resuscitation equipment (should) (should not) be unpacked and ready for use.

17. A baby who was meconium stained and not vigorous at birth had meconium suctioned from the trachea and continued to require supplemental oxygen to keep oxygen saturation as measured by pulse oximetry (SpO$_2$) >85%. As soon as the heart rate is above 100 bpm, this baby should receive (routine) (post-resuscitation) care.

18. When twins are expected, there should be _____(number) people present in the delivery room to form the resuscitation team.

## Key Points

1. Most newly born babies are vigorous. Only about 10% require some kind of assistance and only 1% need major resuscitative measures (intubation, chest compressions, and/or medications) to survive.

2. The most important and effective action in neonatal resuscitation is to ventilate the baby's lungs.

3. Lack of ventilation of the newborn's lungs results in sustained constriction of the pulmonary arterioles, preventing systemic arterial blood from becoming oxygenated. Prolonged lack of adequate perfusion and oxygenation to the baby's organs can lead to brain damage, damage to other organs, or death.

4. When a fetus/newborn first becomes compromised, an initial period of attempted rapid breathing is followed by primary apnea and decreasing heart rate that will improve with tactile stimulation. If compromise continues, secondary apnea ensues, accompanied by a continued fall in heart rate and blood pressure. Secondary apnea cannot be reversed with stimulation; assisted ventilation must be provided.

5. Initiation of effective positive-pressure ventilation during secondary apnea usually results in a rapid improvement in heart rate.

6. Many, but not all, babies who will require neonatal resuscitation can be anticipated by identifying the presence of antepartum and intrapartum risk factors associated with the need for neonatal resuscitation.

7. All newborns require initial assessment to determine whether resuscitation is required.

## Key Points—*continued*

8. Every birth should be attended by at least 1 person whose only responsibility is the baby and who is capable of initiating resuscitation. Either that person or someone else who is immediately available should have the necessary additional skills required to perform a complete resuscitation. When resuscitation is anticipated, additional personnel should be present in the delivery room before the delivery occurs.

9. Resuscitation should proceed rapidly.
   - You have approximately 30 seconds to achieve a response from one step before deciding whether you need to go on to the next.
   - Evaluation and decision making are based primarily on respirations, heart rate, and oxygenation.

10. Behavioral skills such as teamwork, leadership, and effective communication are critical to successful resuscitation of the newborn.

11. The steps of neonatal resuscitation are as follows:
    A. Initial steps.
       - Provide warmth.
       - Position head and clear airway as necessary.*
       - Dry and stimulate the baby to breathe.
       - Evaluate respirations, heart rate, and oxygenation.
    B. Provide positive-pressure ventilation with a resuscitation positive-pressure device and apply pulse oximeter.*
    C. Provide chest compressions as you continue assisted ventilation and insert emergency umbilical venous catheter.*
    D. Administer epinephrine as you continue assisted ventilation and chest compressions.*

    *Consider intubation of the trachea at these points.

## Lesson 1 Review

*(The answers follow.)*

1. About _____% of newborns will require some assistance to begin regular breathing.

2. About _____% of newborns will require extensive resuscitation to survive.

3. Careful identification of risk factors during pregnancy and labor can identify all babies who will require resuscitation. (True) (False).

4. Chest compressions and medications are (rarely) (frequently) needed when resuscitating newborns.

5. Before birth, the alveoli in a baby's lungs are (collapsed) (expanded) and filled with (fluid) (air).

6. The air that fills the baby's alveoli during normal transition contains _____% oxygen.

7. The air in the baby's lungs causes the pulmonary arterioles to (relax) (constrict) so that the oxygen can be absorbed from the alveoli and distributed to all organs.

8. If a baby does not begin breathing in response to stimulation, you should assume she is in _____ apnea and you should provide _____.

9. If a baby enters the stage of secondary apnea, her heart rate will (rise) (fall), and her blood pressure will (rise) (fall).

10. Restoration of adequate ventilation usually will result in a (rapid) (gradual) (slow) improvement in heart rate.

11. Resuscitation (should) (should not) be delayed until the 1-minute Apgar score is available.

12. Premature babies may present unique challenges during resuscitation because of
    A. Fragile brain capillaries that may bleed
    B. Lungs deficient in surfactant, making ventilation difficult
    C. Poor temperature control
    D. Higher likelihood of an infection
    E. All of the above

## Lesson 1 Review—*continued*

**13.** Complete the missing parts of the chart.

A. Apnea or heart rate below _____

B. Provide _____ and apply _____

C. Heart rate below _____

D. Heart rate below _____

E. Insert an _____ and give _____

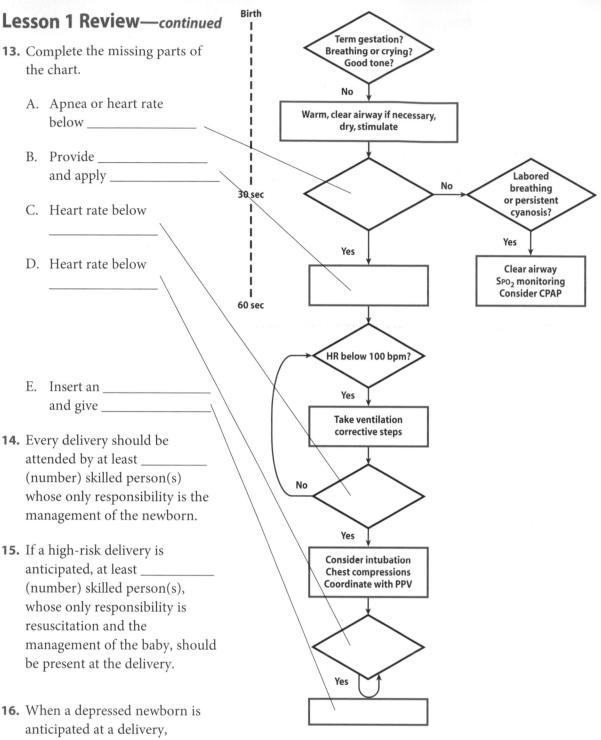

Birth

Term gestation?
Breathing or crying?
Good tone?

No

Warm, clear airway if necessary, dry, stimulate

No → Labored breathing or persistent cyanosis?

30 sec

Yes

60 sec

Yes → Clear airway
SPO₂ monitoring
Consider CPAP

HR below 100 bpm?

Yes

Take ventilation corrective steps

No

Yes

Consider intubation
Chest compressions
Coordinate with PPV

Yes

**14.** Every delivery should be attended by at least _____ (number) skilled person(s) whose only responsibility is the management of the newborn.

**15.** If a high-risk delivery is anticipated, at least _____ (number) skilled person(s), whose only responsibility is resuscitation and the management of the baby, should be present at the delivery.

**16.** When a depressed newborn is anticipated at a delivery, resuscitation equipment (should) (should not) be unpacked and ready for use.

**17.** A baby who was meconium stained and not vigorous at birth had meconium suctioned from the trachea and continued to require supplemental oxygen to keep oxygen saturation as measured by pulse oximetry (SPO₂) >85%. As soon as the heart rate is above 100 bpm, this baby should receive (routine) (post-resuscitation) care.

**18.** When twins are expected, there should be _____(number) people present in the delivery room to form the resuscitation team.

## Lesson 1 Answers to Questions

1. 10%.

2. 1%.

3. False.

4. Chest compressions and medications are **rarely** needed when resuscitating newborns.

5. Before birth, the alveoli are **expanded** and filled with **fluid.**

6. The air that fills the baby's alveoli during normal transition contains **21%** oxygen.

7. Oxygen in the air causes pulmonary arterioles to **relax.**

8. You should assume **secondary apnea** and you should provide **positive-pressure ventilation.**

9. The baby's heart rate will **fall,** and her blood pressure will **fall.**

10. Ventilation usually will result in a **rapid** improvement in heart rate.

11. Resuscitation **should not** be delayed until the 1 minute Apgar score is available.

12. Premature babies have fragile brain capillaries, immature lungs, and poor temperature control, and are more likely to have an infection. Therefore, **all of the above** is the correct answer.

13. A.  Apnea or heart rate below **100 beats per minute.**
    B.  Provide **positive-pressure ventilation** and apply **an oximeter** ($Sp_{O_2}$) **monitor.**
    C.  Heart rate below **60 beats per minute.**
    D.  Heart rate below **60 beats per minute.**
    E.  Insert an **intravenous line (umbilical catheter)** and give **epinephrine IV.**

14. Every delivery should be attended by at least **1** skilled person.

15. At least **2** skilled persons should be present at a high-risk delivery.

16. Equipment **should** be unpacked if a newborn is anticipated to be depressed at delivery.

17. Since the baby required continuous supplemental oxygen, he should receive **post-resuscitation** care.

18. There should be **4** people present in the delivery room to form the resuscitation team prepared to resuscitate (2 for each baby).

## Lesson 1: Equipment Check Performance Checklist

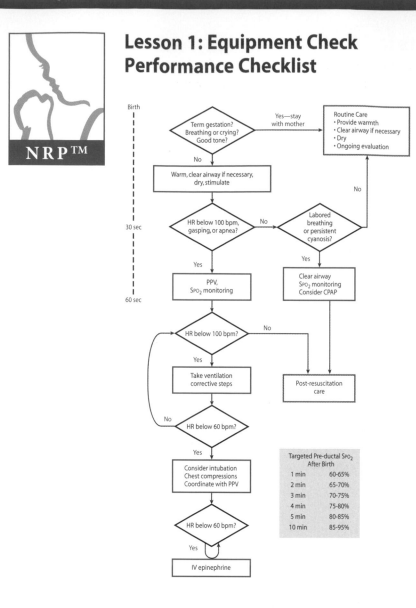

### The Performance Checklist Is a Learning Tool

The learner uses the checklist as a reference during independent practice, or as a guide for discussion and practice with a Neonatal Resuscitation Program (NRP) instructor. When the learner and instructor agree that the learner can perform the skills correctly and smoothly without coaching and within the context of a scenario, the learner may move on to the next lesson's Performance Checklist.

This Equipment Check Performance Checklist includes only the most essential supplies and equipment for neonatal resuscitation. You may wish to add supplies or additional safety checks to meet your unit's standards or protocols. When the learner knows the routine and supplies are present and functioning, the Equipment Check should take approximately 1 minute to complete.

**Knowledge Check**

- Why is it important to have an organized routine for checking the presence and function of resuscitation supplies and equipment prior to every birth?

- Besides checking presence and function of equipment, what other resources should be assembled prior to a birth identified as high-risk?

**Learning Objectives**

1. Demonstrate an organized routine for checking presence and function of supplies and equipment necessary for newborn resuscitation, using the NRP flow diagram interventions as your guide.

2. Identify any additional preparatory routines for high-risk birth specific to this birth setting.

3. Locate the Quick Pre-resuscitation Checklist in the Appendix of this lesson.

**"You are notified that a woman has been admitted to the hospital in active labor. Check your supplies and equipment to prepare for the birth. As you work, say your thoughts and actions aloud so I will know what you are thinking and doing."**

Instructor should check boxes as the learner responds correctly. The learner may refer to this checklist or the Quick Pre-resuscitation Checklist that follows it to ensure the availability and function of essential supplies and equipment.

| Performance Steps | Details |
|---|---|
| **Warm:**<br>☐ Preheat warmer<br>☐ Lay out towels or blankets | Learner begins with equipment needed for initial steps of resuscitation and ends with equipment needed for complex resuscitation. |
| **Clear the airway 3 ways:**<br>☐ Bulb syringe<br>☐ 10F or 12F suction catheter attached to wall suction, set at 80-100 mm Hg<br>☐ Meconium aspirator | Turns on wall suction to "continuous" and occludes suction tubing; adjusts suction to 80-100 mm Hg. |
| **Auscultate**<br>☐ Stethoscope | Picks up stethoscope, places in ears, and taps on diaphragm to ensure function. |

| Performance Steps | Details |
|---|---|
| **Oxygenate**<br>☐ Turn on oxygen flowmeter to 5-10 L/min | If birth is imminent, suction and air/oxygen should be turned on and ready for use. |
| ☐ Adjust blender to hospital standard for initiation of resuscitation | Are air/$O_2$ tanks full, if used in your setting? |
| ☐ Pulse oximeter probe<br>☐ Pulse oximeter | Safety Check: Even if beginning resuscitation with 21% oxygen, the air/oxygen flow should be turned on in the event that supplemental oxygen is needed. A self-inflating bag will work even without gas flow; therefore, turn on air/oxygen so that gas is flowing if blender is turned up to administer supplemental oxygen. |
| **Ventilate**<br>☐ Check presence and function of positive-pressure ventilation (PPV) device<br>☐ Check presence of term- and preterm-size masks<br>☐ 8F feeding tube and 20-mL syringe | It is most important to check that safety features are working to prevent over-inflation of lungs with PPV. <u>Manometers</u> present and functioning? Connected to oxygen/air?<br><u>Self-inflating bag:</u> Pop-off valve working?<br><u>Flow inflating bag:</u> Does it inflate properly (no rips or missing attachments)?<br><u>T-piece:</u> Maximum circuit pressure set appropriately? Peak inspiratory pressure and positive end-expiratory pressure set appropriately? |
| **Intubate**<br>☐ Laryngoscope<br>☐ Size 0 and 1 blades with bright light<br>☐ Stylet (optional)<br>☐ Endotracheal (ET) tubes (2.5, 3.0, 3.5, 4.0)<br>☐ End tidal $CO_2$ detector<br>☐ Laryngeal mask airway and 5-mL syringe | Learner should know how to attach and detach blade from laryngoscope; check laryngoscope light.<br><br>If setting up for intubation, ET tube should stay clean inside its package even if package is open and stylet is inserted. |
| **Medicate**<br>Access to<br>☐ 1:10,000 epinephrine<br>☐ Supplies for administering medications and placing emergency umbilical venous catheter<br>☐ Documentation supplies | Location and protocol for checking emergency medications and supplies for vascular access are specific to each birth unit. |

| Performance Steps | Details |
|---|---|
| **Thermoregulate**<br>For very preterm newborns<br>☐ Plastic wrap or bag<br>☐ Chemically activated warming pad<br>☐ Transport incubator | |
| **Other**<br>Unit-specific items<br>☐<br>☐<br>☐<br>☐ | These items may be specific to your unit.<br>Tailor the Equipment Checklist to meet facility requirements. |

**Instructor asks the learner Reflective Questions to enable self-assessment, such as:**

1. Tell me how using this organized approach to checking resuscitation equipment works for you.

2. If all equipment and supplies were present, how long would it take you to confirm readiness for a birth?

3. Did you notice anything in this Equipment Checklist that is missing, specific to our birth setting? What would you change about this checklist?

### Neonatal Resuscitation Program Key Behavioral Skills

| | |
|---|---|
| Know your environment. | Allocate attention wisely. |
| Anticipate and plan. | Use all available information. |
| Assume the leadership role. | Use all available resources. |
| Communicate effectively. | Call for help when needed. |
| Delegate workload optimally. | Maintain professional behavior. |

# Appendix

### Neonatal Resuscitation Supplies and Equipment

**Suction equipment**

Bulb syringe

Mechanical suction and tubing

Suction catheters, 5F or 6F, 8F, 10F, 12F or 14F

8F feeding tube and 20-mL syringe

Meconium aspirator

**Bag-and-mask equipment**

Device for delivering positive-pressure ventilation, capable of delivering 90% to 100% oxygen

Face masks, newborn and premature sizes (cushioned-rim masks preferred)

Oxygen source

Compressed air source

Oxygen blender to mix oxygen and compressed air with flowmeter (flow rate up to 10 L/min) and tubing

Pulse oximeter and oximeter probe

**Intubation equipment**

Laryngoscope with straight blades, No. 0 (preterm) and No. 1 (term)

Extra bulbs and batteries for laryngoscope

Endotracheal tubes, 2.5-, 3.0-, 3.5-, 4.0-mm internal diameter (ID)

Stylet (optional)

Scissors

Tape or securing device for endotracheal tube

Alcohol sponges

$CO_2$ detector or capnograph

Laryngeal mask airway

**Medications**

Epinephrine 1:10,000 (0.1 mg/mL)—3-mL or 10-mL ampules

Isotonic crystalloid (normal saline or Ringer's lactate) for volume expansion—100 or 250 mL

Dextrose 10%, 250 mL

Normal saline for flushes

**Umbilical vessel catheterization supplies**

Sterile gloves

Scalpel or scissors

Antiseptic prep solution

Umbilical tape

Umbilical catheters, 3.5F, 5F

Three-way stopcock

Syringes, 1, 3, 5, 10, 20, 50 mL

Needles, 25, 21, 18 gauge, or puncture device for needleless system

**Neonatal Resuscitation Supplies and Equipment**—*continued*

**Miscellaneous**

Gloves and appropriate personal protection

Radiant warmer or other heat source

Firm, padded resuscitation surface

Clock with second hand (timer optional)

Warmed linens

Stethoscope (with neonatal head)

Tape, 1/2 or 3/4 inch

Cardiac monitor and electrodes or pulse oximeter and probe (optional for delivery room)

Oropharyngeal airways (0, 00, and 000 sizes or 30-, 40-, and 50-mm lengths)

**For very preterm babies**

Size 00 laryngoscope blade (optional)

Reclosable, food-grade plastic bag (1-gallon size) or plastic wrap

Chemically activated warming pad (optional)

Transport incubator to maintain baby's temperature during move to the nursery

**Neonatal Resuscitation Program Quick Pre-resuscitation Checklist**

**Newborn Resuscitation Supplies and Equipment at Radiant Warmer**

This checklist includes only the most essential supplies and equipment needed at the radiant warmer for most neonatal resuscitations. Tailor this list to meet your unit-specific needs to ensure that supplies and equipment are present and functioning and unit-specific safety checks have been done prior to <u>every</u> birth.

| | |
|---|---|
| **Warm** | Preheat warmer<br>Towels or blankets |
| **Clear airway** | Bulb syringe<br>10F or 12F suction catheter attached to wall suction set at 80-100 mm Hg<br>Meconium aspirator |
| **Auscultate** | Stethoscope |
| **Oxygenate** | Method to give free-flow oxygen (mask, tubing, flow-inflating bag, or T-piece)<br>Gases flowing just prior to birth, 5-10 L/min<br>Blender set per protocol<br>Pulse oximeter probe (detached from oximeter until needed)<br>Pulse oximeter |
| **Ventilate** | Positive-pressure ventilation (PPV) device(s) present with term and preterm masks<br>PPV device(s) functioning<br>Connected to air/oxygen source (blender)<br>8F feeding tube and 20-mL syringe |
| **Intubate** | Laryngoscope<br>Size 0 and Size 1 (and size 00, optional) blades with bright light<br>Endotracheal tubes, sizes 2.5, 3.0, 3.5, 4.0<br>Stylets<br>End tidal $CO_2$ detector<br>Laryngeal mask airway (size 1) and 5-mL syringe |
| **Medicate** | Access to 1:10,000 epinephrine and normal saline<br>Supplies for administering meds and placing emergency umbilical venous catheter<br>Documentation supplies |
| **Thermoregulate** | Plastic bag or plastic wrap<br>Chemically activated warming pad<br>Transport incubator ready |
| **Other** | |

**Apgar Score**

The Apgar score describes the condition of the newborn immediately after birth and, when properly applied, provides a standardized mechanism to record fetal-to-neonatal transition. Each of the 5 signs is awarded a value of 0, 1, or 2. The 5 values are then added, and the sum becomes the Apgar score. Resuscitative interventions modify the components of the Apgar score; therefore, the resuscitative measures being administered at the time the score is assigned should also be registered. A suggested form for completion at deliveries is shown in the following table.

APGAR SCORE  CHRMR            Gestational Age _____ weeks

| SIGN | 0 | 1 | 2 | 1 minute | 5 minutes | 10 minutes | 15 minutes | 20 minutes |
|---|---|---|---|---|---|---|---|---|
| Color | Blue or Pale | Acrocyanotic | Completely Pink | | | | | |
| Heart Rate | Absent | <100 bpm | >100 bpm | | | | | |
| Reflex Irritability | No Response | Grimace | Cry or Active Withdrawal | | | | | |
| Muscle Tone | Limp | Some Flexion | Active Motion | | | | | |
| Respiration | Absent | Weak Cry; Hypoventilation | Good, Crying | | | | | |
| | | | TOTAL | | | | | |

| Comments: | Resuscitation | | | | |
|---|---|---|---|---|---|
| | Minutes | 1 | 5 | 10 | 15 | 20 |
| | Oxygen | | | | | |
| | PPV/NCPAP | | | | | |
| | ETT | | | | | |
| | Chest Compressions | | | | | |
| | Epinephrine | | | | | |

Apgar scores should be assigned at 1 minute and 5 minutes after birth. When the 5-minute score is less than 7, additional scores should be assigned every 5 minutes for up to 20 minutes. These scores should not be used to dictate appropriate resuscitative actions, nor should interventions for depressed newborns be delayed until the 1-minute assessment. The scores should be recorded in the baby's birth record. Complete documentation of the events taking place during a resuscitation also must include a narrative description of interventions performed.

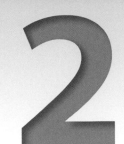

# Initial Steps of Resuscitation

### In Lesson 2 you will learn how to

- Decide if a newborn needs to be resuscitated.
- Open the airway, and provide the other initial steps of resuscitation.
- Resuscitate a newborn when meconium is present.
- Provide free-flow oxygen and/or continuous positive airway pressure when needed.
- Attach an oximeter and interpret oximeter readings.

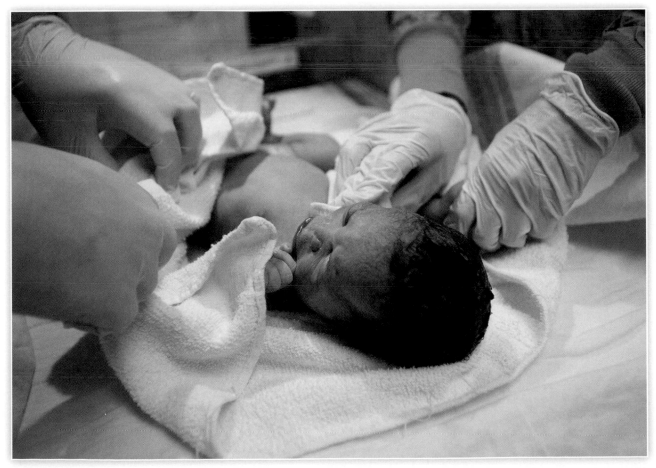

The following 2 cases are examples of how the initial steps of evaluation and resuscitation may be used. As you read each case, imagine yourself as part of the resuscitation team. The details of the initial steps will be described in the remainder of the lesson.

## *Case 1.*
## An uncomplicated delivery

A 24-year-old woman enters the hospital in active labor at term. Membranes ruptured 1 hour before, and the amniotic fluid was clear. Her cervix dilates progressively and, after several hours, a baby girl is born vaginally from the vertex presentation.

The cord is clamped and cut. She begins to cry as she is dried with a warm towel.

She is active and crying, is noted to have good muscle tone, and, therefore, is placed on her mother's chest to remain warm and to continue transition as her color becomes increasingly pink.

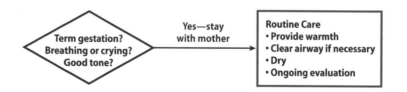

## Case 2.
## Resuscitation in presence of meconium-stained amniotic fluid

A multiparous woman presents at term in early labor. Soon after admission, her membranes rupture, and the fluid is noted to contain meconium. Fetal heart rate monitoring shows a Category II pattern (indeterminate pattern, requiring evaluation and surveillance and possibly other tests to ensure fetal well-being). A judgment is made to allow a vaginal delivery.

Immediately after birth, the baby has poor tone and minimal respiratory efforts. He is placed under a radiant warmer while his oropharynx is cleared of meconium with a large-bore suction catheter. His trachea is intubated and suction is applied to the endotracheal tube as it is slowly withdrawn from the trachea, but no meconium is recovered. The baby still has only weak respiratory efforts.

The baby is dried with a warm towel and stimulated to breathe by flicking the soles of his feet. At the same time, his head is repositioned to open his airway. He immediately begins to breathe more effectively, and the heart rate is measured to be more than 120 beats per minute (bpm). Because he is still cyanotic at more than 5 minutes after birth, he is given supplemental oxygen by holding an oxygen mask close to his face as an oximetry probe is secured on his right hand. The oximetry reading is above the expected value shown in the flow diagram, so the oxygen is gradually withdrawn to bring the values within range.

By 10 minutes after birth, the baby is breathing regularly and his oxygen saturation as measured by pulse oximetry ($SpO_2$) is approaching 90%, so the supplemental oxygen is gradually withdrawn based on oximetry readings. He now has a heart rate of 150 bpm, and remains pink with $SpO_2$ of 90% to 95% without supplemental oxygen. He is placed on his mother's chest, with the oximeter still attached, to continue transition while vital signs and activity are observed closely and monitored frequently for possible deterioration.

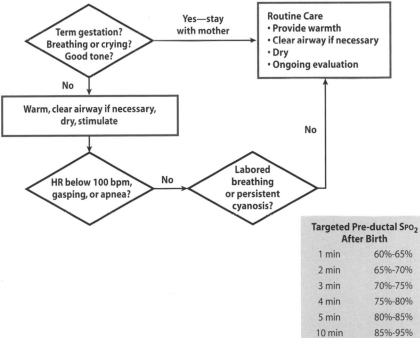

| Targeted Pre-ductal $SpO_2$ After Birth | |
|---|---|
| 1 min | 60%-65% |
| 2 min | 65%-70% |
| 3 min | 70%-75% |
| 4 min | 75%-80% |
| 5 min | 80%-85% |
| 10 min | 85%-95% |

# How do you determine if a baby requires resuscitation?

- Term gestation?
- Breathing or crying?
- Good muscle tone?

- *Was the baby born at term?*

Although more than 90% of babies will complete intrauterine to extrauterine transition without requiring any assistance, the vast majority of these babies will be born at term. If the baby is born preterm, there is a significantly higher likelihood that some degree of resuscitation will be required. For example, preterm babies are more likely to have stiff, underdeveloped lungs, may have insufficient muscle strength to make strong initial respiratory efforts, and have less capacity to maintain body temperature after birth. Because of these additional risk factors, preterm babies should be evaluated, and the initial steps of resuscitation should be carried out under a radiant warmer rather than at the mother's bedside. If the baby is in the late-preterm category (34-36 weeks' gestation) and is judged to have stable vital signs, she can then be returned to her mother's chest within several minutes to complete transition. Details of management of the unstable preterm baby will be covered in Lesson 8.

 **Gasping usually indicates a significant problem and requires the same intervention as no respiratory efforts at all (apnea).**

- *Is the baby breathing or crying?*

Breathing is evident by watching the baby's chest. A vigorous cry also indicates breathing. However, do not be misled by a baby who is gasping. Gasping is a series of deep, single or stacked inspirations that occur in the presence of hypoxia and/or ischemia. It is indicative of severe neurologic and respiratory depression.

- *Is there good muscle tone?*

Healthy term babies should have flexed extremities and be active (Figure 2.1) as opposed to sick or preterm babies, who often will have extended and flaccid extremities (Figure 2.2).

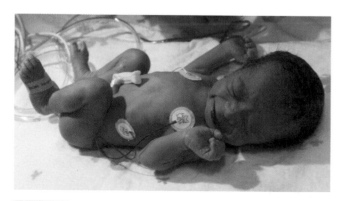

**Figure 2.1.** At-risk newborn: good tone. This baby is slightly preterm and small for gestational age. However, tone is excellent.

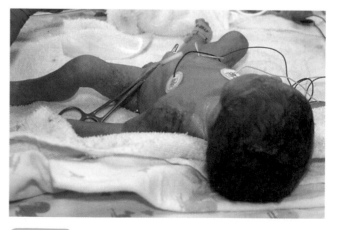

**Figure 2.2.** At-risk newborn: poor tone. This baby's poor tone is worse than one would anticipate from her being born preterm.

## What are the initial steps and how are they administered?

If the baby is term and vigorous, the initial steps may be provided in modified form, as described in Lesson 1 (page 20 under "Routine Care").

Once you decide that resuscitation is required, all the initial steps should be initiated within a few seconds. Although they are listed as "initial" and are given in a particular order, they should be applied throughout the resuscitation process.

- *Provide warmth.*
The baby should be placed under a radiant warmer so that the resuscitation team has easy access to the baby and the radiant heat helps reduce heat loss (Figure 2.3). The baby should not be covered with blankets or towels. Leave the baby uncovered to allow full visualization and to permit the radiant heat to reach the baby. If you suspect that the baby has significant asphyxia, particular care should be taken not to overheat her.

- *Open the airway by slightly extending the neck.*
The baby should be **positioned** on the back or side, with the neck slightly extended in the "sniffing" position. This will bring the posterior pharynx, larynx, and trachea in line and facilitate unrestricted air entry. This alignment in the supine position is also the best position for assisted ventilation with a mask and/or the placement of an endotracheal tube. The goal is to move the baby's nose as far anterior as possible, thus creating the "sniffing" position.

Care should be taken to prevent hyperextension or flexion of the neck, since either may restrict air entry (Figure 2.4).

### Initial Steps

- **Provide warmth**
- **Position; clear airway (as necessary)**
- **Dry, stimulate, reposition**

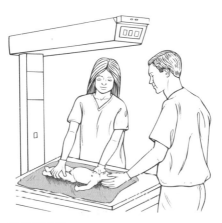

**Figure 2.3.** Radiant warmer for resuscitating newborns

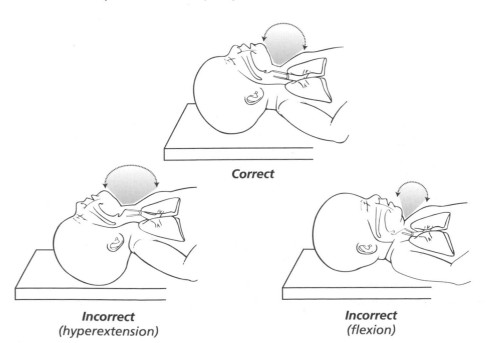

**Correct**

**Incorrect**
**(hyperextension)**

**Incorrect**
**(flexion)**

**Figure 2.4.** Correct and incorrect head positions for resuscitation

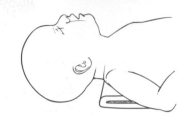

**Figure 2.5.** Optional shoulder roll for maintaining "sniffing" position

To help maintain the correct position, you may place a rolled blanket or towel under the shoulders (Figure 2.5). This shoulder roll may be particularly useful if the baby has a large occiput (back of head) resulting from molding, edema, or prematurity.

- *Clear airway (as necessary).*

After delivery, the appropriate method for clearing the airway further will depend on

1. The presence of meconium on the baby's skin or in the airway.

2. The baby's level of activity as shown in the diagram below.

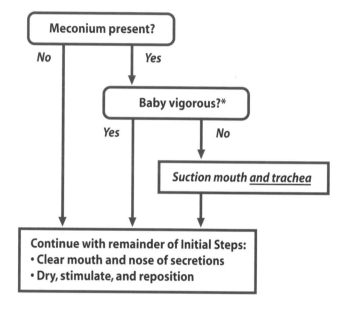

* Vigorous is defined as strong respiratory efforts, good muscle tone, and a heart rate greater than 100 bpm. The technique of determining the heart rate is described later in this lesson.

## What do you do if meconium is present and the baby is *not* vigorous?

If the baby is born through meconium-stained amniotic fluid, has depressed respirations, has depressed muscle tone, and/or has a heart rate below 100 bpm, direct suctioning of the trachea soon after delivery is indicated before many respirations have occurred to reduce the chances of the baby developing meconium aspiration syndrome—a very serious respiratory disorder.

To suction the trachea,

- Insert a laryngoscope and use a 12F or 14F suction catheter to clear the mouth and posterior pharynx so that you can visualize the glottis (Figure 2.6).

- Insert an endotracheal tube into the trachea.

- Attach the endotracheal tube to a suction source. (A special aspirator device will be needed.) (Figure 2.6)

- Apply suction for several seconds when the tube is in the trachea, and continue as the tube is slowly withdrawn. It may help to count, "1-one thousand, 2-one thousand, 3-one thousand, withdraw."

- Repeat as necessary until little additional meconium is recovered, or until the baby's heart rate indicates that resuscitation must proceed without delay (Figure 2.7).

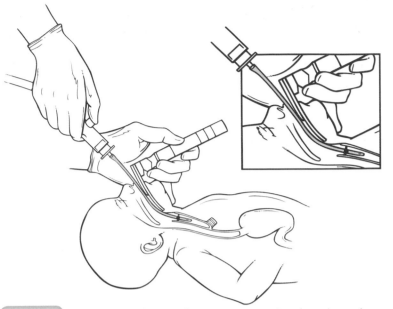

**Figure 2.6.** Visualizing the glottis and suctioning meconium from the trachea using a laryngoscope and endotracheal tube. (See Lesson 5 for details.)

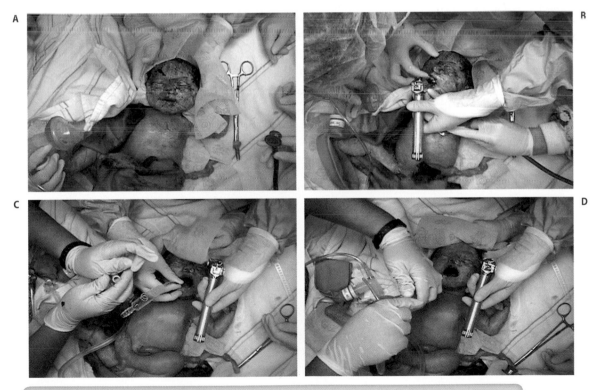

**Figure 2.7.**

A. Limp baby covered with meconium.
B. Resuscitator preparing to intubate.
C. Endotracheal tube has been inserted, a meconium aspiration device has been connected to the tube, and the suction tubing is about to be connected.
D. Suction control port is occluded so that meconium is suctioned from the trachea as tube is withdrawn.

*Details of performing endotracheal intubation and suctioning are described in Lesson 5. Individuals who will initiate resuscitation, but who will not intubate newborns, should still be competent in assisting with endotracheal intubation.*

**Note:** Some previous recommendations have suggested that the need for endotracheal suctioning should be based on whether the meconium has "thick," versus "thin," consistency. While it may be reasonable to speculate that thick meconium is more hazardous than thin, there are currently no clinical studies that warrant basing suctioning guidelines on meconium consistency.

Also, various techniques, such as squeezing the chest, inserting a finger in the baby's mouth, or externally occluding the airway, have been proposed to prevent babies from aspirating meconium. None of these techniques have been subjected to rigorous research evaluation, and all may be harmful to the baby. They are not recommended.

## What do you do if meconium is present and the baby *is* vigorous?

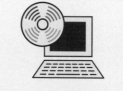

**You are encouraged to view this video on the DVD that accompanies this textbook:** *Using a Meconium Aspirator*

If the baby born with meconium-stained fluid has a normal respiratory effort, normal muscle tone, and a heart rate greater than 100 bpm, simply use a bulb syringe or large-bore suction catheter to clear secretions and any meconium from the mouth and nose as needed. This procedure is described in the next section. This baby may stay with his mother and receive routine care and ongoing evaluation.

**Review**

*(The answers are in the preceding section and at the end of the lesson.)*

1. A newborn who is born at term, has no meconium in the amniotic fluid or on the skin, is breathing well, and has good muscle tone (does) (does not) need resuscitation.

2. A newborn with meconium in the amniotic fluid who **is not vigorous** (will) (will not) need to have his trachea suctioned via an endotracheal tube. A newborn with meconium in the amniotic fluid who **is vigorous** (will) (will not) need to have his trachea suctioned via an endotracheal tube.

3. When deciding which babies need tracheal suctioning, the term "vigorous" is defined by what 3 characteristics?

   (1) _____

   (2) _____

   (3) _____

4. When a suction catheter is used to clear the oropharynx of meconium before inserting an endotracheal tube, the appropriate size is _____F or _____F.

5. Which drawing shows the correct way to position a newborn's head prior to suctioning the airway?

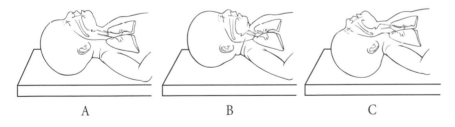

| A | B | C |

6. A newborn is covered with meconium, is breathing well, has normal muscle tone, and has a heart rate of 120 beats per minute. The correct action is to

   _____ Insert an endotracheal tube and suction her trachea.

   _____ Suction the mouth and nose with a bulb syringe or suction catheter.

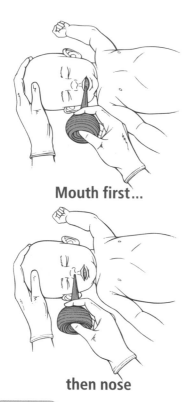

**Mouth first...**

**then nose**

**Figure 2.8.** Suction the mouth and nose: "M" before "N"

## How do you clear the airway if no meconium is present?

Secretions may be removed from the airway by wiping the nose and mouth with a towel or by suctioning with a bulb syringe or suction catheter. If the newborn has copious secretions coming from the mouth, turn the head to the side. This will allow secretions to collect in the cheek where they can be removed more easily.

Use a bulb syringe or a catheter attached to mechanical suction to remove any fluid that appears to be blocking the airway. When using suction from the wall or from a pump, the suction pressure should be set so that, when the suction tubing is blocked, the negative pressure (vacuum) reads approximately 100 mm Hg.

The mouth is suctioned before the nose to ensure that there is nothing for the newborn to aspirate if he should gasp when the nose is suctioned. You can remember "mouth before nose" by thinking "M" comes before "N" in the alphabet (Figure 2.8). If material in the mouth and nose is not removed before the newborn breathes, the material can be aspirated into the trachea and lungs. When this occurs, the respiratory consequences can be serious.

 **Caution: When you suction, particularly when using a catheter, be careful not to suction vigorously or deeply. Stimulation of the posterior pharynx during the first few minutes after birth can produce a vagal response, causing severe bradycardia or apnea. Brief, gentle suctioning with a bulb syringe usually is adequate to remove secretions.**

If bradycardia occurs during suctioning, stop suctioning and reevaluate the heart rate.

Suctioning, in addition to clearing the airway to allow unrestricted air entry to the lungs, also provides a degree of *stimulation.* In some cases, this is all the stimulation needed to initiate respirations in the newborn.

## Once the airway is clear, what should be done to prevent further heat loss and to stimulate breathing?

Often, positioning the baby and suctioning secretions will provide enough stimulation to initiate breathing. Drying will also provide stimulation. Drying the body and head will also help prevent heat loss. If 2 people are present, the second person can be drying the baby while the first person is positioning and clearing the airway.

As part of preparation for resuscitation, you should have several pre-warmed absorbent towels or blankets available. Initially, the baby is placed on one of these towels, which can be used to dry most of the fluid. This towel should then be discarded, and fresh pre-warmed towels or blankets should be used for continued drying and stimulation (Figures 2.9 and 2.10).

While you dry the baby, and thereafter, be sure to keep the head in the "sniffing" position to maintain a good airway.

NOTE: Additional strategies to reduce heat loss in preterm babies will be described in Lesson 8.

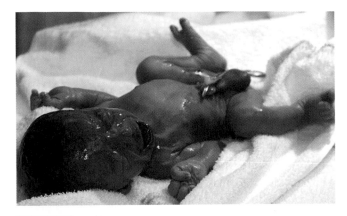

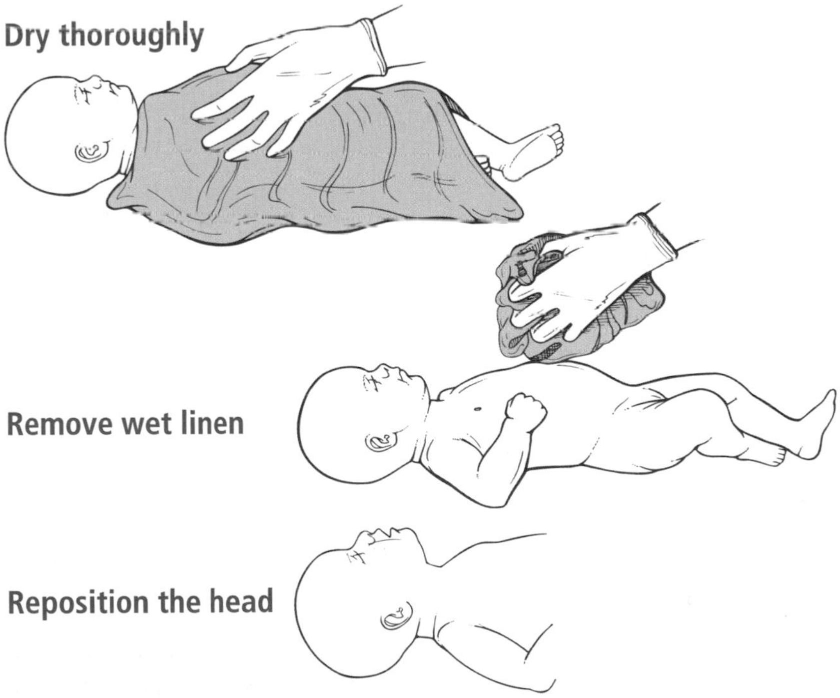

**Figure 2.9.** Newborn immediately following birth. Drying and removing the wet linen will probably stimulate breathing and prevent body cooling.

**Dry thoroughly**

**Remove wet linen**

**Reposition the head**

**Figure 2.10.** Dry and remove wet linen to prevent heat loss, and reposition the head to ensure an open airway

# What other forms of stimulation may help a baby breathe?

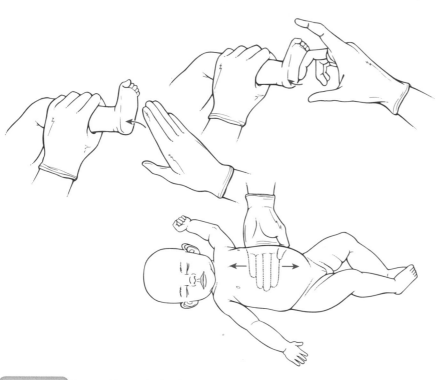

**Figure 2.11.** Acceptable methods of stimulating a baby to breathe

Both drying and suctioning stimulate the newborn. For many newborns, these steps are enough to induce respirations. If the newborn does not have adequate respirations, additional tactile stimulation may be provided *briefly* to stimulate breathing.

It is important to understand the correct methods of tactile stimulation. Stimulation may be useful not only to encourage a baby to begin breathing during the initial steps of resuscitation, but also may be used to stimulate continued breathing after positive-pressure ventilation (PPV).

Safe and appropriate methods of providing additional tactile stimulation include

- Slapping or flicking the soles of the feet
- Gently rubbing the newborn's back, trunk, or extremities (Figure 2.11)

 **Overly vigorous stimulation is not helpful and can cause serious injury. Do not shake the baby.**

Remember, if a newborn is in primary apnea, almost any form of stimulation will initiate breathing. If a baby is in secondary apnea, no amount of stimulation will work. Therefore, 1 or 2 slaps or flicks to the soles of the feet, or rubbing the back once or twice, should be sufficient. If the newborn remains apneic, PPV should be initiated immediately, as described in Lesson 3.

 **Continued use of tactile stimulation in a newborn who is not breathing wastes valuable time. For persistent apnea, give positive-pressure ventilation.**

## What forms of stimulation may be hazardous?

Certain actions that were used in the past to provide tactile stimulation to apneic newborns, such as slapping the back or buttocks or shaking the baby, can harm a baby and should not be used.

 **Review**

*(The answers are in the preceding section and at the end of the lesson.)*

7. In suctioning a baby's nose and mouth, the rule is to first suction the _____ and then the _____.

8. Make a check mark next to the correct ways to stimulate a newborn.

    _____ Slap the back    _____ Slap the sole of foot

    _____ Rub the back    _____ Squeeze the rib cage

9. If a baby is in secondary apnea, stimulation of the baby (will) (will not) stimulate breathing.

10. A newborn is still not breathing after a few seconds of stimulation. The next action should be to administer

    _____ Additional stimulation

    _____ Positive-pressure ventilation

**Now that you have warmed and positioned the baby, cleared the airway, dried and stimulated the baby, and repositioned the baby's head, what do you do next?**

**Evaluate the baby**

Your next step is to evaluate the newborn to determine if further resuscitation actions are indicated. *Remember, the entire resuscitation process up to this point should take no more than 30 seconds* (unless suctioning of meconium from the trachea was required, which may lengthen the initial resuscitation steps). The vital signs that you evaluate are respirations and heart rate.

!  **Remember, gasping respirations are ineffective and require the same intervention as for apnea.**

- *Respirations*

There should be good chest movement, and the rate and depth of respirations should increase after a few seconds of tactile stimulation.

- *Heart rate*

The heart rate should be more than 100 bpm. The easiest and quickest method to determine the heart rate is to feel for a pulse at the base of the umbilical cord, where it attaches to the baby's abdomen (Figure 2.12). However, sometimes the umbilical vessels are constricted so that the pulse is not palpable. Therefore, if you cannot feel a pulse, you should use a stethoscope to listen for the heartbeat over the left side of the chest. If you can feel a pulse or hear the heartbeat, tap it out on the bed so that others will also know the heart rate. If you are unable to detect a heartbeat or cannot assess the heart rate by one of these 2 methods, ask another member of the team to place an oximetry probe or cardiac leads on the baby and quickly connect a pulse oximeter or electronic cardiac monitor, as either of these devices can display the heart rate.

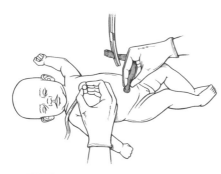

**Figure 2.12.** Determining heart rate by palpating base of cord and listening with a stethoscope

Counting the number of beats in 6 seconds and multiplying by 10 provides a quick estimate of the beats per minute.

## What do you do if the heart rate or respirations are abnormal?

!  **Administering free-flow oxygen or continuing to provide tactile stimulation to a nonbreathing newborn or to a newborn whose heart rate is below 100 bpm is of little or no value and only delays appropriate treatment.**

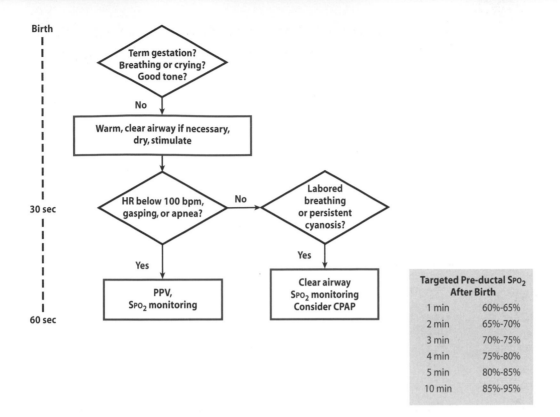

| Targeted Pre-ductal $S_{PO_2}$ After Birth | |
|---|---|
| 1 min | 60%-65% |
| 2 min | 65%-70% |
| 3 min | 70%-75% |
| 4 min | 75%-80% |
| 5 min | 80%-85% |
| 10 min | 85%-95% |

If the baby is not breathing (apnea), or has gasping respirations, or if the heart rate is below 100 bpm, despite stimulation, you should proceed immediately to providing PPV, as will be described in Lesson 3.

> ! **The most effective and important action in resuscitating a compromised newborn is to assist ventilation.**

If the baby *is* breathing and the heart rate is *above* 100 bpm, but the respirations are labored, or if you believe the baby is cyanotic, many clinicians would administer continuous positive airway pressure (CPAP) by face mask, which also will be described later in this lesson. In any of these cases (starting PPV, giving CPAP, or judging the baby to be cyanotic), you should attach an oximeter to assess the efficacy of your action and the possible need for supplemental oxygen.

# How do you assess for cyanosis and use an oximeter to determine if the baby needs supplemental oxygen?

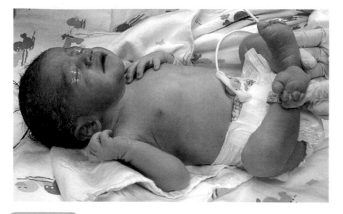

**Figure 2.13.** Acrocyanosis. This baby has acrocyanosis of hands and feet, but trunk and mucous membranes are pink. Supplemental oxygen is not required.

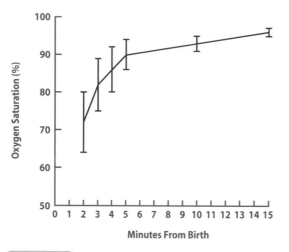

**Figure 2.14.** Pre-ductal oxygen saturation changes following birth (median and interquartile range). (From Mariani G, Dik PB, Ezquer A, et al. Pre-ductal and post-ductal O2 saturation in healthy term neonates after birth: *J Pediatr.* 2007;150:418.)

A baby's skin color, changing from blue to pink, can provide the most rapid and visible indicator of the baby's state of oxygenation. The baby's skin color is best determined by looking at the central part of the body. Cyanosis caused by low oxygen in the blood will appear as a blue hue to the lips, tongue, and torso. Acrocyanosis, which is a blue hue to only the hands and feet (Figure 2.13), is often caused by decreased circulation to the extremities and is not, by itself, an indication of decreased blood oxygen levels in vital organs. Only central cyanosis should be a sign suggesting low blood oxygenation, which may require intervention. **An oximeter should be used to confirm the perception of cyanosis.**

Two factors complicate the use of cyanosis alone to determine the baby's need for supplemental oxygen.

- Studies have shown that clinical assessment of skin color is not very reliable, and varies as a function of skin pigmentation.

- Other studies have documented that babies undergoing normal transition may take several minutes after birth to increase their blood oxygen saturation ($SpO_2$) from approximately 60%, which is the normal intrauterine state, to more than 90%, which is the eventual state of air-breathing healthy newborns. Figure 2.14 shows the time course of $SpO_2$ changes after birth in healthy newborns born at term. Values following cesarean section deliveries are slightly lower than values following vaginal deliveries.

Therefore, it is not unusual for a newborn to appear slightly cyanotic for the first few minutes after birth. If the cyanosis persists, you should attach a pulse oximetry probe to determine if the baby's oxygenation is abnormal. If the levels are low and not increasing, you may need to provide supplemental oxygen.

 **Oximetry can be helpful to assist in judging the accuracy of your assessment, but should not delay your resuscitation actions. Stabilization of ventilation, heart rate, and oxygenation should remain priorities.**

## How does an oximeter work, and how do you use it?

An oximeter (Figure 2.15) measures the color of blood flowing through the capillaries of the skin and compares the color to the known color of blood containing various amounts of oxygen. Oxygen is carried on the hemoglobin contained in red blood cells. Hemoglobin that has no oxygen is a blue color, and hemoglobin fully saturated with oxygen is red. The oximeter analyzes the color and displays a number between 0% (no oxygen) and 100% (fully saturated with oxygen). It is considered to be most accurate when SPO$_2$ values are between approximately 60% and 90%.

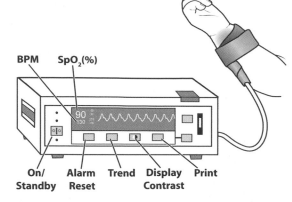

**Figure 2.15.** Oximeter with oximeter probe attached to the baby's right wrist

> **Note: The saturation of hemoglobin with oxygen (SPO$_2$), which is measured by an oximeter, is very different from the PO$_2$, or partial pressure of oxygen dissolved in plasma, which is measured by a blood gas analyzer. Be careful not to confuse the two.**

An oximeter has a probe that contains a small light source and a light detector (Figure 2.6A). The probe is placed on the skin, the light shines through the skin, is reflected off of the red blood cells in the skin capillaries, and is sensed by the detector. The circuitry in the oximeter instrument converts the signal from the detector into a number that is displayed on the monitor and signifies the percent that the hemoglobin is saturated with oxygen. Since the blood in the capillaries is pulsatile, the oximeter also can display an accurate heart rate.

Proper placement of the probe is important for the following reasons:

- The probe must be attached to a sufficiently thin area of skin and tissue, with capillaries sufficiently close to the surface, so that the light source can enter the skin easily and be sensed by the detector. In a baby, the side of the wrist or palm works well.

- The light and the detector must be oriented correctly so that the sensor can detect the reflected light. The probe should wrap around the tissue so that the detector can "see" the light source.

- You want the blood sensed by the oximeter to have the same oxygen saturation as the blood perfusing vital organs, such as the heart muscle and the brain. In newborns, this means placing the oximeter probe on the right arm (Figure 2.16), which receives blood from the aorta before it reaches the ductus arteriosus. Blood in the aorta past the ductus arteriosus may be mixed with blood with low oxygen levels coming from the pulmonary artery across the ductus, which may remain open for hours after birth.

You are encouraged to view this video on the DVD that accompanies this textbook: *Using Pulse Oximetry*

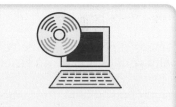

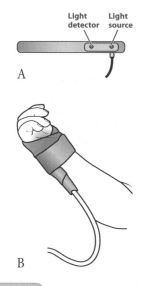

**Figure 2.16.** Oximeter probe (A) attached to a baby's hand on the hypothenar eminence

- To permit the most rapid acquisition of signal, the probe should be attached to the baby before it is connected to the instrument.

> **During a neonatal resuscitation, it is recommended that the oximeter probe be placed on the newborn's right hand or wrist so as to detect pre-ductal saturation.**

| Targeted Pre-ductal SpO₂ After Birth | |
|---|---|
| 1 min | 60%-65% |
| 2 min | 65%-70% |
| 3 min | 70%-75% |
| 4 min | 75%-80% |
| 5 min | 80%-85% |
| 10 min | 85%-95% |

Ranges of pre-ductal oximetry values during the first 10 minutes following birth of uncomplicated babies born at term. The ranges shown are approximations of the interquartile values reported by Dawson et al (*Pediatrics*. 2010;Jun; 125:e1340-1347) and adjusted to provide easily remembered targets.

Once the oximeter sensor is attached to the baby and plugged into the instrument, you should watch the monitor to see that it is detecting a pulse with each heartbeat and that the monitor is reading a saturation percentage. Most instruments will not give a steady saturation reading until a consistent pulse is detected. If this is not happening, you may need to adjust the probe to be sure that the sensor is positioned opposite the light source. In rare cases, the oximeter will not be able to detect the pulse and saturation because of poor perfusion from low blood volume or an absent or very low heartbeat. This complication will be covered in Lessons 6 and 7.

After the oximeter is reading reliably, you should adjust the percentage of inspired oxygen concentration to achieve the target values for saturations shown in Figure 2.14 and summarized in the table. This will require the availability of compressed air and an oxygen blender, as described below. Try to avoid oxygenation that is either too high or too low—either of which can be toxic.

## What do you do if the baby has labored breathing and/or central cyanosis?

If the baby is making respiratory efforts, but is working hard to breathe, has grunting respirations or intercostal retractions, or has persistent central cyanosis or hypoxemia confirmed by oximetry, administration of CPAP by mask may be beneficial, particularly if the baby is preterm. (See Lesson 8.) Continuous positive airway pressure can be delivered only with a flow-inflating bag (Figure 2.17) or with a T-piece resuscitator, as will be described in more detail in Lesson 3. It cannot be given by most brands of self-inflating bags.

Although previous recommendations called for administration of 100% oxygen whenever cyanosis was present or the baby had significant respiratory distress following birth, there is increasing evidence that exposure to excess oxygen during or following a period of insufficient oxygen delivery or poor tissue perfusion may be harmful, particularly in babies born preterm. (See Lesson 8.) In addition, as mentioned previously, assessment of cyanosis as an indication of oxygen levels has

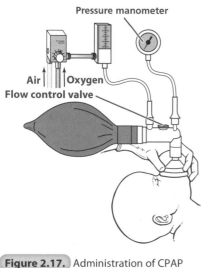

**Figure 2.17.** Administration of CPAP using a flow-inflating bag

been shown to be quite inaccurate. Therefore, if your assessment of skin color suggests cyanosis, you will want to confirm that assessment using an oximeter. If respiratory distress worsens so that heart rate falls below 100 bpm, or saturation cannot be maintained above 90% despite 100% oxygen, you should administer positive-pressure ventilation.

## How do you give supplemental oxygen?

Supplemental oxygen is not routinely needed at the beginning of a resuscitation. However, when a baby appears cyanotic or the oximeter readings are lower than expected during resuscitation, the oxygen levels may increase more quickly if a concentration of oxygen higher than the 21% oxygen in room air is administered. But, administering 100% oxygen is likely to increase the oxygen saturations more quickly than would be experienced by a healthy baby following birth, and may even reach toxic levels. This is particularly likely if the baby is preterm, or if oxygen administration lasts more than a few minutes, even in a term baby. Thus, it is best to use an oxygen concentration that can be varied throughout the range of 21% to 100%. This will require having a compressed air source and an oxygen blender (Figure 2.18). This equipment will be described in more detail in Lesson 3.

Free-flow oxygen can be given to a spontaneously breathing baby by using one of the following delivery methods, some of which you will learn about in more detail in Lesson 3:

- Oxygen mask (Figure 2.19)

- Flow-inflating bag and mask

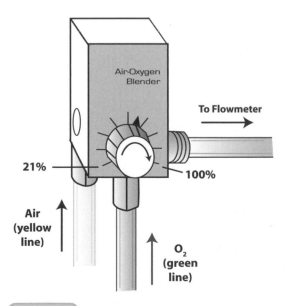

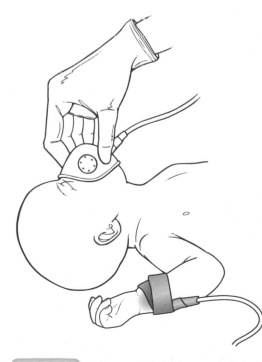

**Figure 2.18.** Mixing oxygen and air with an oxygen blender. The control knob dials in the desired oxygen concentration.

**Figure 2.19.** Oxygen mask held close to the baby's face to give the desired oxygen concentration

- T-piece resuscitator
- Oxygen tubing held close to the baby's mouth and nose (Figure 2.20)

Whichever method you use, the mask should be held close to the face to maintain the concentration of oxygen, but not so tight that pressure builds up within the mask (Figure 2.21).

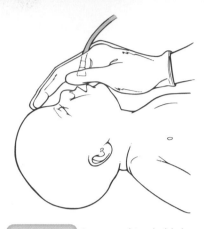

**Figure 2.20.** Oxygen tubing held close to the baby's face with the oxygen concentrated to the face with a cupped hand

**Free-flow oxygen cannot be given reliably by a mask attached to a *self*-inflating bag. (See Lesson 3.)**

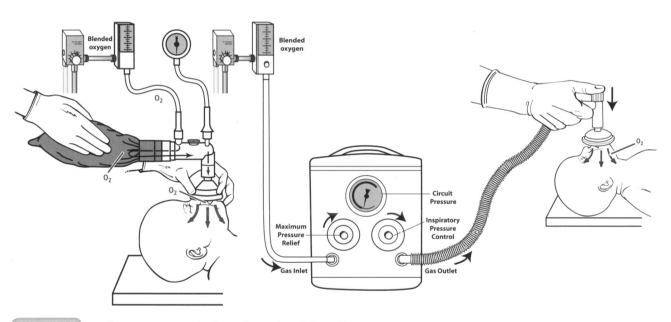

**Figure 2.21.** Free-flow oxygen given by flow-inflating bag (left) and by T-piece resuscitator (right). Note that mask is not held tightly on the face, unless continuous positive airway pressure is being given. A compressed air source and oxygen blender will be required to give a variable concentration of oxygen.

## How do you decide how much supplemental oxygen to give?

There is an ongoing controversy about how much oxygen to use during neonatal resuscitation. The 2010 Guidelines (see back of textbook) recommend that, during resuscitation of newly born babies at term, you start resuscitation with room air and then be guided by oximetry to use the concentration of oxygen necessary to achieve oxygen saturations that approximate those demonstrated by uncompromised term babies undergoing a normal transition. As described earlier in this lesson, those saturations start at the *in utero* value (~60%) and gradually increase over 10 minutes to the neonatal value of over 90%. (See Figure 2.14 and the table in the flow diagram.) If the baby is born preterm (see Lesson 8) or resuscitation can be anticipated, achieving these goals will be facilitated by attaching the oximeter early in the stabilization process and having blended oxygen readily available.

## If the baby continues to require supplemental oxygen, how should it be given?

After the resuscitation, when respirations and heart rate are stable and you have established that the newborn requires ongoing supplemental oxygen, pulse oximetry and arterial blood gas determinations should guide the appropriate oxygen concentration. All babies are vulnerable to injury from excess oxygen, with extremely preterm babies being the most vulnerable.

Oxygen and compressed air that come from a wall source or tank are very cold and dry. To prevent heat loss and drying of the respiratory mucosa, oxygen given to newborns for long periods should be heated and humidified. However, during resuscitation, dry, unheated oxygen may be given for the few minutes required to stabilize the newborn's condition.

Avoid giving unheated and nonhumidified oxygen at high flow rates (above approximately 10 L/min), because convective heat loss can become a significant problem. A flow rate of 5 L/min is usually adequate for free-flow oxygen during resuscitation.

## How do you know when to stop giving free-flow oxygen?

When the newborn no longer has central cyanosis, or oximetry saturations are above 85% to 90%, gradually decrease the amount of supplemental oxygen provided until the newborn can maintain oximetry saturations in the expected normal range while breathing room air. Subsequently, arterial blood gas determinations and oximetry should be used to continue adjusting oxygen levels to the normal range.

If cyanosis or oxygen saturation less than 85% persists despite administration of free-flow oxygen, the baby may have significant lung disease, and a trial of positive-pressure ventilation may be indicated. (See Lesson 3.) If ventilation is adequate and the baby remains cyanotic or oxygen saturation is less than 85%, a diagnosis of cyanotic congenital heart disease or persistent pulmonary hypertension of the newborn should be considered. (See Lesson 7.)

## Review

*(The answers are in the preceding section and at the end of the lesson.)*

11. A newborn has poor tone, labored breathing, and cyanosis. Your initial steps are to *(Check all that are appropriate.)*

    _____ Place the newborn on a radiant warmer.

    _____ Remove all wet linens.

    _____ Suction his mouth and nose.

    _____ Consider giving CPAP or free-flow supplemental oxygen.

    _____ Consider applying a pulse oximetry probe and activating an oximeter.

    _____ Dry and stimulate.

**12.** Which drawings show the correct way to give free-flow oxygen to a baby?

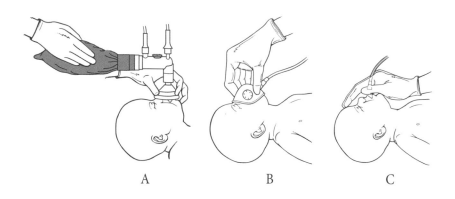

A          B          C

**13.** Check "true" or "false" for each of the following statements about oxygen administration:

**TRUE**       **FALSE**

_____   _____   Oximeters are devices that measure the $P_{O_2}$ of the blood.

_____   _____   In the delivery room, the oximetry probe should always be placed on the baby's right hand or wrist.

_____   _____   Oxygen saturation should be expected to be >90% by 2 minutes of age.

_____   _____   A baby who is cyanotic and apneic should receive free-flow oxygen as the best treatment.

**14.** If you need to give supplemental oxygen for longer than a few minutes, the oxygen should be _____ and _____.

**15.** You have stimulated a newborn and suctioned her mouth. It is now 30 seconds after birth, and she is still apneic and pale. Her heart rate is 80 beats per minute. Your next action is to

_____ Continue stimulation and give free-flow supplemental oxygen.

_____ Provide positive-pressure ventilation.

**16.** You count a newborn's heartbeats for 6 seconds and count 6 beats. You report the heart rate as _____.

**17.** An oximeter will show both $S_{PO_2}$ and _____.

## Key Points

1.  If meconium is present and the newborn *is not vigorous,* suction the baby's trachea before proceeding with any other steps. If the newborn *is vigorous,* suction the mouth and nose only, and proceed with taking the baby to the mother for your further assessment.

2.  "Vigorous" is defined as a newborn who has strong respiratory efforts, good muscle tone, and a heart rate greater than 100 beats per minute.

3.  Open the airway by positioning the newborn in a "sniffing" position.

4.  Appropriate forms of tactile stimulation are
    *   Slapping or flicking the soles of the feet
    *   Gently rubbing the back

5.  Continued use of tactile stimulation in an apneic newborn wastes valuable time. For persistent apnea, begin positive-pressure ventilation promptly.

6.  A fetus has an oxygen saturation of approximately 60%, and it may take up to 10 minutes for a healthy newborn to increase saturation to the normal range of over 90%.

7.  Acceptable methods for administering free-flow oxygen are
    *   Oxygen mask held firmly over the baby's face
    *   Mask from a flow-inflating bag or T-piece resuscitator held closely over the baby's mouth and nose
    *   Oxygen tubing cupped closely over the baby's mouth and nose

8.  Free-flow oxygen cannot be given reliably by a mask attached to a self-inflating bag.

9.  Decisions and actions during newborn resuscitation are based on the newborn's
    *   Respirations
    *   Heart rate
    *   Color (oxygenation)

10. Determine a newborn's heart rate by counting how many beats are in 6 seconds, then multiply by 10. For example, if you count 8 beats in 6 seconds, announce the baby's heart rate as 80 beats per minute.

11. Oxygen should be treated as a drug—either too little or too much can be injurious.

**12.** Use pulse oximetry:
- When resuscitation is anticipated
- When positive-pressure ventilation is required for more than a few breaths
- When central cyanosis is persistent
- When supplemental oxygen is administered
- To confirm your perception of cyanosis

## Lesson 2 Review

*(The answers follow.)*

**1.** A newborn who is born at term, has no meconium in the amniotic fluid or on the skin, is breathing well, and has good muscle tone (does) (does not) need resuscitation.

**2.** A newborn with meconium in the amniotic fluid who **is not vigorous** (will) (will not) need to have his trachea suctioned via an endotracheal tube. A newborn with meconium in the amniotic fluid who **is vigorous** (will) (will not) need to have his trachea suctioned via an endotracheal tube.

**3.** When deciding which babies need tracheal suctioning, the term "vigorous" is defined by what 3 characteristics?

(1) _____

(2) _____

(3) _____

**4.** When a suction catheter is used to clear the oropharynx of meconium before inserting an endotracheal tube, the appropriate size is _____F or _____F.

**5.** Which drawing shows the correct way to position a newborn's head prior to suctioning the airway?

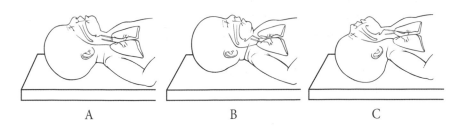

A          B          C

## Lesson 2 Review—*continued*

6. A newborn is covered with meconium, is breathing well, has normal muscle tone, has a heart rate of 120 beats per minute, and is pink. The correct action is to

   _____ Insert an endotracheal tube and suction her trachea.

   _____ Suction the mouth and nose with a bulb syringe or suction catheter.

7. In suctioning a baby's nose and mouth, the rule is to first suction the _____ and then the _____.

8. Make a check mark next to the correct ways to stimulate a newborn.

   _____ Slap the back           _____ Slap the sole of foot

   _____ Rub the back            _____ Squeeze the rib cage

9. If a baby is in secondary apnea, stimulation of the baby (will) (will not) stimulate breathing.

10. A newborn is still not breathing after a few seconds of stimulation. The next action should be to administer

    _____ Additional stimulation

    _____ Positive-pressure ventilation

11. A newborn has poor tone, labored breathing, and cyanosis. Your initial steps are to *(Check all that are appropriate.)*

    _____ Place the newborn on a radiant warmer.

    _____ Remove all wet linens.

    _____ Suction his mouth and nose.

    _____ Consider giving CPAP or free-flow supplemental oxygen.

    _____ Consider applying a pulse oximetry probe and activating an oximeter.

    _____ Dry and stimulate.

## Lesson 2 Review—*continued*

**12.** Which drawings show the correct way to give free-flow oxygen to a baby?

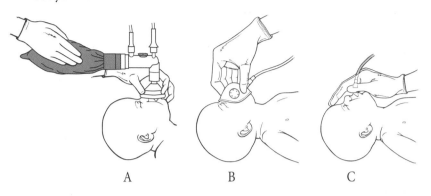

A          B          C

**13.** Check "true" or "false" for each of the following statements about oxygen administration:

**TRUE**      **FALSE**

_____   _____   Oximeters are devices that measure the $Po_2$ of the blood.

                       In the delivery room, the oximetry probe should always be placed on the baby's right hand or wrist.

_____   _____   Oxygen saturation should be expected to be >90% by 2 minutes of age.

_____   _____   A baby who is cyanotic and apneic should receive free-flow oxygen as the best treatment.

**14.** If you need to give supplemental oxygen for longer than a few minutes, the oxygen should be _____ and _____.

**15.** You have stimulated a newborn and suctioned her mouth. It is now 30 seconds after birth, and she is still apneic and pale. Her heart rate is 80 beats per minute. Your next action is to

_____ Continue stimulation and give free-flow supplemental oxygen.

_____ Provide positive-pressure ventilation.

**16.** You count a newborn's heartbeats for 6 seconds and count 6 beats. You report the heart rate as _____.

**17.** An oximeter will show both $Spo_2$ and _____.

## Answers to Questions

1. **Does not** need resuscitation.

2. A newborn with meconium who is not vigorous **will** need to have a laryngoscope inserted and be suctioned with an endotracheal tube. A newborn with meconium who is vigorous **will not** need to have a laryngoscope inserted and be suctioned with an endotracheal tube.

3. "Vigorous" is defined as: **(1) strong respiratory efforts, (2) good muscle tone,** and **(3) heart rate greater than 100 beats per minute.**

4. A **12F** or **14F** suction catheter should be used to suction meconium.

5. The correct head position is **A**, the "sniffing position." B is too flexed and C is overextended.

6. Since the newborn is active, she does not need to have her trachea suctioned, but you should **suction the mouth and nose with a bulb syringe or suction catheter.**

7. First suction the **mouth** and then the **nose.**

8. Stimulate by **slapping the sole of the foot** and/or **rubbing the back.**

9. Stimulation of the baby **will not** stimulate breathing if the baby is in secondary apnea.

10. If not breathing after stimulation, provide **positive-pressure ventilation.**

11. **All actions are appropriate.**

12. **All drawings are correct.**

13. **False** (Oximeters measure $SpO_2$); **True; False** ($SpO_2$ is expected to be >65% at 2 minutes of age); **False** (A baby who is apneic should receive positive-pressure ventilation as the best treatment).

14. The oxygen should be **heated** and **humidified.**

15. She should receive **positive-pressure ventilation.**

16. If you count 6 heartbeats in 6 seconds, report the baby's heart rate as **60 beats per minute (6 × 10 = 60).**

17. An oximeter will show both $SpO_2$ and **heart rate.**

# Lesson 2: Initial Steps Performance Checklist

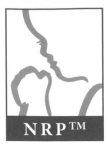

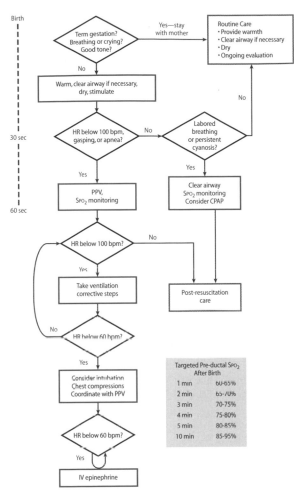

Birth

Term gestation? Breathing or crying? Good tone? → Yes—stay with mother → Routine Care
• Provide warmth
• Clear airway if necessary
• Dry
• Ongoing evaluation

No

Warm, clear airway if necessary, dry, stimulate

30 sec

HR below 100 bpm, gasping, or apnea? → No → Labored breathing or persistent cyanosis?

No →

Yes

Yes

60 sec

PPV, SpO₂ monitoring

Clear airway
SpO₂ monitoring
Consider CPAP

HR below 100 bpm? → No →

Yes

Take ventilation corrective steps

Post-resuscitation care

No

HR below 60 bpm?

Yes

Consider intubation
Chest compressions
Coordinate with PPV

| Targeted Pre-ductal SpO₂ After Birth | |
|---|---|
| 1 min | 60-65% |
| 2 min | 65-70% |
| 3 min | 70-75% |
| 4 min | 75-80% |
| 5 min | 80-85% |
| 10 min | 85-95% |

HR below 60 bpm?

Yes

IV epinephrine

## The Performance Checklist Is a Learning Tool

The learner uses the checklist as a reference during independent practice or as a guide for discussion and practice with a Neonatal Resuscitation Program™ (NRP™) instructor. When the learner and instructor agree that the learner can perform the skills correctly and smoothly without coaching and within the context of a scenario, the learner may move on to the next lesson's Performance Checklist.

## Knowledge Check

- How do you determine if a newborn requires resuscitation?

- How do you manage the baby who is born with meconium-stained amniotic fluid?

- How does pulse oximetry work and what is its function?

**Learning Objectives**

1 Identify the newborn who requires initial steps of resuscitation.

2 Demonstrate correct technique for performing initial steps, including decision making for a baby born with meconium-stained amniotic fluid.

3 Demonstrate correct placement of oximeter probe and interpretation of pulse oximetry.

**"You are called to attend a cesarean birth due to breech presentation. How would you prepare for the birth of this baby? As you work, say your thoughts and actions aloud so your assistant and I will know what you are thinking and doing."**

Instructor should check boxes as the learner responds correctly.

| Participant Name: | | |
|---|---|---|
| | ☐ Obtains relevant perinatal history | Gestational age? Fluid clear? How many babies? Other risk factors? |
| | Performs equipment check<br>☐ If obstetric provider indicates that meconium is present in amniotic fluid, prepares for intubation and meconium aspiration | **Warmer** on and towels to dry, **Clear airway** (bulb syringe, wall suction set at 80-100 mm Hg, meconium aspirator), **Auscultate** (stethoscope), **Oxygenate** (checks oxygen, blender, pulse oximeter and probe), **Ventilate** (checks positive-pressure ventilation [PPV] device), **Intubate** (laryngoscope and blades, endotracheal tubes, stylets, end-tidal $CO_2$ detector), **Medicate** (code cart accessible), **Thermoregulate** |
| **Option 1: Meconium-stained amniotic fluid, vigorous newborn.** | | |
| **"The baby has been born."** | | |
| **Sample Vital Signs** | **Performance Steps** | **Details** |
| Appears term<br>Respiratory rate (RR)-crying<br>Tone-flexed | Completes initial assessment when baby is born.<br>☐ Learner asks 3 questions:<br>• Term?<br>• Breathing or crying?<br>• Good tone? | Initial assessment determines whether or not baby will receive initial steps of resuscitation at the radiant warmer. |
| | ☐ Allows baby to stay with his mother for routine care: Warm, clear airway if necessary, dry, stimulate if necessary, continue evaluation | "Vigorous" meconium-stained baby is defined by<br>• Strong respiratory efforts<br>• Good muscle tone<br>• Heart rate (HR) >100 beats per minute (bpm)<br>Assume that a crying baby with good tone has HR >100 bpm. |

| | Option 2: Meconium-stained amniotic fluid; non-vigorous newborn | |
|---|---|---|
| | **"The baby has been born."** | |
| **Sample Vital Signs** | **Performance Steps** | **Details** |
| Appears term<br>Not breathing<br>Limp | Completes initial assessment when baby is born.<br>☐ Learner asks 3 questions:<br>   • Term?<br>   • Breathing or crying?<br>   • Good tone? | This baby requires initial steps, even without the additional risk factor of meconium-stained amniotic fluid. |
| RR-apneic<br>HR-70 bpm<br>Tone-limp | ☐ Receives at radiant warmer. Does not dry or stimulate to breathe.<br>☐ Assesses breathing, heart rate, tone.<br>☐ Indicates tracheal suctioning would be required. | This is a "non-vigorous" meconium-stained baby.<br><br>Intubation and tracheal suctioning procedure discussed in Lesson 5. |
| | Baby has been intubated and suctioned.<br>Continue with any option below and begin with<br>"Receives baby at radiant warmer." | |
| | **Option 3: Clear fluid, newborn requires initial steps** | |
| | **"The baby has been born."** | |
| Term-yes<br>RR-weak<br>Tone-limp | Completes initial assessment when baby is born<br>☐ Learner asks 3 questions:<br>   • Term?<br>   • Breathing or crying?<br>   • Good tone? | Instructor may tailor scenario to meet learner needs; any or all of the assessment questions may prompt initiation of initial steps. |
| | ☐ **Receives baby at radiant warmer**<br>   • Positions airway<br>   • Suctions mouth and nose<br>   • Dries with towel or blanket<br>   • Removes wet linen<br>   • Stimulates by flicking soles or rubbing back | Learner should move quickly through these steps. |
| RR-cry<br>HR-120 bpm<br>Tone–fair<br>Color-cyanotic | ☐ Assesses breathing and heart rate | If learner believes baby is cyanotic and requires supplemental oxygen, learner should administer free-flow oxygen and immediately connect pulse oximeter to confirm the perception of cyanosis. |
| | **"The baby is now 3 minutes old and appears cyanotic"** | |
| Breathing<br>HR-140 bpm<br>Appears cyanotic | ☐ Begins supplemental oxygen<br>☐ Places oximeter probe on right hand or wrist, then connects oximeter<br>☐ Confirms reliable signal by ensuring audio/pulsing light correlates with baby's actual heart rate | Free-flow oxygen may be given by oxygen mask, flow-inflating bag and mask, T-piece resuscitator, or oxygen tubing. It may not be given through the mask of a self-inflating bag. |

| | | |
|---|---|---|
| $SPO_2$-65% | ☐ Continues free-flow oxygen and weans per oximetry target range for age | Target range for 3 minutes of age = 70%-75%. |
| $SPO_2$-72% | ☐ Does not begin supplemental oxygen and continues to monitor baby's transition | |

**Option 4: Clear fluid, newborn requires initial steps.**

**"The baby has been born."**

| Sample Vital Signs | Performance Steps | Details |
|---|---|---|
| Appears term<br>Weak cry<br>Limp | Completes initial assessment when baby is born<br>☐ Learner asks 3 questions:<br>• Term?<br>• Breathing or crying?<br>• Good tone?<br>☐ Receives baby at radiant warmer<br>• Positions airway<br>• Suctions mouth and nose<br>• Dries with towel or blanket<br>• Removes wet linen<br>• Stimulates by flicking soles or rubbing back | Learner should move through these steps quickly; handle baby gently, do not use bulb syringe aggressively, do not waste time continuing to stimulate baby if unresponsive. |
| RR-labored<br>HR-110 bpm<br>Tone-fair<br>Color-cyanotic | ☐ Assesses breathing, heart rate | Visual perception of cyanosis is unreliable. If newborn seems persistently cyanotic, start supplemental oxygen and confirm cyanosis with pulse oximetry. |
| | ☐ Begins free-flow oxygen<br>☐ Attaches oximeter probe to right hand or wrist; then attaches to oximeter<br>☐ Considers continuous positive airway pressure (CPAP) | Free-flow oxygen may be given by oxygen mask, flow-inflating bag and mask, T-piece resuscitator, or oxygen tubing. It may not be given through the mask of a self-inflating bag.<br><br>CPAP is possible with flow-inflating bag or T-piece resuscitator. |
| RR-40 breaths per minute<br>HR-120 bpm<br>$SPO_2$-74% | ☐ Evaluates oximetry reading in relation to age. | Refers to table of pre-ductal oxygen saturation targets on Neonatal Resuscitation Program flow diagram. |
| RR-40 breaths per minute and unlabored<br>HR-140 bpm<br><br>$SPO_2$-97%<br>or<br>$SPO_2$-65% | At 3 minutes of age:<br><br><br>☐ Weans supplemental oxygen<br><br>☐ Indicates need for PPV | <br><br><br><br>Increases free-flow oxygen concentration and/or indicates need for trial of PPV. |

**Instructor asks the learner Reflective Questions to enable self-assessment, such as:**

1. How did you know if the newborn required
   A. Initial steps at the radiant warmer?
   B. Intubation and suction of meconium from the trachea?
   C. Routine care and could stay with his mother?
   D. Supplemental oxygen?

2. Tell us about how you used pulse oximetry to guide your actions.

3. At what point would you need to call for more help?

4. What went well during this resuscitation?

5. Would you do anything differently when faced with this scenario (indicate which scenario) again?

### Neonatal Resuscitation Program Key Behavioral Skills

| | |
|---|---|
| Know your environment. | Allocate attention wisely. |
| Anticipate and plan. | Use all available information. |
| Assume the leadership role. | Use all available resources. |
| Communicate effectively. | Call for help when needed. |
| Delegate workload optimally. | Maintain professional behavior. |

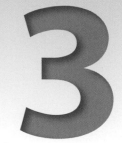

# Use of Resuscitation Devices for Positive-Pressure Ventilation

## In Lesson 3 you will learn

- When to give positive-pressure ventilation

- The similarities and differences among *flow-inflating bags, self-inflating bags,* and *T-piece resuscitators*

- How to assess oxygenation and manage oxygen delivery in babies receiving positive-pressure ventilation

- The correct placement of a mask on the newborn's face

- How to test and troubleshoot devices used to provide positive-pressure ventilation

- How to administer positive-pressure ventilation with a face mask and positive-pressure device and assess effective ventilation

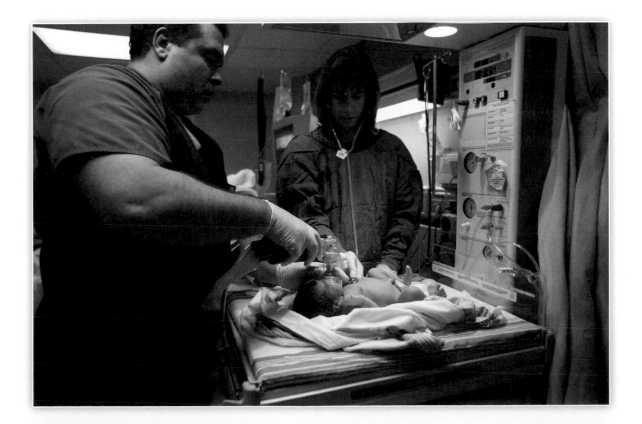

The following case is an example of how positive-pressure ventilation (PPV) is provided during resuscitation. As you read the case, imagine yourself as part of the resuscitation team. The details of how to deliver PPV are then described in the remainder of the lesson.

## Case 3.
# Resuscitation with positive-pressure ventilation using bag and mask

A 20-year-old woman with pregnancy-induced hypertension has labor induced at 38 weeks' gestation. Several late decelerations of fetal heart rate are noted, but labor progresses quickly and a baby boy is soon delivered.

He is limp and apneic and is taken to the radiant warmer, where a nurse appropriately positions his head to open his airway, while his mouth and nose are cleared of secretions with a bulb syringe. He is dried with warm towels, wet linen is removed, his head is repositioned, and he is further stimulated to breathe by flicking the soles of his feet.

No spontaneous respirations are noted after these actions; therefore, positive-pressure ventilation (PPV) is provided with a bag and mask and 21% oxygen (room air). A second person comes to assist; she places an oximeter probe on the baby's right hand, and connects it to a pulse oximeter. The assistant auscultates the chest and reports that the heart rate is 70 beats per minute (bpm) and not rising, oxygen saturation is 63% and not increasing, and breath sounds are not audible on either side of the chest.

The nurse initiates corrective ventilation steps by reapplying the mask to the face and repositioning the baby's head to open the airway. The assistant reports that there is still no chest movement and no audible breath sounds. The nurse stops ventilating and quickly suctions the mouth and nose, opens the baby's mouth, and reattempts PPV; however, there is still no evidence of effective ventilation. The nurse increases inspiratory pressure while her assistant auscultates the newborn's chest, but reports no bilateral breath sounds or chest rise. Pressure is increased again to about 30 cm $H_2O$. The assistant reports bilateral breath sounds and chest movement with each ventilation. The baby is about 2 minutes old; the heart rate is 80 bpm and oxygen saturation is 64%. The assistant increases the oxygen concentration to 40%.

The assistant monitors the baby's respiratory effort, heart rate, and oxygen saturation, while the nurse ventilates the baby effectively for an additional 30 seconds. At this point, the baby has an occasional spontaneous breath, heart rate is 120 bpm, and oxygen saturation is 82% at 3 minutes of age. The oxygen blender is turned down to 25%. The assistant quickly inserts an orogastric tube. The nurse decreases her ventilation rate and watches for improving respiratory efforts while the assistant stimulates the baby to breathe. When the newborn is 4 minutes of age, he is breathing spontaneously, the heart rate is 140 bpm, oxygen saturation is 87%, and PPV is discontinued. Free-flow supplemental oxygen is discontinued as the saturation remains above 85% and the orogastric tube is removed. He is shown to his mother, and she is encouraged to hold him while the next steps are explained. After a few more minutes of observation, the baby is moved to the nursery for post-resuscitation care, where vital signs, oximetry, and the baby's overall status are monitored closely for further problems.

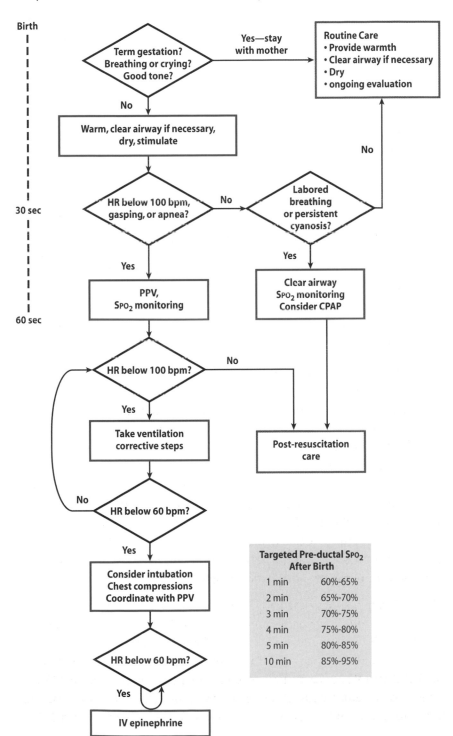

## What will this lesson cover?

In this lesson, you will learn how to prepare and use a resuscitation bag and mask and/or a T-piece resuscitator to deliver PPV. The option of delivering continuous positive airway pressure (CPAP) by mask will be covered in more detail in Lesson 8.

You learned in Lesson 2 how to determine within a few seconds whether some form of resuscitation is required and how to perform the initial steps of resuscitation. You learned that, if the baby is breathing but has persistent central cyanosis, you attach an oximeter to confirm low oxygen saturation and administer free-flow supplemental oxygen.

This lesson will cover what to do next if the baby is not breathing effectively or is bradycardic after you have performed the initial steps.

> **!** Ventilation of the lungs is the single most important and most effective step in cardiopulmonary resuscitation of the compromised newborn.

## What are the indications for positive-pressure ventilation?

If the baby is not breathing (apneic) or is gasping, the heart rate is below 100 beats per minute (bpm) even with breathing, and/or the saturation remains below target values despite free-flow supplemental oxygen being increased to 100%, the next step is to provide PPV.

## What terms do you need to know when giving positive-pressure ventilation?

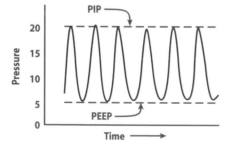

**Figure 3.1.** Pressure tracing during positive-pressure ventilation.
PIP = Peak Inspiratory Pressure;
PEEP = Positive-End Expiratory Pressure.

This lesson will address the following components of PPV (Figure 3.1):

- Peak inspiratory pressure (PIP): This is the pressure delivered with each breath, such as the pressure at the end of a squeeze of a resuscitation bag or at the end of the breath with a T-piece resuscitator.

- Positive end-expiratory pressure (PEEP): This is the gas pressure remaining in the system between breaths, such as occurs during relaxation and before the next squeeze.

- Continuous positive airway pressure (CPAP): This is the same as PEEP, but is the term used when the baby is breathing spontaneously and not receiving positive-pressure breaths. It is the pressure in the system at the end of a spontaneous breath when a mask is held tightly on the baby's face, but the bag is not being squeezed.

- Rate: The number of assisted breaths being administered, such as the number of times per minute that the bag is squeezed.

## What are the different types of resuscitation devices available to ventilate newborns?

Three types of devices are available to ventilate newborns, and they work in different ways.

**1** The *self-inflating bag* fills spontaneously after it has been squeezed, pulling gas (air or oxygen or a mixture of both) into the bag.

**2** The *flow-inflating bag* (also called an anesthesia bag) fills only when gas from a compressed source flows into it and the outlet of the bag is occluded by being placed tightly against a surface (for testing) or against the baby's face with a mask, or is connected to the baby's airway via an endotracheal tube.

**3** The *T-piece resuscitator* provides flow-controlled and pressure-limited breaths and works only when gas from a compressed source flows into it.

Find out what kind of resuscitation device is used in your hospital. If your hospital uses the T-piece resuscitator in the delivery area, you should still learn the details of whichever of the 2 types of bags are commonly used outside of the delivery area.

A self-inflating bag should be readily available as a backup wherever resuscitation may be needed, in case a compressed gas source fails or the T-piece device malfunctions. Details of all 3 devices are found in the Appendix to this lesson. You should read those section(s) of the Appendix that apply to the device(s) used in your hospital.

The *self-inflating bag,* as its name implies, inflates automatically without a compressed gas source (Figure 3.2). It remains inflated at all times, unless being squeezed. The concentration of oxygen being delivered using a self-inflating bag may not be consistent unless a reservoir is attached to the gas inlet. Peak inspiratory pressure (ie, peak inflation pressure) is controlled by how hard the bag is squeezed. Positive end-expiratory pressure can be administered only if an additional valve is attached to the self-inflating bag. Continuous positive airway pressure cannot be delivered reliably with a self-inflating bag. To help ensure that appropriate pressure is used when providing PPV in a newborn, you should use a self-inflating bag that has an integral *pressure gauge or, if there is a site for attaching a pressure gauge (manometer), you should make sure one is attached.*

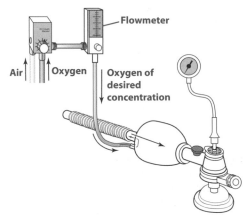

**Figure 3.2.** Self-inflating bag remains inflated without gas flow and without having the mask sealed on the face

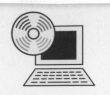

**You are encouraged to view this video on the DVD that accompanies this textbook:** *CPAP Administration*

The *flow-inflating bag* is collapsed like a deflated balloon when not in use (Figure 3.3). It inflates only when a gas source is forced into the bag and the opening of the bag is sealed, as when the mask is placed tightly on a baby's face, or when the baby has been intubated and the bag is attached to the endotracheal tube. Peak inspiratory pressure is controlled by the flow rate of incoming gas, adjustment of the flow-control valve, and how hard the bag is squeezed. Positive end-expiratory pressure or CPAP is controlled by an adjustable flow-control valve.

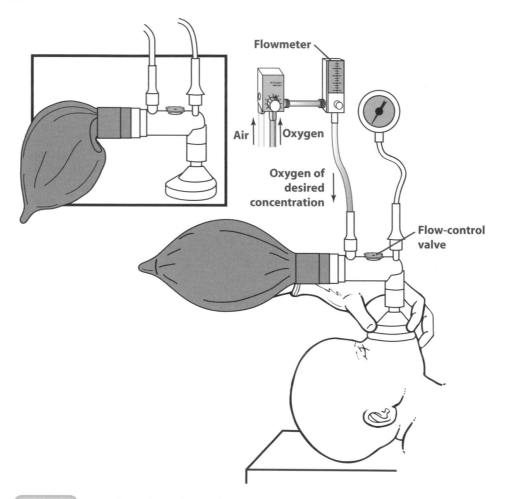

**Figure 3.3.** Flow-inflating bag inflates only with a compressed gas source and with mask sealed on face; otherwise, the bag remains deflated (inset)

The ***T-piece resuscitator*** (Figure 3.4) is flow controlled and pressure limited. Like the flow-inflating bag, this device requires a compressed gas source. Peak inspiratory pressure and positive end-expiratory pressure (PEEP or CPAP), if desired, are set manually with adjustable controls. Breaths are delivered when the operator alternately occludes and opens the aperture on the device connected to the mask or endotracheal tube.

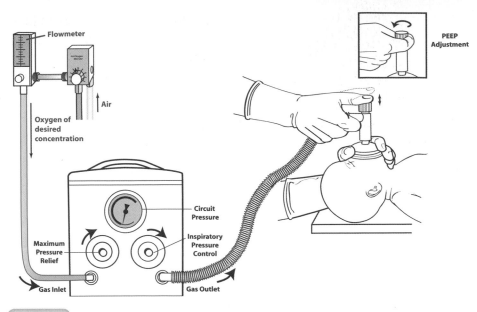

**Figure 3.4.** Flow-controlled, pressure-limited device (T-piece resuscitator). Pressures are pre-set by adjusting controls on the device and are delivered by occluding and opening the aperture in the PEEP cap.

## What are the advantages and disadvantages of each assisted-ventilation device?

The ***self-inflating bag*** (Figure 3.5) is found more commonly in the hospital delivery room and resuscitation cart than the flow-inflating bag. It often is considered easier to use because it reinflates completely after being squeezed; this happens even if it is not attached to a compressed gas source and even if its mask is not on a patient's face. The disadvantage of this is that you will be less likely to know if you have achieved a good seal between the mask and the baby's face, which is required for the pressure from the squeezed bag to result in effective gas flow delivered to the baby's lungs. It cannot be used to administer free-flow or "blow-by" oxygen reliably through the mask and cannot be used to deliver CPAP.

When a self-inflating bag is not being squeezed, the amount of gas or oxygen flow that comes out of the patient outlet depends on the relative resistance and leaks in valves within the bag. Even when the self-inflating bag is connected to a 100% oxygen source, most of the oxygen is directed out of the back of the bag, and an unpredictable amount is directed toward the patient unless the bag is being squeezed.

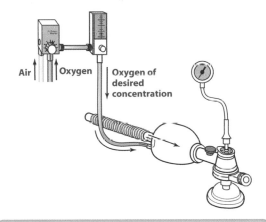

**Figure 3.5.** Self-inflating bag

**Advantages**
- Will always refill after being squeezed, even with no compressed gas source
- Pressure-release valve makes overinflation less likely

**Disadvantages**
- Will inflate even if there is not a seal between the mask and the patient's face
- Requires oxygen reservoir to provide high concentration of oxygen
- Cannot be used to deliver free-flow oxygen reliably through the mask
- Cannot be used to deliver continuous positive airway pressure (CPAP) and can deliver positive end-expiratory pressure (PEEP) only when a PEEP valve is added and pressurized gas is entering the bag

Therefore, the self-inflating bag cannot be used to deliver free-flow oxygen through the mask. In addition, as was described in Lesson 2, the self-inflating bag must have an oxygen reservoir attached to deliver a high concentration of oxygen, even while PPV is being provided.

In some situations, providers may want to deliver PEEP to a baby who is receiving PPV, or CPAP to a spontaneously breathing baby. Positive end-expiratory pressure can be delivered with a self-inflating bag if a special "PEEP valve" is used, but there must be pressurized gas entering the bag to generate the PEEP. Also, CPAP cannot be administered with a self-inflating bag, even if a PEEP valve is present.

As a safety precaution, most self-inflating bags have a pressure-release valve (pop-off valve) that limits the peak inspiratory pressure that can be delivered. However, the pressure at which the valve "pops off" can vary considerably from the manufacturer's specifications; therefore, the only reliable way to monitor the pressure being delivered to the baby and to prevent the use of excessive pressures is to attach a pressure gauge (manometer) to the bag. You should use a self-inflating bag that has an integral *pressure gauge or, if there is a site for attaching a pressure gauge (manometer), you should make sure one is attached.*

The *flow-inflating bag* (Figure 3.6) requires a compressed gas source for inflation. When the gas flows into the device, it will take the path of least resistance and either flow out the patient outlet or into the bag. To make the bag inflate, you need to keep the gas from escaping by having the face mask sealed tightly against the newborn's face. Therefore, when a newborn is being resuscitated, the bag will not fill unless there is gas flow **and** the mask is tightly sealed over the baby's mouth and nose, or the device is attached to an endotracheal tube inserted into the baby's airway. Absent or partial inflation of the flow-inflating bag indicates that a tight seal has not been established.

In addition, because the oxygen concentration that exits a flow-inflating bag is the same as that which enters the bag, the flow-inflating bag can reliably be used to deliver free-flow oxygen at any concentration up to 100% oxygen if desired.

The main disadvantage of using a flow-inflating bag is that it takes more practice to use it effectively. In addition, because a compressed gas source is required to inflate the bag, it is sometimes not available for use as quickly as a self-inflating bag. This may become an issue when the need for resuscitation is unanticipated.

Because most flow-inflating bags do not have a safety valve, it is important to watch for the degree of chest movement with each assisted breath to avoid underinflation or overinflation of the lungs. The pressure being delivered can be adjusted using the flow-control valve. The use of a pressure gauge is recommended to provide a more

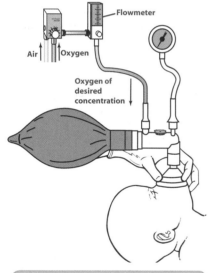

**Figure 3.6.** Flow-inflating bag

**Advantages**
- Can deliver up to 100% oxygen, depending on the source
- Easy to determine when there is a seal on the patient's face
- Can be used to deliver free-flow oxygen at concentrations up to 100%, depending on the source

**Disadvantages**
- Requires a tight seal between the mask and the patient's face to remain inflated
- Requires a gas source to inflate
- Requires use of a pressure gauge to monitor pressure being delivered with each breath

objective assessment of peak inspiratory pressure and to help maintain consistency of each assisted breath.

The *T-piece resuscitator* (Figure 3.7) has many similarities to the flow-inflating bag, with the added feature of mechanically controlling airway pressures. Like the flow-inflating bag, the T-piece resuscitator requires gas flow from a compressed gas source and has an adjustable flow-control valve to regulate the desired amount of CPAP or PEEP. The T-piece resuscitator also requires a tight mask-to-face seal to deliver a breath and can deliver up to 100% free-flow oxygen. The device also requires some preparation time for set-up prior to use, and pressure limits must be estimated based on the expected needs of the newborn.

The T-piece resuscitator differs from the flow-inflating bag in that the peak inspiratory pressure is controlled by a mechanical adjustment instead of by the amount of squeeze on the bag. Gas flow is directed to the baby or the environment when you alternately occlude and open the aperture in the PEEP cap with your finger or thumb. The T-piece resuscitator provides more consistent pressure with each breath than either the self-inflating or flow-inflating bag, and is not subject to operator fatigue that may occur while squeezing a bag. However, there is a risk of delivering breaths with a longer than desired inspiratory time if the operator does not monitor the duration of occlusion of the PEEP cap with each breath.

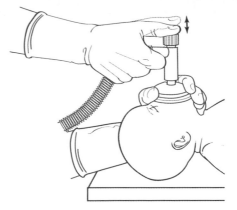

**Figure 3.7.** T-piece resuscitator

**Advantages**
- Consistent pressure
- Reliable control of peak inspiratory pressure and positive end-expiratory pressure
- Reliable delivery of 100% oxygen
- Operator does not become fatigued from bagging

**Disadvantages**
- Requires compressed gas supply
- Requires pressures to be set prior to use
- Changing inflation pressure during resuscitation is more difficult
- Risk of prolonged inspiratory time

## What are important characteristics of resuscitation devices used to ventilate newborns?

The equipment used should be specifically designed for newborns. Consideration should be given to the following:

### Appropriate-sized masks
A variety of masks appropriate for babies of different sizes should be available at every delivery, because it may be difficult to determine the required size before birth. The mask should rest on the chin and cover the mouth and nose, but not the eyes, while still being small enough to create a tight seal on the face.

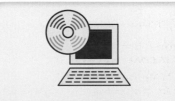

**You are encouraged to view this video on the DVD that accompanies this textbook:** *Using the T-piece Resuscitator*

| Targeted Pre-ductal $S_{PO_2}$ After Birth | |
|---|---|
| 1 min | 60%-65% |
| 2 min | 65%-70% |
| 3 min | 70%-75% |
| 4 min | 75%-80% |
| 5 min | 80%-85% |
| 10 min | 85%-95% |

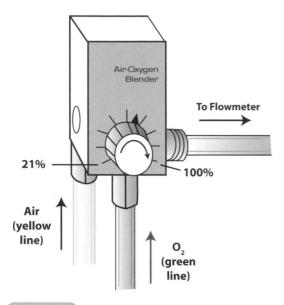

**Figure 3.8A.** Mixing oxygen and air with an oxygen blender. The control knob dials in the desired oxygen concentration.

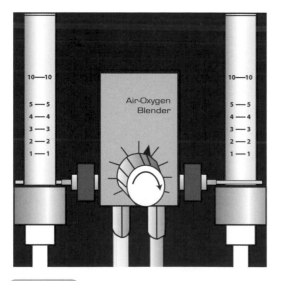

**Figure 3.8B.** Mixing oxygen and air with an oxygen blender with double output for 2 flowmeters. One flowmeter can be connected to a bag-and-mask device, while the other can be connected to oxygen tubing used to give free-flow oxygen.

## Capability to deliver variable oxygen concentrations during resuscitation

As described in Lesson 2, when PPV or supplemental oxygen is used, you should use an oximeter to judge the baby's state of oxygenation and to guide you in the concentration of oxygen to use. The recommended target to achieve is an oxygen saturation ($S_{PO_2}$) similar to that of a healthy term baby following birth.

You will need the following equipment to deliver variable oxygen concentrations during resuscitation:

• *Compressed air and oxygen source*
You will need a source of compressed air (either from a built-in wall source or compressed gas tank) to mix with a 100% oxygen source to achieve oxygen concentrations between 21% (room air) and 100%.

• *Oxygen blender* (Figure 3.8A and 3.8B)
An oxygen blender is needed to deliver an oxygen concentration between 21% and 100%. High-pressure hoses run from the oxygen and air sources to the blender, which has a dial that adjusts the gas mixture to achieve oxygen levels between 21% and 100% oxygen. The blender then connects to an adjustable flowmeter so that gas flow rates of 0 to 20 L/min of the desired oxygen concentration can be delivered directly to the baby or to the positive-pressure device. Management of oxygen delivery will be discussed later in this lesson.

**Capability to control peak pressure, end-expiratory pressure, and inspiratory time**

Establishing adequate ventilation is the most important step in resuscitating newborns. The amount of positive pressure required will vary, based on the state of the newborn's lungs. Delivery of excessive positive pressure can injure the lung, while use of inadequate pressure may delay establishment of effective ventilation. Adding PEEP when assisting ventilation with intermittent positive pressure, or administering CPAP to babies who are breathing spontaneously, may be helpful in establishing effective lung inflation, especially in babies with immature lungs, as will be discussed in Lesson 8. The presence of a pressure gauge is helpful to monitor the peak and end-expiratory pressures being delivered.

The duration of the inspiratory time is one factor that contributes to inflating the lungs. Increasing the inspiratory time is accomplished by squeezing a flow-inflating bag for a longer time or by keeping your finger on the PEEP cap of the T-piece resuscitator longer. However, the optimum inspiratory time to use during resuscitation of a newborn has not been determined.

**Appropriate-sized bag**

Bags used for newborns should have a minimum volume of about 200 mL and a maximum of 750 mL. Term newborns require only 10 to 25 mL with each ventilation (4 to 6 mL/kg). Bags larger than 750 mL, which are designed for older children and adults, make it difficult to provide such small volumes and deliver controlled peak pressure. Bags that are too small will not adequately reinflate between breaths when rates of 40 to 60 breaths/minute are used.

**Safety features**

To minimize complications resulting from high ventilation pressures, resuscitation devices should have certain safety features to prevent or guard against inadvertent use of high pressures. These features will be different for each type of device.

## What safety features prevent the pressure in the device from getting too high?

You will attach a resuscitation device to a mask, which will be held tightly against the patient's face, or to an endotracheal tube, which will be in the patient's trachea. In either case, if you ventilate with high pressure and/or rate, the lungs could become overinflated, causing rupture of the alveoli and a resulting air leak, such as a pneumothorax.

*Self-inflating bags* should have a pressure-release valve (commonly called a **pop-off valve**) (Figure 3.9), which generally is set by the manufacturer to 30 to 40 cm $H_2O$. If peak inspiratory pressures greater than 30 to 40 cm $H_2O$ are generated, the valve opens, limiting the pressure being transmitted to the newborn. There may be wide variation in the point at which a pressure-release valve opens. The make and age of the bag as well as the method with which a non-disposable bag has been cleaned affect the opening pressure of the valve.

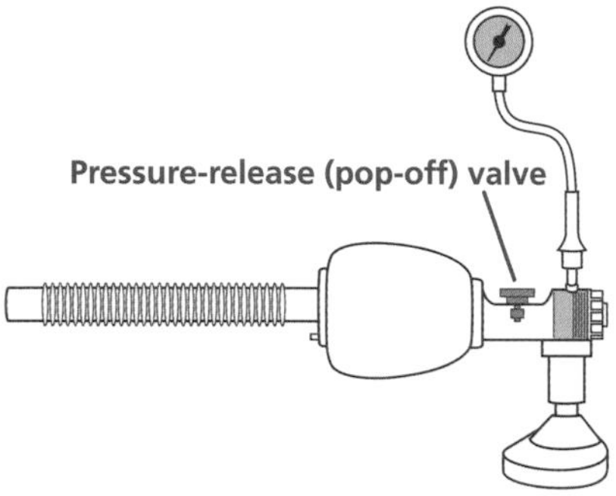

In some self-inflating bags, the pressure-release valve can be temporarily occluded or bypassed to allow higher pressures to be administered. This usually is not necessary, but can be done to ventilate a newborn's non-aerated lungs when the usual pressures are not effective, especially with the first few breaths. Care must be taken not to use excessive pressure while the pressure-release valve is bypassed.

Self-inflating bags also should be equipped with a pressure gauge (manometer) or a port to attach a pressure gauge to allow you to monitor the peak inspiratory pressure as you squeeze the bag.

*Flow-inflating bags* have a flow-control valve (Figure 3.10), which can be adjusted to deliver the desired PEEP. If the flow-control valve is adjusted incorrectly, it is possible to overinflate the baby's lungs inadvertently. An attached pressure gauge should be used to avoid giving excessive pressures.

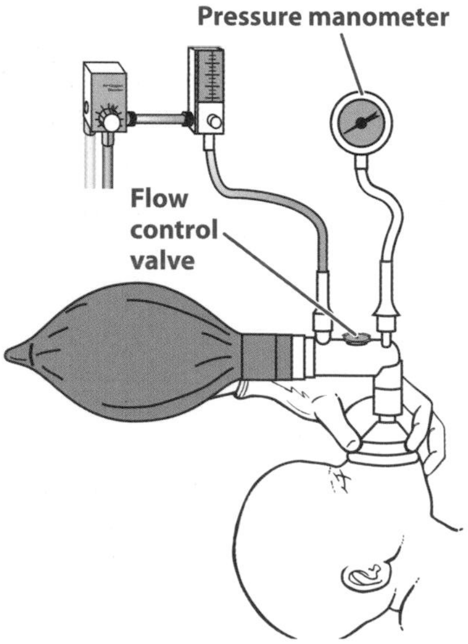

**Pressure-release (pop-off) valve**

**Figure 3.9.** Self-inflating bag with pressure-release (pop-off) valve

**Pressure manometer**

**Flow control valve**

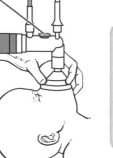

**Figure 3.10.** Flow-inflating bag with flow-control valve and attached manometer

> **!** Be certain to connect the oxygen supply line to the correct connection site as indicated by the bag's manufacturer. Connection of the oxygen supply line to the pressure gauge port has been reported to result in inadvertent high-inflating pressures being delivered to the patient and may result in a pneumothorax.

*T-piece resuscitators* have 2 controls to adjust the inspiratory pressure. The *inspiratory pressure* control sets the amount of pressure delivered during a normal assisted breath. The *peak inspiratory pressure* control is a safety feature that prevents the pressure from exceeding a preset value (usually 40 cm $H_2O$, but adjustable*). Excessive pressure also can be avoided by watching the circuit pressure gauge (Figure 3.11).

* Note: Some manufacturers recommend that the maximum relief control be adjusted to an institution-defined limit when the device is put into original service and not be readjusted during regular use.

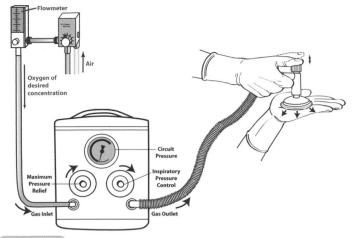

**Figure 3.11.** Maximum pressure relief and inspiratory pressure controls on T-piece resuscitator

**Table 3-1. Features of devices used for positive-pressure ventilation during neonatal resuscitation**

| Characteristic | Self-Inflating Bag | Flow-Inflating Bag | T-piece Resuscitator |
|---|---|---|---|
| **Appropriate-sized Masks** | Available | Available | Available |
| **Oxygen Concentration:**<br>• 90% 100% capability<br>• Variable concentration | • Only with reservoir<br>• Only with blender plus reservoir<br>• Amount of oxygen delivered with no reservoir attached unpredictable | • Yes<br>• Only with blender | • Yes<br>• Only with blender |
| **Peak Inspiratory Pressure** | Amount of squeeze measured by the recommended pressure gauge | Amount of squeeze measured by pressure gauge | Peak inspiratory pressure determined by adjustable mechanical setting |
| **Positive End-expiratory Pressure (PEEP)** | No direct control (unless optional PEEP valve attached) | Flow-control valve adjustment | PEEP control |
| **Inspiratory Time** | Duration of squeeze | Duration of squeeze | Duration that PEEP cap is occluded |
| **Appropriate-sized Bag** | Available | Available | Not applicable |
| **Safety Features** | • Pop-off valve<br>• Pressure gauge | • Pressure gauge | • Maximum pressure relief valve<br>• Pressure gauge |

Each of these characteristics will be described in the Appendix, under the detailed description of each device.

## Review

*(The answers are in the preceding section and at the end of the lesson.)*

1. Flow-inflating bags (will) (will not) work without a compressed gas source.

2. A baby is born apneic and cyanotic. You clear her airway and stimulate her. Thirty seconds after birth, she has not improved. The next step is to (stimulate her more) (begin positive-pressure ventilation).

3. The single most important and most effective step in neonatal resuscitation is (stimulation) (ventilating the lungs).

4. Label these bags "flow-inflating," "self-inflating," or "T-piece resuscitator."

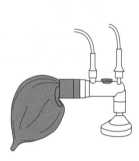 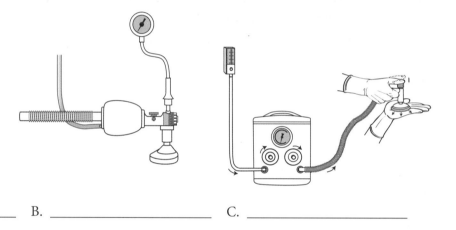

A. _____     B. _____     C. _____

5. Masks of different sizes (do) (do not) need to be available at every delivery.

6. Self-inflating bags require the attachment of a(n)_____ to deliver a high concentration of oxygen.

7. T-piece resuscitators (will) (will not) work without a compressed gas source.

8. Neonatal ventilation bags are (much smaller than) (the same size as) adult ventilation bags.

9. List the principal safety features for each of the following devices:

   Self-inflating bag: _____ and _____

   Flow-inflating bag: _____

   T-piece resuscitator: _____ and _____

## How do I assess the effectiveness of positive-pressure ventilation?

Rising heart rate is the most important indicator of successful resuscitation efforts. Every time PPV is initiated, heart rate is assessed first, along with oxygen saturation, if pulse oximetry is functioning.

If heart rate is not rising with PPV, you will assess for effective ventilation by listening for bilateral breath sounds and looking for chest movement with each positive-pressure breath. Positive-pressure ventilation that achieves bilateral breath sounds and chest movement is considered effective, even if the baby does not respond with rising heart rate and improved oxygen saturation.

However, most newborns respond to effective ventilation with a rising heart rate that exceeds 100 bpm, improvement in oxygen saturation, and, finally, spontaneous respiratory effort.

If you watch for these important signs, PPV can be provided effectively with any of the positive-pressure devices described in this lesson. The choice of which one(s) to employ should be determined by individual facilities.

> **!** The most important indicator of successful positive-pressure ventilation is rising heart rate.

## What concentration of oxygen should be used when giving positive-pressure ventilation during resuscitation?

Several recent studies suggest that resuscitation of term newborns with 21% oxygen (room air) is just as successful as resuscitation with 100% oxygen. There is also some evidence that exposure to 100% oxygen during and following perinatal asphyxia may be harmful. However, since asphyxia involves deprivation of oxygen to body tissues, and pulmonary blood flow improves when oxygen concentration is increased, there is a theoretical possibility that using supplemental oxygen during resuscitation of newborns with asphyxia will result in more rapid restoration of tissue oxygen and, perhaps, less permanent tissue damage and improved blood flow to the lungs.

As described in Lesson 2, in an attempt to balance the hazards possibly associated with these 2 extremes of oxygenation, this program recommends that your goal during and following resuscitation of a newborn should be to achieve an oxyhemoglobin saturation as measured by pulse oximetry that closely mimics the saturation measured in uncompromised babies born at term as they establish air breathing during the first few minutes of extrauterine life.

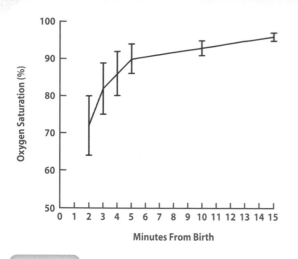

**Figure 3.12.** Pre-ductal oxygen saturation changes following birth (median and interquartile range). (From Mariani G, Dik PB, Ezquer A, et al. Pre-ductal and post-ductal $O_2$ saturation in healthy term neonates after birth. *J Pediatr.* 2007;150:418-421.)

| Targeted Pre-ductal $S_{PO_2}$ After Birth | |
|---|---|
| 1 min | 60%-65% |
| 2 min | 65%-70% |
| 3 min | 70%-75% |
| 4 min | 75%-80% |
| 5 min | 80%-85% |
| 10 min | 85%-95% |

Before birth and throughout intrauterine development, the fetus lives in an environment that results in a blood oxygen saturation that remains consistently at approximately 60%. After the first breath of room air is taken and the umbilical cord is cut, the normal newborn delivered at term gradually increases his or her oxygen saturation to greater than 90% (Figure 3.12). However, even healthy newborns may take 10 minutes or longer to reach this normal extrauterine saturation.

To match this normal gradual increase of saturation when resuscitating a baby who is compromised at birth, you will need to attach an oximeter as soon as possible, to help guide you in how much supplemental oxygen to use, if any. While the oximeter is being attached, you can begin resuscitation with 21% oxygen in term newborns; preterm newborns may achieve normal oxygen saturations more quickly if you start with a somewhat higher oxygen concentration. If you have had adequate time to prepare for the resuscitation (such as with a baby being born preterm), you may decide to start with an intermediate concentration to help you achieve the desired saturation more quickly, without resulting in periods of too low or too high a saturation.

> ! **Ventilation of the lungs is the single most important and most effective step, regardless of the concentration of oxygen being used.**

Once the oximeter is giving a reliable reading, as indicated by the monitor's pulse light, adjust the blender up or down to try to achieve an $S_{PO_2}$ reading in the saturation range shown in the table.

# Can you give free-flow oxygen using a resuscitation device?

### Self-inflating bag:

*Free-flow oxygen cannot be given via the mask of a **self-inflating bag-and-mask device** (Figure 3.13).*

The oxygen flow entering a self-inflating bag will, normally, be diverted to the air inlet, through its attached oxygen reservoir, and then evacuated either out the end of the oxygen reservoir or out a valve that is attached to the reservoir. The amount of oxygen sent to the patient will depend on the relative resistance of the various valves and, therefore, may not reach the patient unless the bag is being squeezed. If your hospital is equipped with self-inflating bags, you may need to have a separate setup available for delivering free-flow oxygen, as described in Lesson 2.

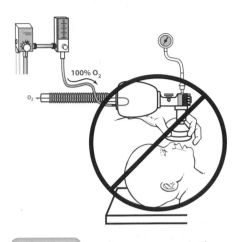

**Figure 3.13.** Free-flow oxygen cannot be given reliably by self-inflating bag; bag must be squeezed for reliable oxygen delivery so a separate set-up may be necessary to deliver free-flow oxygen

### Flow-inflating bag/T-piece resuscitator:

*A **flow-inflating bag or T-piece resuscitator** can be used to deliver free-flow oxygen (Figure 3.14).*

The mask should be placed loosely on the face, allowing some gas to escape around the edges. If the mask is held tightly to the face, pressure will build up in the bag or in the T-piece device and be transmitted to the newborn's lungs in the form of CPAP or PEEP. If a flow-inflating bag is used, the bag should not inflate when used to provide free-flow oxygen. An inflated bag indicates that the mask is tight against the face and positive pressure is being provided.

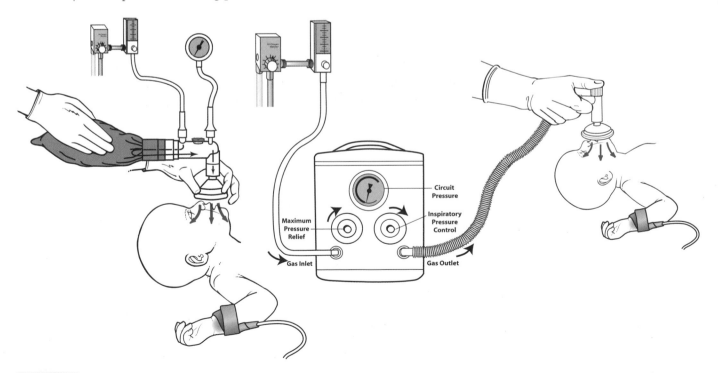

**Figure 3.14.** Free-flow oxygen given by flow-inflating bag (left) and by T-piece resuscitator (right). Note that mask is not held tightly on the face. Administration of less than 100% oxygen will require compressed air and a blender.

## What characteristics of face masks make them effective for ventilating newborns?

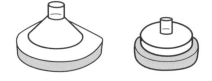

**Figure 3.15.** Face masks with rims

Masks come in a variety of shapes, sizes, and materials. Selection of a mask for use with a particular newborn depends on how well the mask fits and conforms to the newborn's face. The correct mask will achieve a tight seal between the mask and the newborn's face.

The rim on masks for newborns is cushioned (Figure 3.15) and is made from either a soft, flexible material, such as foam rubber, or an air-inflated ring. The rim conforms to the shape of the newborn's face, making it easier to form a seal.

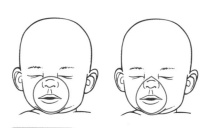

**Figure 3.16.** Round (left) and anatomically shaped (right) face masks

Masks also come in 2 shapes—round and anatomically shaped (Figure 3.16). Anatomically shaped masks are shaped to fit the contours of the face. They are made to be placed on the face with the most pointed part of the mask fitting over the nose.

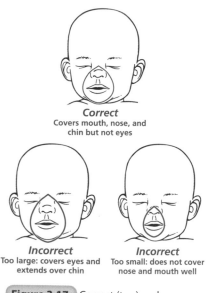

**Correct**
Covers mouth, nose, and chin but not eyes

**Incorrect**
Too large: covers eyes and extends over chin

**Incorrect**
Too small: does not cover nose and mouth well

**Figure 3.17.** Correct (top) and incorrect (bottom) mask sizes

Masks also come in several sizes. Masks suitable for small premature babies as well as for term babies should be available for use.

If the mask is the correct size, the rim will cover the tip of the chin, the mouth, and the nose, but not the eyes (Figure 3.17).

- Too large—may cause eye damage and will not seal well

- Too small—will not cover the mouth and nose and may occlude the nose

> **!** **Be sure to have various-sized masks available. Effective ventilation of a preterm baby with a term-newborn size mask is impossible.**

## How do you prepare the resuscitation device for an anticipated resuscitation?

### Assemble the equipment

Estimate the size of the baby and be sure you have appropriate-sized masks. The PPV device should be assembled and connected to a blender that has both an oxygen and an air supply. The oxygen blender enables you to provide any concentration of oxygen from 21% (room air) up to 100% oxygen, if needed. If a self-inflating bag is used, be sure the oxygen reservoir is attached. Prepare the oximeter and be certain that a neonatal-sized probe is available. (Note: If an oxygen blender and pulse oximeter are not immediately available, start PPV with 21% oxygen [room air] while you are obtaining an air-oxygen source and an oximeter.)

### Test the equipment

Once the equipment has been selected and assembled, check the device and mask to be sure they function properly. Bags that have cracks or holes, valves that stick or leak, devices that do not function properly, or defective masks must not be used. The equipment should be checked when rooms are stocked, and again before each delivery. The operator should check it again just before its use. There is a specific checklist for each of the devices, as described in the respective appendices.

> **!** **Be very familiar with the type of resuscitation device(s) you are using. Know exactly how to check it quickly to determine whether it is functioning properly.**

## Review

*(The answers are in the preceding section and at the end of the lesson.)*

10. Free-flow oxygen can be delivered reliably through the mask attached to a (flow-inflating bag) (self-inflating bag) (T-piece resuscitator).

11. When giving free-flow oxygen with a flow-inflating bag and mask, it is necessary to place the mask (securely) (loosely) on the baby's face to allow some gas to escape around the edges of the mask.

12. Before an anticipated resuscitation, the ventilation device should be connected to a(n) _____, which enables you to provide oxygen in any concentration, from room air up to 100% oxygen.

13. Resuscitation of the term newborn may begin with _____% oxygen. The oxygen concentration used during resuscitation is guided by the use of _____, which measures oxygen saturation.

# What do you need to do before beginning positive-pressure ventilation?

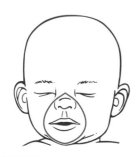

**If you are alone, call for a second person to provide assistance.**
Your assistant applies the pulse oximeter and monitors heart rate and breath sounds with a stethoscope.

**Select the appropriate-sized mask.**
Remember, the mask should cover the mouth, nose, and tip of the chin, but not the eyes (Figure 3.18).

**Figure 3.18.** Correct-sized mask covers mouth, nose, and tip of chin, but not the eyes

**Be sure there is a clear airway.**
You may want to suction the mouth and nose to be certain there will be no obstruction to PPV that you will be delivering. When the baby is apneic, airway obstruction may not be clinically apparent.

**Position the baby's head.**
As described in Lesson 2, the baby's neck should be slightly extended (but not overextended) into the "sniffing position" to maintain an open airway. One way to accomplish this is to place a rolled towel or small blanket under the shoulders (Figure 3.19).

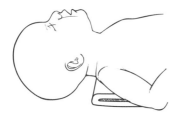

**Figure 3.19.** Correct position for assisted ventilation

**Position yourself at the bedside.**
You will need to position yourself at the baby's side or head to use a resuscitation device effectively (Figure 3.20). Both positions leave the chest and abdomen unobstructed for visual monitoring of the baby, for chest compressions, and for vascular access via the umbilical cord, should these procedures become necessary. If you are right-handed, you probably will feel most comfortable controlling the resuscitation device with your right hand and the mask with your left hand. If you are left-handed, you probably will want to control the resuscitation device with your left hand and hold the mask with your right hand. The mask may be swiveled to orient it properly.

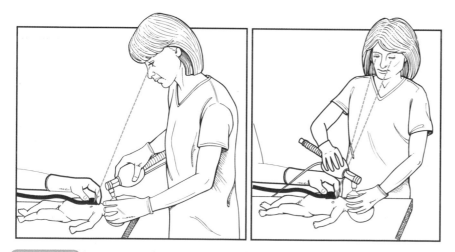

**Figure 3.20.** Two correct positions for visualizing chest movement during assisted ventilation

## How do you position the mask on the face?

The mask should be placed on the face so that it covers the nose and mouth, and the tip of the chin rests within the rim of the mask. You may find it helpful to begin by cupping the chin in the mask and then covering the nose (Figure 3.21).

Anatomically shaped masks should be positioned with the pointed end over the nose. Once the mask is positioned, an airtight seal can be formed by using light downward pressure on the rim of the mask and/or gently squeezing the mandible up toward the mask (Figure 3.22).

The mask usually is held on the face with the thumb, index, and/or middle finger encircling much of the rim of the mask, while the ring and fifth fingers lift the chin forward to maintain a patent airway.

Care should be taken in holding the mask. Observe the following precautions:

• Do not "jam" the mask down on the face. Too much pressure can bruise the face and inadvertently flex the baby's neck.

• Be careful not to rest your fingers or hand on the baby's eyes.

• Recheck the position of the mask and the baby's head at intervals while providing PPV to make sure they are still correctly positioned

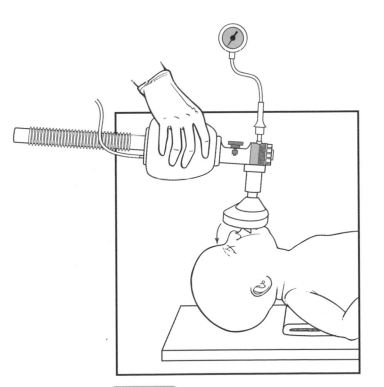

**Figure 3.21.** Cup the chin in the mask and then cover the nose

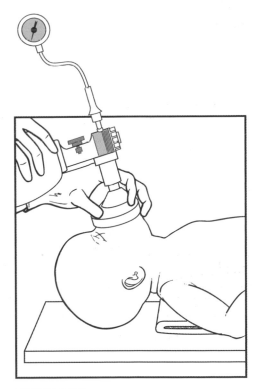

**Figure 3.22.** Correctly positioned mask on face. Light pressure on the mask will help create a seal. Anterior pressure on the posterior rim of the mandible (not shown) may also help.

## Why is establishing a seal between the mask and the face so important?

An airtight seal between the rim of the mask and the face is essential to achieve the positive pressure required to inflate the lungs *with any of the resuscitation devices.*

Although a self-inflating bag will remain inflated despite an inadequate seal, you will not be able to generate pressure to inflate the lungs when you squeeze the bag.

A flow-inflating bag will not inflate without a good mask-to-face seal and, therefore, you will not be able to squeeze the bag to create the desired pressure.

A T-piece resuscitator will not deliver positive pressure unless there is a good mask-to-face seal.

Remember,

- A tight seal is required for a flow-inflating bag to inflate.
- A tight seal is required for each of the resuscitation devices to generate positive pressure to inflate the lungs.

## How do you know how much inflation pressure to deliver?

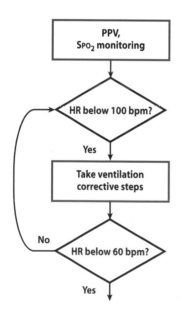

The lungs of a fetus are filled with fluid, but the lungs of a newborn must be filled with air. The first few breaths may need to be delivered with higher than usual pressures to fill the lungs with air. However, excessively high lung volumes and airway pressures can cause lung injury; therefore, it is important to squeeze the resuscitation bag just enough so that heart rate and oxygen saturation increase.

Start with an inspiratory pressure of about 20 cm $H_2O$. Rising heart rate (along with rising oxygen saturation if pulse oximetry is functional at this point) and audible bilateral breath sounds are the best indicators that inflation pressures are adequate.

Each breath might move the baby's chest; however, it is possible to provide adequate ventilation without visible chest movement, especially if the newborn is preterm.

 The best indication that the mask is sealed and the lungs are being adequately inflated is rising heart rate and audible bilateral breath sounds. When pulse oximetry has a reliable signal, oxygen saturation should also rise, and you will likely see chest movement with ventilation.

If the baby appears to be taking very deep breaths during PPV, the lungs are being overinflated. You are using too much pressure, and there is danger of producing a pneumothorax. Remember that the volume of a normal breath in a term newborn is much smaller than the amount of gas in your resuscitation bag: one-tenth of a 240-mL self-inflating bag or one-thirtieth of a 750-mL flow-inflating bag (Figure 3.23). Preterm babies require even smaller gas volumes to inflate the lungs and avoid injury (Chapter 8).

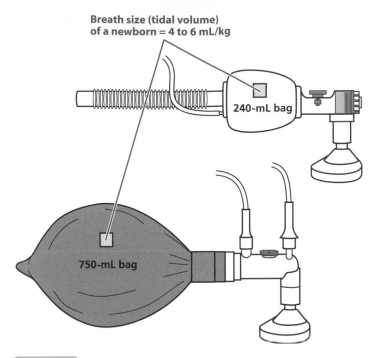

Breath size (tidal volume) of a newborn = 4 to 6 mL/kg

240-mL bag

750-mL bag

## What do you do if the baby's heart rate and oxygen saturation are not rising and you do not hear bilateral breath sounds or see chest movement?

**Figure 3.23.** Relative sizes of normal breath and common resuscitation bags

The recommended steps are summarized in Table 3.2. You have squeezed the bag or set the T-piece resuscitator to deliver 20 cm H$_2$O pressure. If heart rate and oximetry do not improve quickly **(within the first 5 to 10 breaths),** look for the presence of chest movement with each positive-pressure breath and ask your assistant to listen with a stethoscope for bilateral breath sounds. Be careful not to mistake abdominal movement because of air entering the stomach for effective ventilation of the lungs.

If the chest is not moving with each breath and there are poor breath sounds, begin the ventilation corrective sequence. There are 3 possible reasons for ineffective ventilation:

• An inadequate seal between the mask and the baby's face.

• The baby's airway is blocked.

• Not enough pressure is being used to inflate the lungs.

### Inadequate seal
If you hear or feel air escaping from around the mask, or if the 4 signs are not improving, reapply the mask to the face to form a better seal. Use a little more pressure on the rim of the mask and lift the jaw a little more forward. Do not press down hard on the baby's face. The most common place for a leak to occur is between the cheek and bridge of the nose (Figure 3.24).

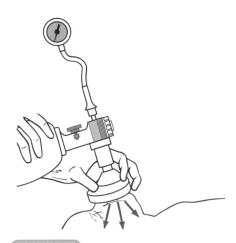

**Figure 3.24.** Inadequate seal of mask on face may result in poor chest movement

**Blocked airway**

Another possible reason for insufficient ventilation of the baby's lungs is a blocked airway. To correct this,

• Reposition the baby's head.

• Check the mouth, oropharynx, and nose for secretions; suction the mouth and nose if necessary.

• Try ventilating with the baby's mouth slightly open (especially helpful in extremely small premature babies with very small nares).

Repositioning the mask on the face to ensure a good seal and readjusting the baby's head to ensure an open airway usually solves the problem. The next attempt to ventilate the newborn usually results in effective ventilation.

**Not enough pressure**

Increasing the amount of positive pressure to 30 cm $H_2O$ or greater is occasionally necessary if no improvement occurs. The use of a pressure gauge makes it easier to avoid high lung volumes and airway pressure, to assess compliance of the lungs, and to guide selection of subsequent ventilator settings, if necessary.

• Gradually increase the pressure every few breaths until there are bilateral breath sounds and visible chest movement with each breath. With chest movement, the heart rate and oxygen saturation also should improve. Remember to adjust the oxygen concentration to meet the target saturations in the table. Note the amount of pressure required to achieve improvements in heart rate, $SpO_2$ and color, breath sounds, and perceptible chest movement.

• When using a self-inflating bag, if the pressure-release valve "pops off" or releases before 40 cm $H_2O$ is achieved, it is possible to occlude the pressure-release valve to achieve higher pressure. Do so, and cautiously increase the pressure up to a maximum of 40 cm $H_2O$.

• If you cannot achieve chest movement and an increase in heart rate, you should consider inserting a more effective airway—either an endotracheal tube or a laryngeal mask airway. (See Lesson 5.) This may require calling for help from a colleague with the necessary expertise.

Once the gaseous volume (functional residual capacity) has been established in the newborn's lungs, lower pressures can be used for subsequent breaths. Cautiously reduce the inspiratory pressure as long as chest movement is adequate and clinical condition remains stable. Adjust oxygen concentration to meet the target saturations in the table printed with the flow diagram.

**Table 3-2.** Technique for improving positive-pressure ventilation by mask

*Consider using the acronym "MR SOPA" to recall the ventilation corrective steps. The first 2 steps (M-R) should be addressed first, then the next 2 steps (S-O). Then if there is not adequate chest movement, move to the next 2 (P-A).*

| | Corrective Steps | Actions |
|---|---|---|
| M | Mask adjustment. | Be sure there is a good seal of the mask on the face. |
| R | Reposition airway. | The head should be in the "sniffing" position. |
| S | Suction mouth and nose. | Check for secretions; suction if present. |
| O | Open mouth. | Ventilate with the baby's mouth slightly open and lift the jaw forward. |
| P | Pressure increase. | Gradually increase the pressure every few breaths, until there are bilateral breath sounds and visible chest movement with each breath. |
| A | Airway alternative. | Consider endotracheal intubation or laryngeal mask airway. |

> **!** **If you still are unable to obtain physiologic improvement and adequate chest movement with mask ventilation techniques, you will need to use an alternative airway, such as an endotracheal tube, or, if that is not possible, a laryngeal mask airway.**

## What ventilation rate should you provide during positive-pressure ventilation?

During the initial stages of neonatal resuscitation, breaths should be delivered at a rate of **40 to 60 breaths per minute,** or slightly less than once a second. Faster rates often result in less effective breaths and should be consciously avoided.

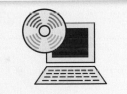

You are encouraged to view this video on the DVD that accompanies this textbook: *MR SOPA: Ventilation Corrective Steps*

Breathe . . . . . . . . . Two . . . . . . . . . Three . . . . . . . . . Breathe . . . . . . . . . Two . . . . . . . . Three . . . . .
(squeeze)       (release . . . . . . . . . . . . . . )       (squeeze)       (release . . . . . . . . . . . . . . )

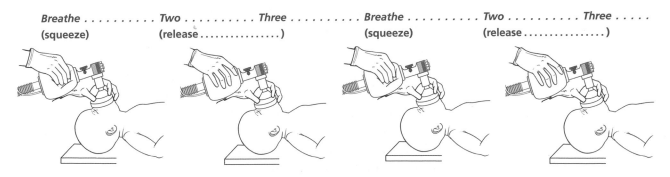

**Figure 3.25.** Count out loud to help maintain a rate of 40 to 60 breaths per minute. Say "Breathe" as you squeeze the bag or occlude the PEEP cap of the T-piece resuscitator, and release while you say "Two, Three."

## Review

*(The answers are in the preceding section and at the end of the lesson.)*

14. Which baby is positioned properly for positive-pressure ventilation?

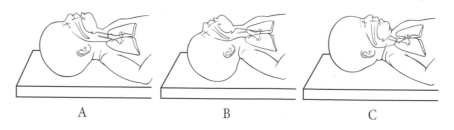

A          B          C

15. Which illustration(s) shows the correct position for assisting positive-pressure ventilation?

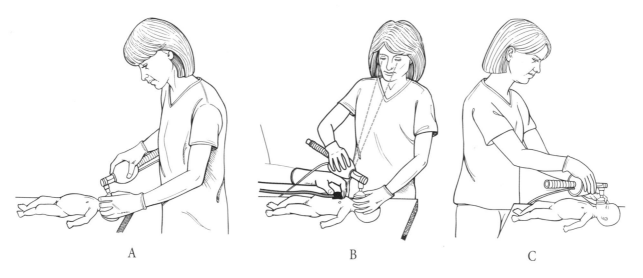

A          B          C

16. You must hold the resuscitation device so that you can see the newborn's _____ and _____.

17. An anatomically shaped mask should be positioned with the (pointed) (rounded) end over the newborn's nose.

18. If you notice that the baby's chest looks as if he is taking deep breaths, you are (overinflating) (underinflating) the lungs, and it is possible that a pneumothorax may occur.

19. When ventilating a baby, you should provide positive-pressure ventilation at a rate of _____ to _____ breaths per minute.

20. Begin positive-pressure ventilation with an initial inspiratory pressure of ___ cm $H_2O$.

**21.** "MR SOPA" stands for:

M = _____
R = _____
S = _____
O = _____
P = _____
A = _____

**22.** Your assistant assesses effectiveness of positive-pressure ventilation by first assessing the _____ and _____ along with listening for _____ _____. If these signs are not acceptable, you should look for _____ movement.

**23.** Which mask is correctly placed on the newborn's face?

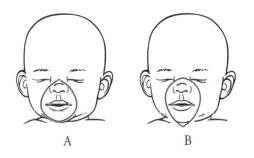

A          B

**24.** You have started positive-pressure ventilation on an apneic newborn. The heart rate is not rising, oxygen saturation is not improving, and your assistant does not hear bilateral breath sounds. List 3 possibilities of what may be wrong.

(1) _____

(2) _____

(3) _____

**25.** If, after performing the ventilation corrective sequence and making appropriate adjustments, you are unable to obtain a rising heart rate or bilateral breath sounds or see chest movement with positive-pressure ventilation, you usually will have to insert a(n)

_____ or _____.

# What do you do if the baby is not improving?

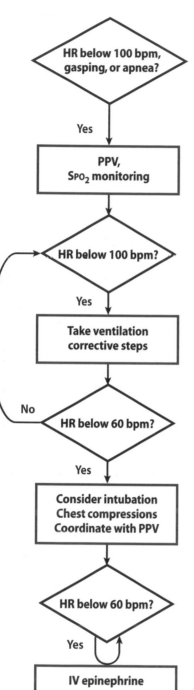

This is what you have done so far:

- Initiated PPV with an inspiratory pressure of about 20 cm $H_2O$, at a rate of 40 to 60 breaths per minute.

- Called for assistance.

- Your assistant attached a pulse oximeter probe to the baby's right hand or wrist, and then listened for rising heart rate and assessed for improving oxygen saturation. If those signs were not evident, your assistant listened for bilateral breath sounds and looked for chest movement with each positive-pressure breath.

- If this was not immediately evident in the first 5 to 10 breaths, you initiated the ventilation corrective steps (MR SOPA).

**If the baby's condition continues to deteriorate or fails to improve, and the heart rate is below 60 bpm despite 30 seconds of effective PPV** (defined by audible bilateral breath sounds and chest movement with ventilation), your next step will be to begin chest compressions. This will be described in Lesson 4. When chest compressions begin, increase the oxygen concentration to 100%. When the heart rate rises above 60 bpm and the pulse oximeter is available and reliable, adjust the oxygen concentration to meet the target saturation range indicated in the table shown below the flow diagram.

**If the heart rate is more than 60 bpm but less than 100 bpm,** continue to administer PPV as long as the baby is showing steady improvement.

- Monitor oxygen saturation and adjust the oxygen concentration to meet the target saturation range indicated in the table shown below the flow diagram.

- Consider inserting an orogastric tube if ventilation continues (discussed in the next section).

- Consider decreasing inspiratory pressure if chest expansion now seems too much.

- As ventilation continues, reassess respiratory effort, heart rate, and oxygen saturation continuously, or at least every 30 seconds.

**If the heart rate is more than 60 bpm but less than 100 bpm,**

- **Ensure effective ventilation.**

- Call for additional expertise.

- Consider that other complications, such as a pneumothorax or hypovolemia, also may be present. These will be described in Lessons 6 and 7.

| Targeted Pre-ductal $S_{PO_2}$ After Birth | |
|---|---|
| 1 min | 60%-65% |
| 2 min | 65%-70% |
| 3 min | 70%-75% |
| 4 min | 75%-80% |
| 5 min | 80%-85% |
| 10 min | 85%-95% |

> **!** Establishing effective ventilation
> is the key to nearly all successful
> neonatal resuscitations.

## What else should you do if positive-pressure ventilation with a mask is to be continued for more than several minutes?

If a newborn requires PPV with a mask for longer than several minutes, consider placing an orogastric tube and leaving it in place.

During PPV with a mask, gas is forced into the oropharynx where it can enter both the trachea and the esophagus. Proper positioning of the newborn will transmit most of the air into the trachea and the lungs. However, some gas may enter the esophagus and be forced into the stomach (Figure 3.26).

Gas forced into the stomach interferes with ventilation in the following ways:

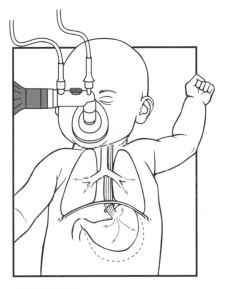

• A stomach distended with gas puts upward pressure on the diaphragm, preventing full expansion of the lungs.

• Gas in the stomach may cause regurgitation of gastric contents, which may then be aspirated into the lungs during PPV.

The problems related to gastric/abdominal distention and aspiration of gastric contents can be reduced by inserting an orogastric tube, suctioning gastric contents, and leaving the gastric tube in place and uncapped, to act as a vent for stomach gas throughout the remainder of the resuscitation.

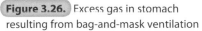

**Figure 3.26.** Excess gas in stomach resulting from bag-and-mask ventilation

## How do you insert an orogastric tube?

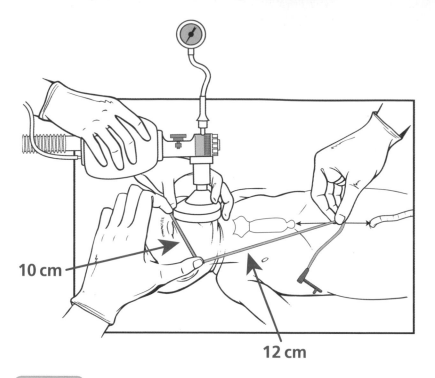

10 cm

12 cm

**Figure 3.27.** Measuring the correct distance for inserting an orogastric tube. In this example, the orogastric tube should be inserted 10 + 12 = 22 cm.

The equipment needed to place an orogastric tube during ventilation includes

- 8F feeding tube

- 20-mL syringe

One member of the team should prepare and place the orogastric tube while the other members of the team continue to provide PPV and assess the baby's heart rate, oxygen saturation, and appearance of spontaneous respirations every 30 seconds.

The major steps are as follows:

1. First, measure the amount of tube you want to insert. It must be long enough to reach the stomach but not so long as to pass beyond it. The length of the inserted tube should be equal to *the distance from the bridge of the nose to the earlobe and from the earlobe to a point halfway between the xiphoid process (the lower tip of the sternum) and the umbilicus.* Note the centimeter mark at this place on the tube (Figure 3.27).

   To minimize interruption of ventilation, measurement of the orogastric tube can be approximated with the mask in place.

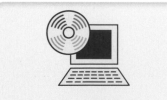

**You are encouraged to view this video on the DVD that accompanies this textbook:**
***Orogastric Tube Placement***

**2** Insert the tube through the ***mouth*** rather than the nose (Figure 3.28A). The nose should be left open for ventilation. Ventilation can be resumed as soon as the tube has been placed.

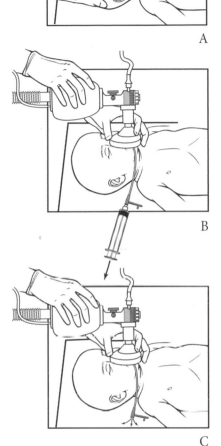

A

**3** Once the tube is inserted the desired distance, attach a syringe and quickly, but gently, remove the gastric contents (Figure 3.28B).

B

**4** Remove the syringe from the tube and leave the end of the tube *open* to provide a vent for air entering the stomach (Figure 3.28C).

C

**5** Tape the tube to the baby's cheek to ensure that the tip remains in the stomach and is not pulled back into the esophagus (Figure 3.28D).

The tube will not interfere with the mask-to-face seal if an 8F feeding tube is used and the tube exits from the side of the mask over the soft area of the baby's cheek. A larger tube may make it difficult to obtain a seal, particularly in premature newborns. A smaller tube can become occluded by secretions easily.

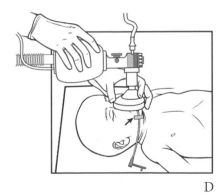

D

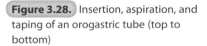

**Figure 3.28.** Insertion, aspiration, and taping of an orogastric tube (top to bottom)

## How do you know if the baby has improved enough that you can stop positive-pressure ventilation?

As the heart rate increases toward normal, continue ventilating the baby at a rate of 40 to 60 bpm. With improvement, the baby's $Spo_2$ should gradually improve. Continue to monitor the movement of the chest and breath sounds to avoid overinflation or underinflation of the lungs.

When the heart rate is above 100 bpm and stable, reduce the rate and pressure of PPV while observing for effective spontaneous respirations and stimulating the baby to breathe effectively. Positive-pressure ventilation may be discontinued when the baby has

- A heart rate continuously over 100 bpm

- Sustained spontaneous breathing

Once the oximetry reading is in the target range, supplemental oxygen, if used, also can be weaned as tolerated.

## Review

*(The answers are in the preceding section and at the end of the lesson.)*

26. You have administered positive-pressure ventilation (with bilateral breath sounds and chest movement) for 30 seconds. What do you do if the newborn's heart rate is now
    - Below 60 beats per minute: _____
    - More than 60 beats per minute and less than 100 beats per minute but steadily improving with effective positive-pressure ventilation: _____
    - More than 60 beats per minute and less than 100 beats per minute and not improving with effective positive-pressure ventilation: _____

27. Assisted ventilation may be discontinued when
    1. _____
    2. _____

28. If you must continue positive-pressure ventilation with a mask for more than several minutes, a(n) _____ should be inserted to act as a vent for the gas in the stomach during the remainder of the resuscitation.

29. How far should this orogastric catheter be inserted? _____ cm

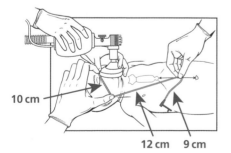

10 cm

12 cm   9 cm

## Key Points

1. Ventilation of the lungs is the single most important and most effective step in cardiopulmonary resuscitation of the compromised newborn.

2. Indications for positive-pressure ventilation are
   - Apnea/gasping
   - Heart rate below 100 beats per minute even if breathing
   - Persistent central cyanosis and low $SpO_2$ despite free-flow supplemental oxygen increased to 100%

3. Resuscitation of term newborns may begin with 21% oxygen (room air); resuscitation of preterm newborns may begin with a somewhat higher oxygen concentration. Pulse oximetry is used to help adjust the amount of supplemental oxygen to avoid giving too much or too little oxygen.

4. Self-inflating bags
   - Fill spontaneously after they are squeezed, pulling oxygen or air into the bag
   - Remain inflated at all times
   - Must have a tight mask-to-face seal to inflate the lungs
   - Can deliver positive-pressure ventilation (PPV) without a compressed gas source; user must be certain the bag is connected to an oxygen source for the purpose of neonatal resuscitation
   - Require attachment of an oxygen reservoir to deliver high oxygen concentration
   - Cannot be used to administer free-flow oxygen reliably through the mask and cannot be used to deliver continuous positive airway pressure (CPAP)
   - Should have an integral pressure gauge, or, if there is a site for attaching a pressure gauge (manometer), it should be attached

5. Flow-inflating bags
   - Fill only when gas from a compressed source flows into them
   - Depend on a compressed gas source
   - Must have a tight mask-to-face seal to inflate
   - Use a flow-control valve to regulate pressure/inflation
   - Should have a pressure gauge (manometer)
   - Look like a deflated balloon when not in use
   - Can be used to administer free-flow oxygen and CPAP

6. The flow-inflating bag will not work if
   - The mask is not properly sealed over the newborn's nose and mouth.
   - There is a hole in the bag.
   - The flow-control valve is open too far.
   - The pressure gauge is missing or the port is not occluded.

7. T-piece resuscitators
   - Depend on a compressed gas source.
   - Must have a tight mask-to-face seal to inflate the lungs.
   - Require selection of a maximum pressure, peak inspiratory pressure, and positive-end expiratory pressure (PEEP).
   - May require adjustment of peak inspiratory pressure during resuscitation to achieve physiologic improvement, audible breath sounds, and perceptible chest movements.
   - Provide positive pressure when operator alternately occludes and opens the aperture in the PEEP cap.
   - Can be used to deliver free-flow oxygen and CPAP.

8. An oxygen reservoir must be attached to deliver high concentrations of oxygen using a self-inflating bag. Without the reservoir, the bag delivers a maximum of only about 40% oxygen, which may be insufficient for neonatal resuscitation.

9. The PPV device should be assembled and connected to a blender so that any concentration of oxygen from 21% (room air), up to 100% oxygen, can be provided.

10. If an oxygen blender and pulse oximeter are not immediately available, start PPV with 21% oxygen (room air) while you obtain an air-oxygen source and an oximeter.

11. Using pulse oximetry, supplemental oxygen concentration should be adjusted to achieve the target values for pre-ductal saturations summarized in the table on the Neonatal Resuscitation Program™ (NRP™) flow diagram.

12. If you cannot detect audible bilateral breath sounds and see no perceptible chest expansion during assisted ventilation, check or correct the following:
    - **M:** Mask adjustment.
    - **R:** Reposition airway.
    - **S:** Suction mouth and nose.
    - **O:** Open mouth.
    - **P:** Pressure increase.
    - **A:** Airway alternative.

13. The most important indicator of successful PPV is rising heart rate.

14. Effective ventilation is defined by the presence of
    - Bilateral breath sounds
    - Chest movement (heart rate may rise without visible chest movement, especially in preterm newborns)

15. Signs that PPV has been effective, and indications that PPV may be discontinued, are
    - Heart rate rises to over 100 breaths per minute
    - Improvement in oxygen saturation
    - Onset of spontaneous respirations

## Lesson 3 Review

*(The answers follow.)*

1. Flow-inflating bags (will) (will not) work without a compressed gas source.

2. A baby is born apneic and cyanotic. You clear her airway and stimulate her. Thirty seconds after birth, she has not improved. The next step is to (stimulate her more) (begin positive-pressure ventilation).

3. The single most important and most effective step in neonatal resuscitation is (stimulation) (ventilating the lungs).

4. Label these bags "flow-inflating," "self-inflating," or "T-piece resuscitator."

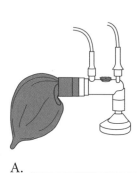 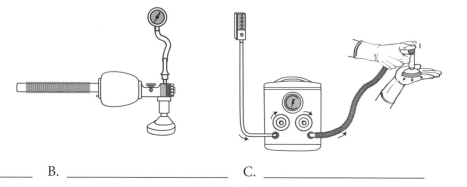

A. _____   B. _____   C. _____

5. Masks of different sizes (do) (do not) need to be available at every delivery.

6. Self-inflating bags require the attachment of a(n)_____ to deliver a high concentration of oxygen.

7. T-piece resuscitators (will) (will not) work without a compressed gas source.

8. Neonatal ventilation bags are (much smaller than) (the same size as) adult ventilation bags.

9. List the principal safety feature for each of the following devices:

   Self-inflating bag: _____ and _____

   Flow-inflating bag: _____

   T-piece resuscitator: _____ and _____

## Lesson 3 Review—*continued*

10. Free-flow oxygen can be delivered reliably through the mask attached to a (flow-inflating bag) (self-inflating bag) (T-piece resuscitator).

11. When giving free-flow oxygen with a flow-inflating bag and mask, it is necessary to place the mask (securely) (loosely) on the baby's face to allow some gas to escape around the edges of the mask.

12. Before an anticipated resuscitation, the ventilation device should be connected to a(n) _____, which enables you to provide oxygen in any concentration, from room air up to 100% oxygen.

13. Resuscitation of the term newborn may begin with _____% oxygen. The inspired oxygen concentration used during resuscitation is guided by the use of a(n) _____, which measures oxygen saturation.

14. Which baby is positioned properly for positive-pressure ventilation?

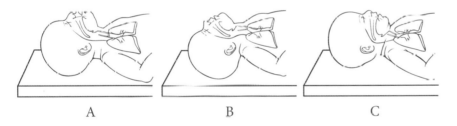

|  A  |  B  |  C  |

15. Which illustration(s) shows the correct position for assisting positive-pressure ventilation?

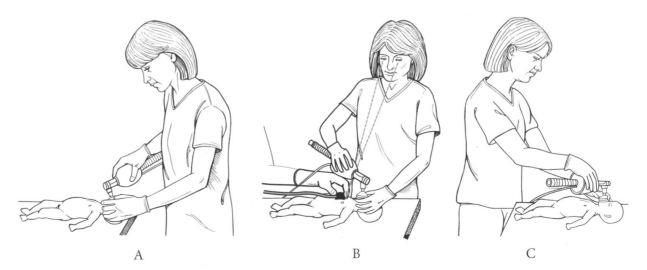

|  A  |  B  |  C  |

## Lesson 3 Review—*continued*

16. You must hold the resuscitation device so that you can see the newborn's _____ and _____.

17. An anatomically shaped mask should be positioned with the (pointed) (rounded) end over the newborn's nose.

18. If you notice that the baby's chest looks as if he is taking deep breaths, you are (overinflating) (underinflating) the lungs, and it is possible that a pneumothorax may occur.

19. When ventilating a baby, you should provide positive-pressure ventilation at a rate of _____ to _____ breaths per minute.

20. Begin positive-pressure ventilation with an initial inspiratory pressure of ___ cm H$_2$O.

21. "MR SOPA" stands for:
    M = _____
    R = _____
    S = _____
    O = _____
    P = _____
    A = _____

22. Your assistant assesses effectiveness of positive-pressure ventilation by first assessing the _____ and _____ along with listening for _____ _____. If these signs are not acceptable, you should look for _____ movement.

23. Which mask is correctly placed on the newborn's face?

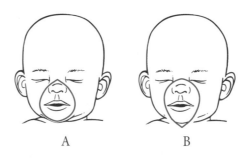

A              B

## Lesson 3 Review—*continued*

**24.** You have started positive-pressure ventilation on an apneic newborn. The heart rate is not rising, oxygen saturation is not improving, and your assistant does not hear bilateral breath sounds. List 3 possibilities of what may be wrong.

1. _____

2. _____

3. _____

**25.** If, after performing the ventilation corrective sequence and making appropriate adjustments, you are unable to obtain a rising heart rate or bilateral breath sounds or see chest movement with positive-pressure ventilation, you usually will have to insert a(n) _____ or a(n) _____.

**26.** You have administered positive-pressure ventilation (with bilateral breath sounds and chest movement) for 30 seconds. What do you do if the baby's heart rate is now
- Below 60 beats per minute? _____
- More than 60 beats per minute and less than 100 beats per minute but steadily improving with effective positive-pressure ventilation? _____
- More than 60 beats per minute and less than 100 beats per minute and not improving with effective positive-pressure ventilation? _____

**27.** Assisted ventilation may be discontinued when

1. _____

2. _____

**28.** If you must continue positive-pressure ventilation with a mask for more than several minutes, a(n) _____ should be inserted to act as a vent for the gas in the stomach during the remainder of the resuscitation.

**29.** How far should this orogastric catheter be inserted? _____ cm

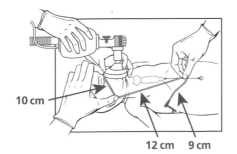

10 cm

12 cm    9 cm

## Lesson 3 Answers to Questions

1. Flow-inflating bags **will not** work without a compressed gas source.

2. The next step is to **begin positive-pressure ventilation.**

3. **Ventilating the lungs** is the most important and effective step in neonatal resuscitation.

4. A. **flow-inflating;** B. **self-inflating;** C. **T-piece resuscitator**

5. Masks of different sizes **do** need to be at every delivery.

6. Self-inflating bags require the attachment of an **oxygen reservoir** to deliver a concentration of oxygen greater than approximately 40%.

7. T-piece resuscitators **will not** work without a compressed gas source.

8. Neonatal ventilation bags are **much smaller than** adult ventilation bags.

9. Self-inflating bag: **Pop-off valve** and **pressure gauge**

   Flow-inflating bag: **Pressure gauge**

   T-piece resuscitator: **Maximum pressure relief control** and **pressure gauge**

10. Free-flow oxygen can be delivered reliably with a **flow-inflating bag and T-piece resuscitator,** but not through the mask of a self-inflating bag.

11. When giving free-flow oxygen, place the mask **loosely** on the baby's face to allow some gas to escape around the edges of the mask.

12. The device should be connected to a **blender** to enable adjustment of inspired oxygen from 21% to 100%.

13. Resuscitation of the baby born at term may be started with **21%** oxygen. Subsequent oxygen concentration should be guided by an **oximeter,** which measures oxygen saturation.

14. Position **A** is the correct position. B and C are overextended and underextended, respectively.

15. **Illustrations A and B** are both correct.

16. You should be able to see the newborn's **chest** and **abdomen.**

## Answers to Questions—*continued*

**17.** An anatomically shaped mask should be positioned with the **pointed** end over the newborn's nose.

**18.** You are **overinflating** the lungs, and there is danger you will produce a pneumothorax.

**19.** Squeeze the resuscitation bag at a rate of **40** to **60** breaths per minute.

**20.** Begin positive-pressure ventilation with an initial inspiratory pressure of **20** cm $H_2O$.

**21.** M = **Mask adjustment**
R = **Reposition airway**
S = **Suction mouth and nose**
O = **Open mouth**
P = **Pressure increase**
A = **Airway alternative**

**22.** Your assistant should note improvement in **heart rate** and **oximetry** and listen for **breath sounds.** You should look for **chest** movement.

**23.** Mask **A** is positioned correctly.

**24. There may be an inadequate seal of the mask on the face, the head may need to be repositioned to open the airway,** or **secretions may need to be suctioned.**

**25.** You usually will have to insert an **endotracheal tube** or a **laryngeal mask airway.**

**26.** Below 60 beats per minute: **Begin chest compressions and consider intubation.**

Between 60 beats per minute and 100 beats per minute and improving: **Adjust oxygen, gradually decrease pressure as heart rate improves, insert orogastric tube, continue monitoring.**

Between 60 beats per minute and 100 beats per minute and not improving: **Repeat MR SOPA and consider intubation.**

**27.** Discontinue assisted ventilation when the **heart rate is above 100 breaths per minute** and the **baby is breathing.**

**28.** An **orogastric tube** should be inserted to act as a vent for the gas in the stomach.

**29.** The orogastric catheter should be inserted **22** cm (10 cm + 12 cm).

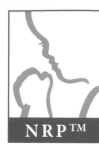

## Lesson 3: Positive-Pressure Ventilation Performance Checklist

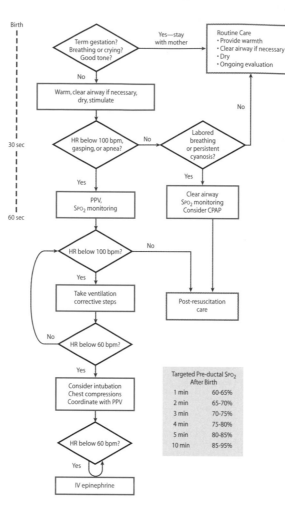

| Targeted Pre-ductal SpO₂ After Birth | |
|---|---|
| 1 min | 60-65% |
| 2 min | 65-70% |
| 3 min | 70-75% |
| 4 min | 75-80% |
| 5 min | 80-85% |
| 10 min | 85-95% |

### The Performance Checklist Is a Learning Tool

The learner uses the checklist as a reference during independent practice, or as a guide for discussion and practice with a Neonatal Resuscitation Program™ (NRP™) instructor. When the learner and instructor agree that the learner can perform the skills correctly and smoothly without coaching and within the context of a scenario, the learner may move on to the next lesson's Performance Checklist.

If the institution policy is that a T-piece resuscitator normally is used in the delivery room, the learner should demonstrate proficiency with that device. However, he or she also should demonstrate ability to use a bag and mask.

**Knowledge Check**

- How will you check the function of the positive-pressure ventilation (PPV) device you will use?

- What are the indicators for beginning PPV?

- What is the correct ventilation rate?

- Which 2 indicators are evaluated when you first begin PPV? If those 2 indicators are not improving, what 2 indicators are next in evaluating effective ventilation?

- How is pulse oximetry used during PPV?

- What are the ventilation corrective steps (MR SOPA)?

- What is the purpose of an orogastric tube and when is it placed?

- What are the indications for stopping PPV?

**Learning Objectives**

1. Identify the newborn who requires PPV.

2. Demonstrate correct technique for PPV, including placement of mask on the newborn's face, rate and pressure, and corrective steps (MR SOPA).

3. Demonstrate correct placement and interpretation of pulse oximetry.

4. Recognize improvement during PPV by first assessing for increasing heart rate and oxygen saturation; if those are not improving, recognize the need to perform ventilation corrective steps and achieve audible breath sounds and chest movement with ventilation.

5. Identify signs that PPV may be discontinued.

6. Demonstrate pertinent key behavioral skills to optimize team performance.

**"You are called to attend the birth of a baby because of failure to progress and maternal fever. How would you prepare for the resuscitation of this baby? As you work, say your thoughts and actions aloud so your assistant and I will know what you are thinking and doing."**

Instructor should check boxes as the learner responds correctly.

| Participant Name: | | |
|---|---|---|
| | ☐ Obtains relevant perinatal history | Gestational age? Fluid clear? How many babies? Other risk factors? |
| | ☐ Performs equipment check<br>☐ Ensures correct size mask, and depending on device, checks function and inspiratory pressure, turns on gas flow 5-10 L/min, sets oxygen blender setting per hospital protocol<br>☐ If obstetric (OB) provider indicates that meconium is present in amniotic fluid, prepares for intubation and tracheal suctioning | **Warm, Clear airway, Auscultate, Oxygenate, Ventilate** (check PPV device), **Intubate, Medicate, Thermoregulate** |

| | "The baby has been born." | |
|---|---|---|

| Sample Vital Signs | Performance Steps | Details |
|---|---|---|
| Gestational age as indicated<br>Apneic<br>Limp | Completes initial assessment when baby is born<br>☐ Learner asks 3 questions<br>• Term?<br>• Breathing or crying?<br>• Good tone? | Initial assessment determines whether or not baby will receive initial steps of resuscitation at the radiant warmer. |
| | ☐ Receives newborn at radiant warmer | |
| | ☐ Meconium management (optional) | Intubation and suction indicated if meconium-stained and not vigorous. |
| | ☐ Performs initial steps | Warm, position airway, suction mouth and nose, dry, remove wet linen, stimulate. |
| Respiratory Rate (RR)-apneic<br>Heart Rate (HR)-40 beats per minute (bpm) | ☐ Evaluates breathing and heart rate | Auscultate or palpate umbilical pulse. |
| | ☐ Applies mask correctly and starts PPV at 20 cm $H_2O$; rate 40-60 bpm | Begin PPV with ____% oxygen per hospital protocol. |
| | ☐ Calls for additional help | PPV requires 2 resuscitators. |
| | ☐ Requests pulse oximetry | Assistant places probe on right hand or wrist, then plugs into oximeter. Oximeter has no signal. |
| HR-40 bpm<br>$SpO_2$ - - - - | ☐ Requests HR and saturation response within 5-10 breaths | Assistant auscultates chest and monitors oximetry. |
| Poor breath sounds; no chest movement | ☐ Assesses bilateral breath sounds and chest movement | |

| Sample Vital Signs | Performance Steps | Details |
|---|---|---|
| | Ventilation Corrective Steps | Instructor may indicate chest movement and breath sounds at any step along sequence. |
| | **M**ask adjustment<br>**R**eposition head<br>**S**uction mouth and nose<br>**O**pen mouth<br>Increase **P**ressure<br><br><br><br><br>Consider **A**lternative airway | Do **M, R** first and reattempt PPV<br><br>If no breath sounds or chest movement, do **S and O** and reattempt PPV.<br>If no breath sounds or chest movement, gradually increase **P**ressure every few breaths, until there are bilateral breath sounds and chest movement with each breath, up to maximum of 40 cm $H_2O$ pressure.<br>If no breath sounds or chest movement, consider endotracheal intubation or laryngeal mask airway. (Lesson 5 notes limitations of the laryngeal mask airway.) |
| | After achieving breath sounds and chest movement<br>☐ Administers effective PPV for 30 seconds | Monitor for overinflation of lungs as functional residual capacity is established with first effective breaths. |
| | ☐ Assesses HR and $Sp_{O_2}$ | Instructor chooses from options below. |
| **Option 1** | | |
| HR-70 bpm<br>RR-4 breaths per minute (gasping)<br>$Sp_{O_2}$-67% | ☐ Continues effective PPV as long as HR is rising<br>☐ If HR not rising, repeats all ventilation corrective steps (MR SOPA) to ensure effective ventilation<br>☐ Adjusts oxygen per oximetry<br>☐ Considers intubation if HR continues >60 bpm and <100 bpm | If HR rises >100 bpm, proceed to Option 2.<br><br>Learner demonstrates continuous assessment of HR and $Sp_{O_2}$ and ability to problem solve based on newborn's response. |
| **Option 2** | | |
| HR-120 bpm<br>RR-10 breaths per minute (weak cry)<br>$Sp_{O_2}$-74% | ☐ Stimulates newborn to breathe spontaneously and slows PPV rate as breathing becomes effective<br>☐ Adjusts oxygen per oximetry | |
| HR-140 bpm<br>RR-60 breaths per minute (grunting)<br>$Sp_{O_2}$-97% | ☐ Monitors newborn's respiratory effort, HR, and $Sp_{O_2}$<br>☐ Gradually withdraws PPV and adjusts oxygen as $Sp_{O_2}$ rises and then discontinues free-flow oxygen | |
| | ☐ Updates family<br>☐ Directs post-resuscitation care | |

| Sample Vital Signs | Performance Steps | Details |
|---|---|---|
| **Option 3** | | |
| HR-40 bpm<br>RR-apneic<br>$SPO_2$ - - - | ☐ Quickly assesses reasons why baby may not be responding<br>☐ If no apparent reason for poor response, indicate need to intubate and begin chest compressions | Consider equipment malfunction, oxygen concentration, need for orogastric tube, or other problem (pneumothorax, hypovolemia). Oximeter—no signal. |

**Instructor asks the learner reflective questions to enable self-assessment, such as,**

1. How did you know the newborn required
   a. Initial steps at the radiant warmer?
   b. Positive-pressure ventilation?
   c. Corrective steps (MR SOPA)?
   d. Supplemental oxygen?

2. Tell me about how you used pulse oximetry to guide your actions.

3. At what point would you need to call for more help?

4. What are some examples of the Key Behavioral Skills you used to communicate clearly with your assistant?

5. What went well during this resuscitation?

6. Would you do anything differently when faced with this scenario (indicate which scenario) again?

**Neonatal Resuscitation Program Key Behavioral Skills**

Know your environment.        Allocate attention wisely.
Anticipate and plan.          Use all available information.
Assume the leadership role.   Use all available resources.
Communicate effectively.      Call for help when needed.
Delegate workload optimally.  Maintain professional behavior.

# Appendix

*Read the section(s) that refers to the type of device used in your hospital.*

## A. Self-inflating resuscitation bags

### What are the parts of a self-inflating bag?

There are 7 basic parts to a self-inflating bag (Figure 3A.1).

1. Air inlet and attachment site for oxygen reservoir

2. Oxygen inlet

3. Patient outlet

4. Valve assembly

5. Oxygen reservoir

6. Pressure-release (pop-off) valve

7. Pressure gauge (some devices incorporate the gauge into the body of the device)

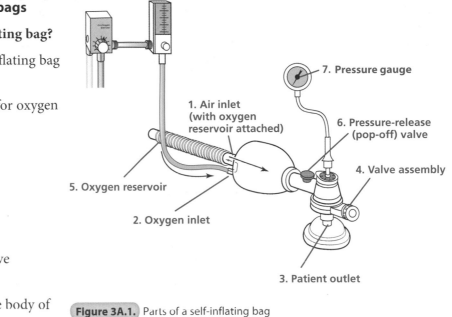

**7. Pressure gauge**

**1. Air inlet (with oxygen reservoir attached)**

**6. Pressure-release (pop-off) valve**

**5. Oxygen reservoir**

**4. Valve assembly**

**2. Oxygen inlet**

**3. Patient outlet**

**Figure 3A.1.** Parts of a self-inflating bag

As the bag re-expands following compression, gas is drawn into the bag through a one-way valve that may be located at either end of the bag, depending on the design. This valve is called the ***air inlet.***

Every self-inflating bag has an ***oxygen inlet,*** which usually is located near the air inlet. The oxygen inlet is a small nipple or projection to which oxygen tubing is attached. In the self-inflating bag, an oxygen tube does not need to be attached for the bag to function. The oxygen tube should be attached when the bag is to be used for neonatal resuscitation.

The ***patient outlet*** is where gas exits from the bag to the baby and where the mask or endotracheal tube attaches.

Most self-inflating bags have a ***pressure-release valve*** that prevents excessive pressure buildup in the bag. To help ensure that appropriate pressure is used when providing positive-pressure ventilation (PPV) in a newborn, you should use self-inflating bags that have an integral ***pressure gauge (manometer), or, if there is a site for attaching a pressure gauge, you should make sure one is attached.*** The attachment site usually consists of a small hole or projection close to the patient outlet. Care should be taken to avoid connecting the oxygen inflow tubing to the site for attaching the pressure gauge, if present. High pressure may be generated in the baby and cause a pneumothorax or other air leak. Attach the oxygen tubing and pressure gauge according to manufacturer instructions.

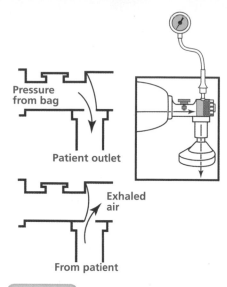

**Figure 3A.2.** Principle of valve assembly of a self-inflating bag

## Appendix—*continued*

Self-inflating bags have a ***valve assembly*** positioned between the bag and the patient outlet (Figure 3A.2). When the bag is squeezed during ventilation, the valve opens, releasing oxygen/air to the patient. When the bag reinflates (during the exhalation phase of the cycle), the valve is closed. This prevents the patient's exhaled air from entering the bag and being re-breathed. You should become familiar with the valve assembly—what it looks like and how it responds as you squeeze and release the bag. If it is missing or malfunctioning, the bag should not be used.

### Why is an oxygen reservoir necessary on a self-inflating bag?

Some babies who require resuscitation with assisted ventilation at birth also may benefit from administration of supplemental oxygen. The amount of supplemental oxygen to use during PPV should be determined by pulse oximetry.

If a self-inflating bag is connected to a 100% oxygen source, the oxygen enters the bag through tubing connected between an oxygen source and the oxygen inlet port on the bag. However, each time the bag reinflates after you squeeze it, air (oxygen concentration 21%) is drawn into the bag through the air inlet. The air dilutes the concentration of oxygen in the bag. Therefore, even though you may have 100% oxygen flowing through the oxygen inlet, it is diluted by the air that enters each time the bag reinflates. As a result, the concentration of oxygen actually received by the patient is reduced and the exact concentration is unpredictable (Figure 3A.3). (The actual concentration will depend on the flow rate of oxygen coming from the source and how frequently the bag is squeezed.)

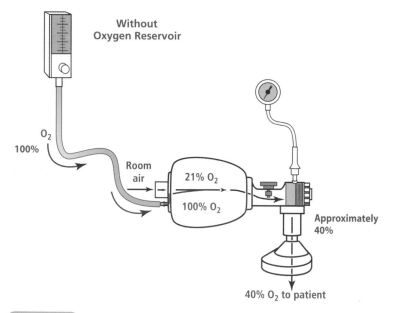

**Figure 3A.3.** Self-inflating bag without an oxygen reservoir and with an oxygen line connected to a 100% oxygen source. This system will deliver only approximately 40% oxygen to the patient and only when the bag is squeezed.

## Appendix—*continued*

Concentrations of oxygen higher than is present in room air are most reliably delivered by using a blender and an *oxygen reservoir.* An oxygen reservoir is an appliance that can be placed over the bag's air inlet (Figure 3A.4). The reservoir allows the gas coming from the blender to collect at the inlet, thus preventing the gas from the blender from being diluted with room air. However, the flow of oxygen is delivered reliably to the patient only when the bag is squeezed. When the bag is not being squeezed, the gas escapes from the open end of the reservoir and never reaches the baby.

Several different types of oxygen reservoirs are available, but they all perform the same function. Some have open ends and others have a valve that allows some air to enter the reservoir (Figure 3A.5). When using these devices, the concentration of oxygen achieved with a self-inflating bag with an oxygen reservoir attached will be close to the concentration set on the blender.

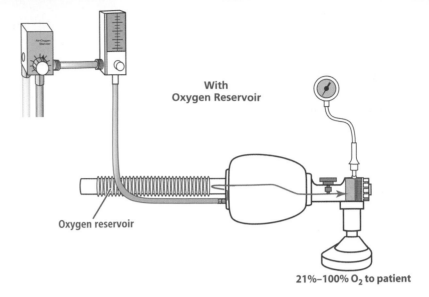

**With Oxygen Reservoir**

Oxygen reservoir

21%–100% O$_2$ to patient

**Figure 3A.4.** Self-inflating bag with oxygen reservoir delivers from 21% to 100% oxygen to the patient, depending on setting on blender

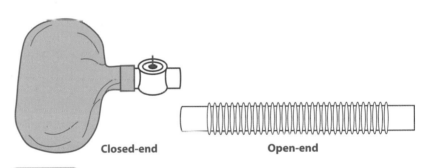

**Closed-end**          **Open-end**

**Figure 3A.5.** Different types of oxygen reservoirs for self-inflating bags

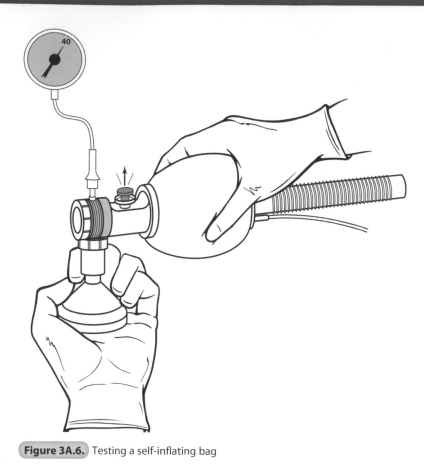

**Figure 3A.6.** Testing a self-inflating bag

## Appendix—*continued*

### How do you test a self-inflating bag before use?

First, be certain that the oxygen tubing and oxygen reservoir are connected. Adjust the flow to 5 to 10 L/min.

To check the operation of a self-inflating bag, block the mask or patient outlet with the palm of your hand and squeeze the bag (Figure 3A.6).

- Do you feel pressure against your hand?

- Can you force the pressure-release valve open?

- Does the pressure gauge (if present) register 30 to 40 cm $H_2O$ pressure when the pressure-release valve opens?

If not,

- Is there a crack or leak in the bag?

- Is the pressure gauge missing, resulting in an open attachment site?

- Is the pressure-release valve missing or stuck closed?

- Is the patient outlet sufficiently blocked?

If your bag generates adequate pressure and the safety features are working while the mask-patient outlet is blocked,

- Does the bag reinflate quickly when you release your grip?

Self-inflating bags usually have more parts than flow-inflating bags. During cleaning, parts may be left out or assembled incorrectly. If parts remain moist after cleaning, they may stick together. If there is any problem with the bag, obtain a new one.

## Appendix—*continued*

### How do you control pressure in a self-inflating bag?

The amount of pressure delivered by a self-inflating bag is not dependent on the flow of oxygen entering the bag. When you seal the mask on the baby's face (or connect the bag to an endotracheal tube), there will be no change in the inflation of a self-inflating bag. The amount of pressure and volume delivered with each breath depends on the following 3 factors:

- How hard you squeeze the bag

- Any leak that may be present between the mask and the baby's face

- The set-point of the pressure-release valve

## Review—Appendix A

*(The answers are in the preceding section and at the end of the Appendix.)*

**A-1.** A self-inflating bag with a pressure gauge site will work only if a pressure gauge is connected to the site or if the connection site is (left open) (plugged).

**A-2.** A self-inflating bag connected to a 100% oxygen source will deliver up to 100% oxygen (by itself) (only when an oxygen reservoir is attached).

**A-3.** A self-inflating bag connected to 100% oxygen, but without an oxygen reservoir attached to it, delivers only about _____% oxygen.

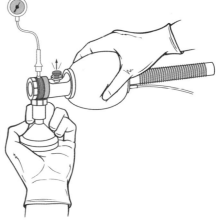

**A-4.** You are testing a resuscitation bag. When you squeeze the bag, you (should) (should not) feel pressure against your hand.

**A-5.** What number should the pressure gauge read in the illustration at the right when you squeeze the bag?

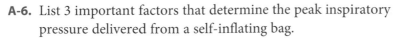

**A-6.** List 3 important factors that determine the peak inspiratory pressure delivered from a self-inflating bag.

1. _____

2. _____

3. _____

## Appendix—*continued*

### B. Flow-inflating resuscitation bags

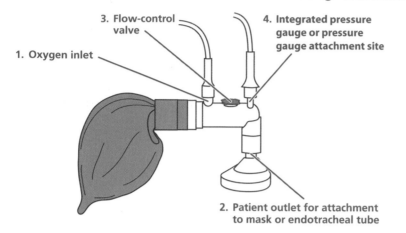

3. Flow-control valve

4. Integrated pressure gauge or pressure gauge attachment site

1. Oxygen inlet

2. Patient outlet for attachment to mask or endotracheal tube

**Figure 3B.1.** Parts of a flow-inflating bag

## What are the parts of a flow-inflating bag?

There are 4 parts to a flow-inflating bag (Figure 3B.1).

1. Oxygen inlet (from blender)

2. Patient outlet

3. Flow-control valve

4. Pressure gauge attachment site

Oxygen from a compressed source (or an oxygen-air mixture from a blender) enters the bag at the *oxygen inlet.* The inlet is a small projection designed to fit into the end of the tubing from the gas supply. The inlet may be at either end of the device, depending on the brand and model you use.

Oxygen (at whatever concentration entered at the inlet) exits from the bag to the patient at the *patient outlet,* where the mask or endotracheal tube attaches to the device. Remember that, even if you plan to use 21% oxygen (ie, air) for positive-pressure ventilation (PPV), you must have a compressed gas source to fill the flow-inflating bag.

The *flow-control* valve provides an adjustable leak that allows you to regulate the pressure in the bag when the bag is connected to an endotracheal tube or the mask is held tightly on the patient's face. The adjustable opening provides an additional outlet for the incoming gas and allows excess gas to escape rather than overinflate the bag or be forced into the patient.

Flow-inflating bags usually have a *site for attaching a pressure gauge* (Figure 3B.2). The attachment site usually is close to the patient outlet. The pressure gauge registers the amount of pressure you are using to ventilate the newborn. If your flow-inflating bag has a connecting site for a pressure gauge, a gauge must be attached to the site, or the attachment site must be occluded with a plug. If not, the site will be a source of leak and the bag will not inflate properly.

**Figure 3B.2.** Flow-inflating bag attached to oxygen source and pressure gauge

## Appendix—*continued*

### How does a flow-inflating bag work?

For a flow-inflating bag to work properly, there must be adequate gas flow from the source and a sealed system. The bag will not inflate adequately if (Figure 3B.3)

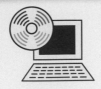

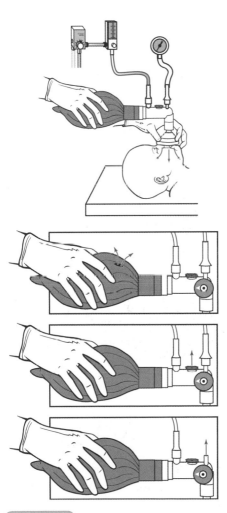

- The mask is not properly sealed against the baby's face.
- The flow from the source is insufficient.

- There is a rip in the bag.

- The flow-control valve is open too far.

- The pressure gauge is not attached, or the tubing from the gas supply has become disconnected or occluded.

**Figure 3B.3.** Reasons for failure of the flow-inflating bag to inflate

## Appendix—*continued*

### How do you test a flow-inflating bag before use?

To check a flow-inflating bag, attach it to a gas source. Adjust the flowmeter to 5 to 10 L/min. Block the patient outlet to make sure the bag fills properly (Figure 3B.4). Do this by making a seal between the mask and the palm of your hand. Adjust the flow-control valve so that the bag is not over-distended. Watch the pressure gauge, and adjust the valve so that there is approximately 5 cm $H_2O$ pressure when the bag is not being squeezed (PEEP), and 30 to 40 cm $H_2O$ peak inflation pressure when the bag is squeezed firmly (peak pressure).

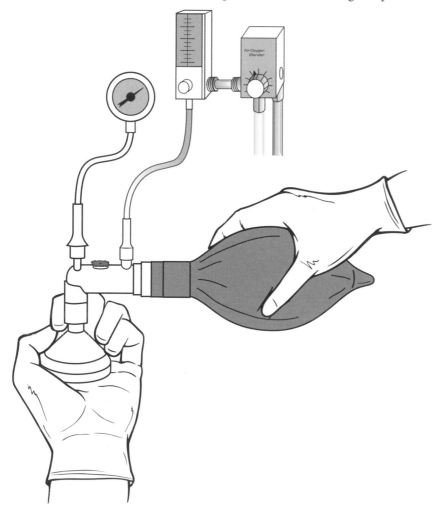

Does the bag fill properly? If not,

- Is there a crack or tear in the bag?

- Is the flow-control valve open too far?

- Is the pressure gauge attached?

- Is the oxygen line connected securely?

- Is the patient outlet sufficiently blocked?

If the bag fills, squeeze the bag.

- Do you feel pressure against your hand?

- Does the pressure gauge register 5 cm $H_2O$ pressure when not squeezed, and 30 to 40 cm $H_2O$ when squeezed firmly?

During this test, squeeze the bag at a rate of 40 to 60 times per minute and a pressure of 40 cm $H_2O$. If the bag does not fill rapidly enough, readjust the flow-control valve or increase the gas flow from the flowmeter.

**Figure 3B.4.** Testing the integrity of a flow-inflating bag

Then, check to be sure that the pressure gauge still reads 5 cm $H_2O$ pressure of positive-end expiratory pressure (PEEP) when the bag is not being squeezed. You may need to make further adjustments in the flow-control valve to avoid excessive PEEP.

If the bag still does not fill properly or does not generate adequate maximum pressure, get another bag and begin again.

# Appendix—*continued*

### How do you adjust the oxygen flow, concentration, and pressure in a flow-inflating bag?

When using a flow-inflating bag, you inflate the bag with compressed gas (ie, an oxygen-air mixture from a blender) (Figure 3B.5). The flow from the flowmeter should be adjusted to 5 to 10 L/min and may need to be increased if the bag does not fill sufficiently. Once the gas enters the bag, it is not diluted as it is in a self-inflating bag without a reservoir. Therefore, whatever concentration of oxygen enters the bag is the same concentration delivered to the patient.

Once the mask is properly positioned on the baby's face (or the bag is connected to an endotracheal tube, as you will learn in Lesson 5), most of the gas coming from the wall or blender will be directed to the bag (and thus to the patient), with some coming out the flow-control valve. This will cause the bag to inflate (Figure 3B.6). There are 2 ways that you can adjust the pressure in the bag and thus the amount of inflation of the bag:

- By adjusting the flowmeter, you regulate how much gas enters the bag.

- By adjusting the flow-control valve, you regulate how much gas escapes from the bag.

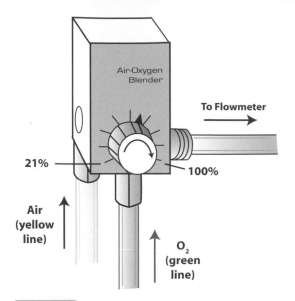

**Figure 3B.5.** Mixing oxygen and air with an oxygen blender. There is a control knob to dial in the desired oxygen concentration.

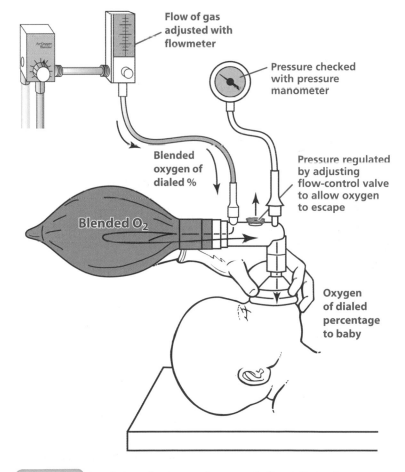

**Figure 3B.6.** Regulation of oxygen and pressure in flow-inflating bag

## Appendix—*continued*

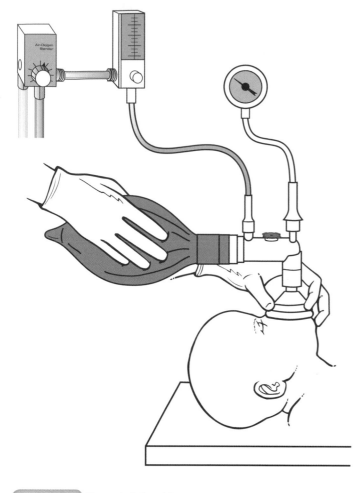

The flowmeter and flow-control valve should be set so that the bag is inflated to the point where it is comfortable to handle and does not completely deflate with each ventilation (Figure 3B.7).

An overinflated bag is difficult to manage and may deliver high pressure to the baby; a pneumothorax or other air leak may develop. An underinflated bag makes it difficult to achieve the desired inflation pressure (Figure 3B.8). With practice, you will be able to make the necessary adjustments to achieve a balance. If there is an adequate seal between the baby's face and the mask, you should be able to maintain the appropriate amount of inflation with the flowmeter set at 5 to 10 L/min.

**Figure 3B.7.** Correctly inflated bag

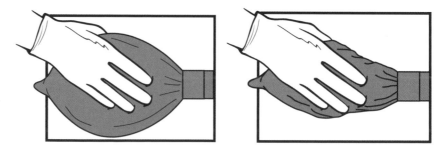

**Figure 3B.8.** Resuscitation bags that are overinflated (left) and underinflated (right)

## Review—Appendix B

*(The answers are in the preceding section and at the end of the Appendix.)*

**B-1.** List 4 reasons why the flow-inflating bag may fail to ventilate the baby.

1. _____

2. _____

3. _____

4. _____

**B-2.** Which flow-inflating bag is being used properly?

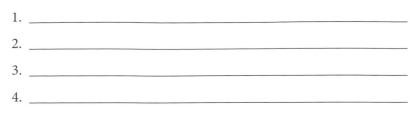

A            B            C

**B-3.** To regulate the pressure of the oxygen going to the baby with a flow-inflating bag, you may adjust either the flowmeter on the wall or the (flow-control valve) (pressure gauge).

**B-4.** If the gas flow through the flow-inflating bag is too high, there (is) (is not) an increased risk for pneumothorax.

## Appendix—*continued*

### C. T-piece Resuscitator

**What are the parts of a T-piece resuscitator?**

There are 6 parts to a flow-controlled, pressure-limited T-piece resuscitator (Figure 3C.1).

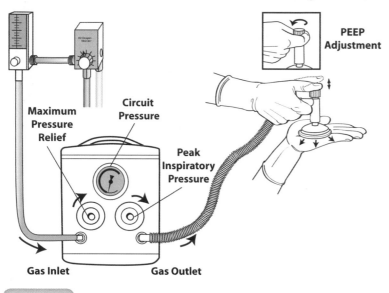

1. Gas inlet

2. Patient (gas) outlet

3. Maximum pressure relief control

4. Circuit pressure gauge

5. Peak inspiratory pressure

6. Patient T-piece with positive end-expiratory pressure (PEEP) cap

**Figure 3C.1.** Parts of the T-piece resuscitator

Gas from a compressed source enters the T-piece resuscitator at the *gas inlet.* The inlet is a small projection designed to fit oxygen tubing and is located under the *maximum pressure relief control.* The desired maximum pressure is set after occluding the PEEP cap and turning the maximum pressure relief control (see following text) to the maximum pressure limit. The manufacturer of one device has set the default level of 40 cm $H_2O$; however, this is adjustable. It should be set about 10 mm Hg higher than the maximum anticipated peak inspiratory pressure, thus about 40 mm Hg for term newborns, and about 30 mm Hg for preterm newborns.

Oxygen exits from the T-piece resuscitator *patient (gas) outlet* by the *gas supply line* to the *patient T-piece,* where the mask or endotracheal tube attaches.

The *peak inspiratory pressure* control is used to set the desired **peak inspiratory pressure.**

The *PEEP cap* is used to set the PEEP.

The *circuit pressure gauge* is used to set and monitor **peak inspiratory pressure,** PEEP, and maximum circuit pressure.

**How does a T-piece resuscitator work?**

The T-piece resuscitator is specially designed for neonatal resuscitation. Pressure controls for maximum pressure, desired **peak inspiratory pressure,** and PEEP must be set by the operator before use (see following text). When the PEEP valve is occluded by the operator, the preset **peak inspiratory pressure** is delivered to the patient for as long as the PEEP valve is occluded.

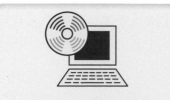

**You are encouraged to view this video on the DVD that accompanies this textbook:**
*Using the T-piece Resuscitator*

## Appendix—*continued*

**How do you prepare the T-piece resuscitator for use?**

*First,* assemble the parts of the T-piece resuscitator as instructed by the manufacturer.

*Second,* attach a test lung to the patient outlet. The test lung is an inflatable balloon that should have been provided by the device manufacturer. Alternatively, the outlet can be occluded during testing, although the inflation time will be shorter than when in clinical use.

*Third,* connect the device to a gas source. This will be a tubing from a blender that permits adjustment of oxygen concentration from 21% (ie, air) to 100%.

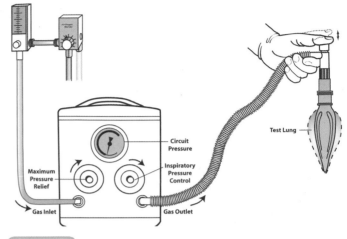

**Figure 3C.2.** Setting up a T-piece resuscitator

*Fourth,* adjust the pressure settings as follows:

- Adjust the flowmeter to regulate how much gas flows into the T-piece resuscitator (5 to 15 L/min recommended).

- Set the maximum circuit pressure by occluding the PEEP cap with your finger and adjusting the maximum pressure relief dial to a selected value (40 cm $H_2O$ is the recommended maximum for term newborns, with a lower value for preterm newborns, as described in Chapter 8) (Figure 3C.2).*

- Set the desired **peak inspiratory pressure** by occluding the PEEP cap with your finger and adjusting the inspiratory pressure control to a selected **peak inspiratory pressure** (Figure 3C.3).

- Set the PEEP by removing your finger from the PEEP cap and adjusting the PEEP cap to the desired setting (2 to 5 cm $H_2O$ is recommended). (See Lesson 8.)

- Remove the test lung and attach the patient T-piece resuscitator to a face mask or be prepared to attach it to an endotracheal tube after the trachea has been intubated. (See Lesson 5.)

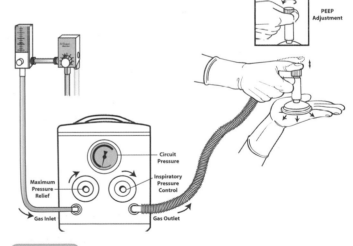

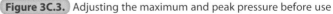

**Figure 3C.3.** Adjusting the maximum and peak pressure before use

When the device is used to ventilate the baby, either by applying the mask to the baby's face or by connecting the device to an endotracheal tube, you control the respiratory rate by intermittently occluding the hole in the PEEP cap during the "breathe" portion of your "breathe-two-three" cadence.

* Note: Some manufacturers recommend that the maximum relief control is adjusted to an institution-defined limit when the device is put into original service and not be readjusted during regular use.

## Appendix—*continued*

If you want to change the peak inspiratory pressure, you will need to readjust the **peak inspiratory pressure** control. This can be done while you are ventilating the patient and will not require reattaching the test lung.

### How do you adjust the concentration of oxygen in a T-piece resuscitator?

The concentration of oxygen delivered to the T-piece resuscitator is the same as that delivered to the baby. Therefore, if the T-piece resuscitator is connected to a source of 100% oxygen, 100% oxygen will be delivered to the baby. To deliver less than 100%, you will have to have a source of compressed air and have the device connected to an oxygen blender. The blender then can be adjusted to provide any concentration of oxygen between 21% and 100%.

### What may be wrong if the baby does not improve or the desired peak pressure is not reached?

- The mask may not be properly sealed on the baby's face.

- The gas supply may not be connected or flow may be insufficient.

- The maximum circuit pressure, **peak inspiratory pressure,** or PEEP may be incorrectly set.

### Can you give free-flow oxygen using a T-piece resuscitator?

Free-flow oxygen can be given reliably with a T-piece resuscitator (Figure 3C.4) if you occlude the PEEP cap and hold the mask loosely on the face. The flow rate of oxygen or gas entering the T-piece resuscitator is the same flow rate that exits the patient T-piece toward the baby when the PEEP cap is occluded. When the mask is held loosely on the face, the flow is maintained without generating pressure as the oxygen or gas diffuses into the environment around the mouth and nares.

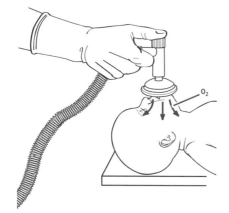

**Figure 3C.4.** Free-flow oxygen given by a T-piece resuscitator

## Review—Appendix C

*(The answers are in the preceding section and at the end of the Appendix.)*

**C-1.** What pressures must be set before using a T-piece resuscitator?

- _____

- _____

- _____

**C-2.** The flow rate on a T-piece resuscitator may need to be (increased) (decreased) if the desired peak inspiratory pressure cannot be obtained.

**C-3.** Free-flow oxygen administered through a T-piece resuscitator requires the PEEP cap to be (open) (occluded).

**C-4.** T-piece resuscitators (will) (will not) work without a compressed gas source.

## Answers to Questions in Appendix

**A-1.** For a self-inflating bag to work, either the pressure gauge must be connected or the connection site must be **plugged.**

**A-2.** A self-inflating bag can deliver 100% oxygen **only when an oxygen reservoir is attached to it.**

**A-3.** Without an oxygen reservoir, a self-inflating bag can deliver a maximum of only about **40%** oxygen.

**A-4.** When you squeeze the bag, you **should** feel pressure against your hand.

**A-5.** The pressure gauge should read **30 to 40 cm $H_2O$** because the pop-off valve is releasing.

**A-6.** The pressure delivered from a self-inflating bag is determined by (1) **how hard you squeeze the bag,** (2) **any leak that may be present between the mask and the baby's face,** and (3) **the set-point of the pressure-release valve.**

**B-1.** The flow-inflating bag may fail to ventilate the baby because of (1) **an inadequate seal between the mask and the face,** (2) **a tear in the bag,** (3) **the flow-control valve is open too far,** and/or (4) **the pressure gauge is not attached or the oxygen tubing is disconnected or occluded.**

**B-2.** Illustration **C** is correct.

**B-3.** Pressure may be regulated by adjusting either the flowmeter or the **flow-control valve.**

**B-4.** If the gas flow through the flow-inflating bag is too high, there **is** an increased risk for pneumothorax.

**C-1.** The pressures set on a T-piece resuscitator are
  - **Maximum circuit pressure**
  - **Peak inspiratory pressure**
  - **Positive end-expiratory pressure**

**C-2.** The flow set on a T-piece resuscitator may need to be **increased** if the desired peak inspiratory pressure cannot be obtained.

**C-3.** Free-flow oxygen administered through a T-piece resuscitator requires the PEEP cap to be **occluded.**

**C-4.** T-piece resuscitators **will not** work without a compressed gas source.

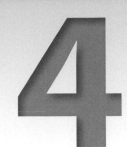
# Chest Compressions

## In Lesson 4 you will learn

- When to begin chest compressions during a resuscitation
- How to administer chest compressions
- How to coordinate chest compressions with positive-pressure ventilation
- When to stop chest compressions

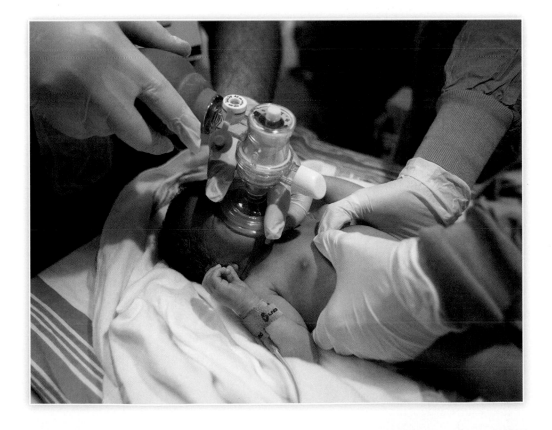

The following case is an example of how chest compressions are delivered during a more extensive resuscitation. As you read the case, imagine yourself as part of the resuscitation team. The details of the chest compressions step will be described in the remainder of the lesson.

## Case 4.
## Resuscitation with positive-pressure ventilation and chest compressions

A pregnant woman contacts her obstetrician after noticing a pronounced decrease in fetal movements at 34 weeks' gestation.

She is admitted to the labor and delivery unit where persistent fetal bradycardia is noted. Additional skilled personnel are called to the delivery room, the radiant warmer is turned on, and resuscitation equipment is prepared. An emergency cesarean section is performed, and a limp, apneic baby is transferred to the neonatal team.

The team positions the baby's head, suctions her mouth and nose, stimulates her with drying and flicking the soles of her feet, and removes the wet linen. However, 30 seconds after birth, the baby is still limp, cyanotic, and without spontaneous respirations.

One member of the team begins positive-pressure ventilation (PPV) with a bag and mask, while a second team member feels the umbilical cord for the pulse and listens with a stethoscope for breath sounds. At the same time, a third member of the team places an oximetry probe on the baby's right hand. The heart rate remains below 60 beats per minute (bpm) despite the presence of breath sounds and a gentle rise and fall of the chest with each manual breath. After 30 seconds of PPV, the baby has a very low heart rate (20 to 30 bpm) and remains cyanotic and limp. The oximeter is not registering a heart rate or saturation.

Because the heart rate has not increased, a member of the team checks to make sure that the mask is fitting properly on the face, the ventilation rate is 40 to 60 breaths per minute, the airway is clear, the head is positioned correctly, and the chest is rising slightly with each breath. Despite increasing the pressure on the bag to increase the chest rise, the heart rate remains below 60 bpm, so the team leader intubates the trachea to ensure effective ventilation. The team begins chest compressions coordinated with PPV using a 3:1 ratio of compressions to ventilations and increasing the oxygen concentration to 100% since the oximeter is still not registering.

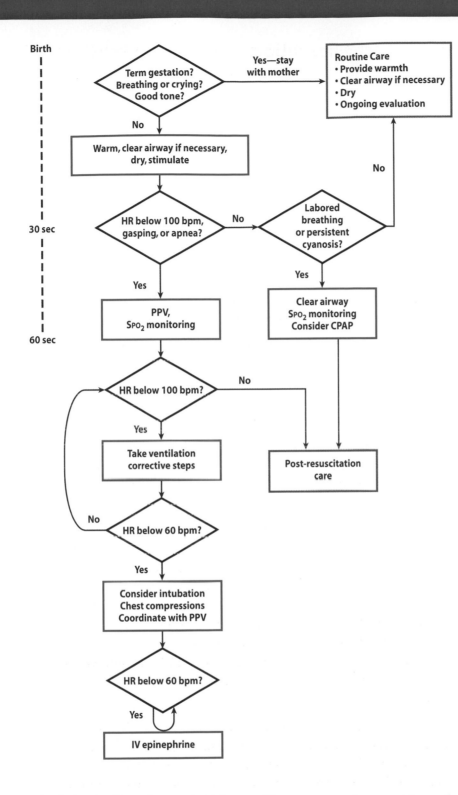

The baby finally makes an initial gasp. Chest compressions are stopped when the heart rate rises above 60 bpm. The team continues PPV, and the heart rate rises to more than 100 bpm as now recorded by the oximeter. The inspired oxygen concentration is adjusted based on pulse oximetry readings. After spontaneous respirations are observed, she is moved to the special care nursery for monitoring and further management.

## What are the indications for beginning chest compressions?

 Chest compressions are indicated whenever the heart rate is below 60 beats per minute, despite at least 30 seconds of effective positive-pressure ventilation (PPV).

## Why perform chest compressions?

 Endotracheal intubation at this time may help ensure adequate ventilation and facilitate the coordination of ventilation and chest compressions.

Babies who have a heart rate below 60 bpm, despite stimulation and 30 seconds of PPV, are likely to have very low blood oxygen levels and significant acidosis. As a result, myocardial function is depressed and the heart is unable to contract strongly enough to pump blood to the lungs to pick up the oxygen that you have now ensured is in the lungs by providing PPV. Therefore, you will need to mechanically pump blood through the heart while you simultaneously continue to ventilate the lungs until the myocardium becomes sufficiently oxygenated to recover adequate spontaneous function. This process also will help restore oxygen delivery to the brain. Although chest compressions can be delivered while ventilations are being administered with bag and mask, endotracheal intubation at this point will make ventilation more effective.

## What are chest compressions?

Chest compressions consist of rhythmic compressions of the sternum that

- Compress the heart against the spine.

- Increase the intrathoracic pressure.

- Circulate blood to the vital organs of the body.

The heart lies in the chest between the lower third of the sternum and the spine. Compressing the sternum compresses the heart and increases the pressure in the chest, causing blood to be pumped into the arteries (Figure 4.1).

When pressure on the sternum is released, blood enters the heart from the veins.

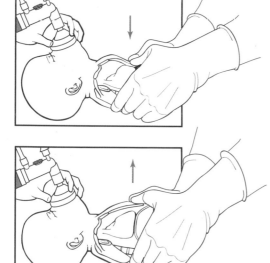

**Figure 4.1.** Compression (top) and release (bottom) phases of chest compressions

## How many people are needed to administer chest compressions, and where should they stand?

Remember that chest compressions are of little value unless the lungs are also being ventilated. Therefore, 2 people are required to administer effective chest compressions—one to compress the chest and one to continue ventilation. This second person may be the same person who came to monitor heart rate and breath sounds during PPV.

The person performing chest compressions must have access to the chest and be able to position his or her hands correctly. The person assisting ventilation should be positioned at the baby's head to be able to maintain an effective mask-face seal (or to stabilize the endotracheal tube) and watch for effective chest movement with ventilation (Figure 4.2). Other team members will be needed to ensure adequate functioning of the oximeter, and to prepare for vascular access and administration of medications, in case the heart rate does not improve with ventilation and chest compressions alone. (See Lesson 6.) To provide more room for another team member to insert an emergency umbilical venous catheter, the person administering chest compressions may need to move to the head of the bed, next to the team member giving ventilations.

## How do you position your hands on the chest to begin chest compressions?

You will learn 2 different techniques for performing chest compressions. These techniques are

- *Thumb technique*, where the 2 thumbs are used to depress the sternum, while the hands encircle the torso and the fingers support the spine (Figure 4.3A). This is the preferred technique.

- *2-finger technique*, where the tips of the middle finger and either the index finger or ring finger of one hand are used to compress the sternum, while the other hand is used to support the baby's back (Figure 4.3B).

## Why is the thumb technique preferred?

The thumb technique is preferred because you can control the depth of compression better than with the 2-finger technique and you can provide pressure that is more consistent. The thumb technique also

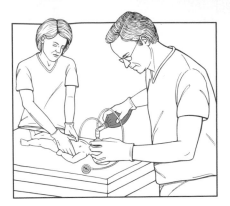

**Figure 4.2.** Two people are required when chest compressions are given

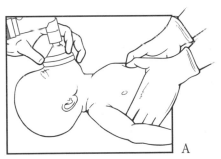

**Preferred technique**

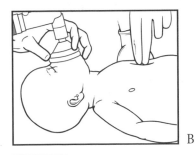

**Figure 4.3.** Two techniques for giving chest compressions: thumb (A) and 2-finger (B)

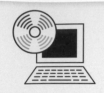

You are encouraged to view this video on the DVD that accompanies this textbook: *Chest Compressions: Head of Infant Positioning*

appears to be superior in generating peak systolic and coronary arterial perfusion pressure. It also is preferable for individuals with long fingernails. Thus, the thumb technique should be used in most situations.

Although the 2-finger technique has been used to permit a colleague easier access to the umbilicus for insertion of an umbilical catheter, with practice, the 2 people delivering compressions and ventilations can both position themselves at the head of the bed, allowing the more effective thumb technique to be used throughout the resuscitation. Performing chest compressions at the head of the bed is most easily accomplished if the trachea has been intubated.

The 2 techniques have the following things in common:

- Position of the baby
  - Firm support for the back is needed
  - Neck slightly extended
- Compressions
  - Location, depth, and rate of compressions

## Where on the chest should you position your thumbs or fingers?

When chest compressions are performed on a newborn, pressure is applied to the lower third of the sternum, which lies between the xiphoid and a line drawn between the nipples (Figure 4.4). The xiphoid is the small projection where the lower ribs meet at the midline. You can quickly locate the correct area on the sternum by running your fingers along the lower edge of the rib cage until you locate the xiphoid. Then, place your thumbs or fingers immediately above the xiphoid. Care must be used to avoid putting pressure directly on the xiphoid.

## How do you position your hands using the thumb technique?

The thumb technique is accomplished by encircling the torso with both hands. The thumbs are placed on the sternum and the fingers are under the baby's back, supporting the spine (Figure 4.5).

The thumbs can be placed side by side or, on a small baby, one over the other (Figure 4.5).

The thumbs are used to compress the sternum, while your fingers provide the support needed for the back. The thumbs should be flexed at the first joint, and pressure should be applied vertically to compress the heart between the sternum and the spine (Figure 4.6).

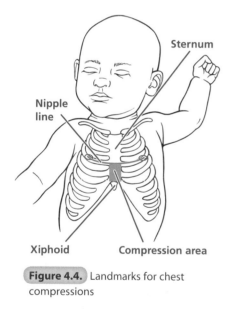

**Figure 4.4.** Landmarks for chest compressions

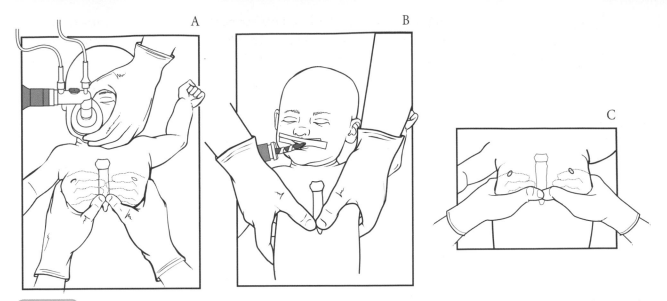

**Figure 4.5.** Thumb technique of chest compressions administered from the bottom (A), from the top (B), and for small chests, with thumbs overlapped (C)

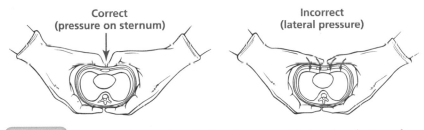

Correct
(pressure on sternum)

Incorrect
(lateral pressure)

**Figure 4.6.** Correct and incorrect application of pressure with thumb technique of chest compressions

The thumb technique has some minor disadvantages. It cannot be used effectively if the baby is large or your hands are small. The required position of the rescuer's body also makes access to the umbilical cord somewhat more difficult when medications become necessary, unless the person administering compressions moves to the head of the bed.

## How do you position your hands using the 2-finger technique?

In the 2-finger technique, the tips of your middle finger and either the index or ring finger of one hand are used for compressions (Figure 4.7). You probably will find it easier to use your right hand if you are right-handed (or your left hand if you are left-handed). Position the 2 fingers perpendicular to the chest as shown, and press with your fingertips. If you find that your nails prevent you from using your fingertips, you should ventilate the newborn while your partner compresses the chest,

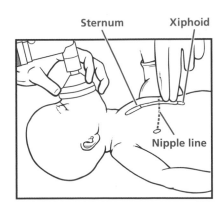

Sternum    Xiphoid

Nipple line

**Figure 4.7.** Correct finger position for 2-finger technique

139

or you could use the preferred thumb technique for performing chest compressions.

When using the 2-finger technique, your other hand must be placed flat under the center of the newborn's back so that the heart is more effectively compressed between the sternum and spine. With the second hand supporting the back, you also can more easily judge the pressure and the depth of compressions.

When compressing the chest, only the 2 fingertips should rest on the chest. This way, you can best control the pressure you apply to the sternum and the spine (Figure 4.8A).

As with the thumb technique, you should apply pressure vertically to compress the heart between the sternum and the spine (Figure 4.8A).

You may find the 2-finger technique to be more tiring than the thumb technique if chest compressions are required for a prolonged period.

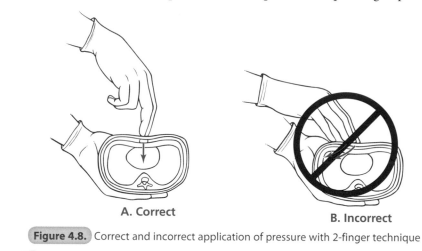

**A. Correct**       **B. Incorrect**

**Figure 4.8.** Correct and incorrect application of pressure with 2-finger technique

 **Review**

*(The answers are in the preceding section and at the end of the lesson.)*

1. A newborn is apneic and bradycardic. Her airway is cleared, and she is stimulated. At 30 seconds, positive-pressure ventilation is begun. At 60 seconds, her heart rate is 80 beats per minute. Chest compressions (should) (should not) be started. Positive-pressure ventilation (should) (should not) continue.

2. A newborn is apneic and bradycardic. She remains apneic, despite having her airway cleared, being stimulated, receiving 30 seconds of positive-pressure ventilation, and ensuring that all ventilation techniques are optimal. Nevertheless, her heart rate is only 40 beats per minute. Chest compressions (should) (should not) be started. Positive-pressure ventilation (should) (should not) continue.

3. The heart rate is 40 beats per minute as determined by auscultation and the oximeter has stopped working. Chest compressions have begun, but the baby is still receiving room air oxygen. What should be done about oxygen delivery? (continue room air) (increase the oxygen concentration to 100%)

4. During the compression phase of chest compressions, the sternum compresses the heart, which causes blood to be pumped from the heart into the (veins) (arteries). In the release phase, blood enters the heart from the (veins) (arteries).

5. Mark the area on this baby (see illustration at right) where you would apply chest compressions.

6. The preferred method of delivering chest compressions is the (thumb) (2-finger) technique.

7. If you anticipate that the baby will need medication by the umbilical route, you can continue chest compressions by one of the following actions:

_____ or _____

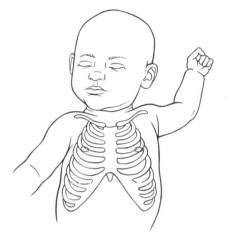

## How much pressure do you use to compress the chest?

Controlling the pressure used in compressing the sternum is an important part of the procedure.

With your fingers and hands correctly positioned, use enough pressure to depress the sternum *to a depth of approximately one-third of the anterior-posterior diameter of the chest* (Figure 4.9), and then release

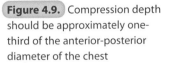 **Figure 4.9.** Compression depth should be approximately one-third of the anterior-posterior diameter of the chest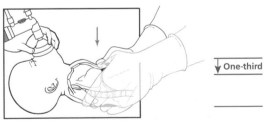

One-third

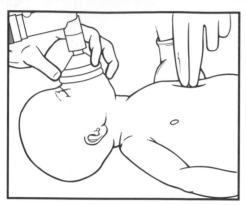

**Figure 4.10.** *Correct* method of chest compressions (fingers remain in contact with chest on release)

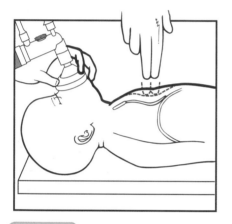

**Figure 4.11.** *Incorrect* method of chest compressions (fingers lose contact with chest on release)

the pressure to allow the heart to refill. One compression consists of the downward stroke plus the release. The actual distance compressed will depend on the size of the baby.

The duration of the downward stroke of the compression also should be somewhat shorter than the duration of the release for generation of maximum cardiac output.

Your thumbs or the tips of your fingers (depending on the method you use) should remain in contact with the chest at all times during both compression *and* release (Figure 4.10). Allow the chest to fully expand by lifting your thumbs or fingers sufficiently during the release phase to permit blood to reenter the heart from the veins. However, *do not* lift your thumbs or fingers off the chest between compressions (Figure 4.11). If you take your thumbs or fingers completely off the sternum after compressions,

- You waste time relocating the compression area.

- You lose control over the depth of compression.

- You may compress the wrong area, producing trauma to the chest or underlying organs.

## Are there dangers associated with administering chest compressions?

Chest compressions can cause trauma to the baby.

Two vital organs lie within the rib cage—the heart and lungs. The liver lies partially under the ribs, although it is in the abdominal cavity. As you perform chest compressions, you must apply enough pressure to compress the heart between the sternum and spine without damaging underlying organs. Pressure applied too low, over the xiphoid, can cause laceration of the liver (Figure 4.12).

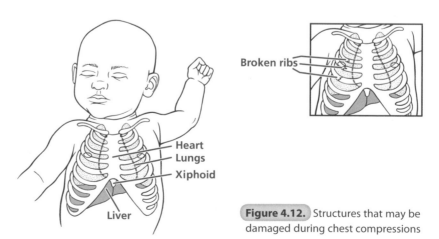

**Figure 4.12.** Structures that may be damaged during chest compressions

Also, the ribs are fragile and can be broken easily.

By following the procedure outlined in this lesson, the risk of these injuries can be minimized.

## How often do you compress the chest and how do you coordinate compressions with ventilation?

During cardiopulmonary resuscitation, chest compressions must always be accompanied by PPV. Avoid giving a compression and a ventilation simultaneously, because one will decrease the efficacy of the other. Therefore, the 2 activities must be coordinated, with one ventilation interposed after every third compression, for a total of 30 breaths and 90 compressions per minute (Figure 4.13).

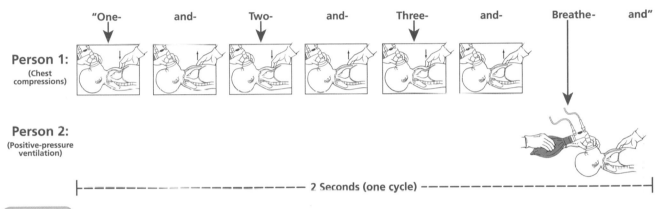

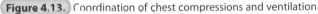

**Figure 4.13.** Coordination of chest compressions and ventilation

The person doing the compressions takes over the counting out loud from the person who is doing the ventilating. The compressor counts "One-and-Two-and-Three-and-Breathe-and" while the person ventilating squeezes during "Breathe-and" and releases during "One-and." Note that exhalation occurs during the downward stroke of the next compression. Counting the cadence will help develop a smooth and well-coordinated procedure.

One *cycle of events* consists of 3 compressions plus 1 ventilation.

- There should be approximately 120 "events" per 60 seconds (1 minute)—90 compressions plus 30 breaths.

Note that, during chest compressions, the ventilation rate is actually 30 breaths per minute rather than the rate you previously learned for PPV, which was 40 to 60 breaths per minute. This lower ventilatory rate is needed to provide an adequate number of compressions and avoid simultaneous compressions and ventilation. To ensure that the process can be coordinated, it is important to practice with another person and to practice the roles of both the compressor and the ventilator.

## How can you practice the rhythm of chest compressions with ventilation?

Imagine that you are the person giving chest compressions. Repeat the words several times while you move your hand to compress the chest on "One-and," "Two-and," "Three-and." Do not press when you say, "Breathe-and." Do not remove your fingers from the surface you are pressing, but be sure to relax your pressure on the chest to permit adequate ventilation during the breath.

Now time yourself to see if you can say and do these 5 cycles of events in 10 seconds. Remember not to press on the "Breathe-and."

Practice saying the words and compressing the chest.

*One-and-Two-and-Three-and*-Breathe-and-*One-and-Two-and-Three-and*-Breathe-and-

*One-and-Two-and-Three-and*-Breathe-and-*One-and-Two-and-Three-and*-Breathe-and-

*One-and-Two-and-Three-and*-Breathe-and

Now imagine that you are the person administering positive-pressure ventilation. This time you want to squeeze your hand when you say "Breathe-and" but not when you say "One-and," "Two-and," "Three-and."

Now time yourself to see if you can say and do these 5 events in 10 seconds. Remember, squeeze your hand only when you say "Breathe-and."

One-and-Two-and-Three-and-*Breathe-and*-One-and-Two-and-Three and-*Breathe-and*-

One-and-Two-and-Three-and-*Breathe-and*-One-and-Two-and-Three and-*Breathe-and*-

One-and-Two-and-Three-and-*Breathe-and*

In a real situation, there will be 2 team members performing resuscitation, with one doing the compressions and one doing the bagging. The person compressing will be speaking "One-and-Two-and-..." out loud. Therefore, it is helpful to practice with a partner, taking turns in each of the roles.

## When do you stop chest compressions?

Although you were told earlier to reassess the effects of your actions approximately every 30 seconds, studies have shown that return of spontaneous circulation may take a minute or so after chest compressions are started. Also, any interruption of chest compressions required to check the heart rate may result in a decrease of perfusion pressure in the coronary arteries. Studies in adults and with animals suggest that there may be a delay of 45 seconds or longer after the compressions are resumed before the coronary perfusion pressure returns to its previous value. Therefore, you may want to wait at least 45 to 60 seconds after you have established well-coordinated chest compressions and ventilation before pausing briefly to determine the heart rate again. Use of an oximeter and a cardiac monitor may be helpful in assessing the heart rate without interrupting compressions; however, if perfusion is very low, the pulse oximeter may not detect a consistent pulse. You should stop administering chest compressions when the heart rate is greater than 60 bpm and concentrate on delivering effective ventilation at the higher rate of 40 to 60 breaths per minute.

### *If the heart rate increases to above 60 bpm while compressions are being provided,*

You can discontinue chest compressions, but continue PPV at the rate of 40 to 60 breaths per minute rate. You should not continue chest compressions, since the cardiac output is probably adequate and the compressions may decrease the effectiveness of the PPV.

Once the heart rate rises above 100 bpm, if the baby begins to breathe spontaneously, you should gradually slow the rate and decrease the pressure of PPV, as described in Lesson 3, and move the baby to the nursery for post-resuscitation care.

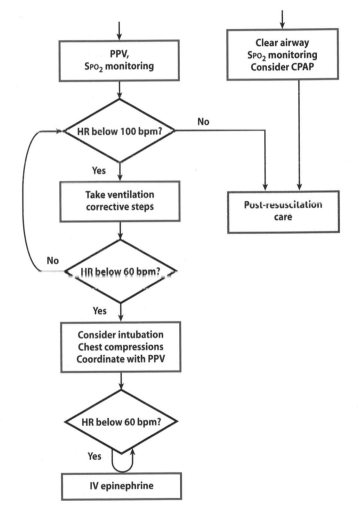

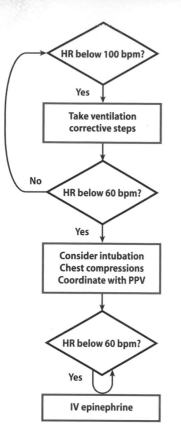

## What do you do if the baby is *not* improving?

While continuing to administer chest compressions and coordinated ventilation, ask yourself the following questions:

- Is ventilation adequate? (Have you performed the ventilation corrective steps? Have you performed endotracheal intubation? If so, is the endotracheal tube in the correct position?)

- Is supplemental oxygen being given?

- Is the depth of chest compression approximately one-third of the diameter of the chest?

- Are the chest compressions and ventilation well coordinated?

***If the heart rate remains below 60 bpm, then you should insert an umbilical catheter and give epinephrine, as described in Lesson 6.***

As illustrated in Case 4 at the beginning of this lesson, you likely will have wanted to intubate the baby's trachea by this point in a resuscitation. Therefore, if intubation is not within your scope of practice, you will need to call for someone trained in endotracheal intubation to come to the delivery room as soon as you recognize that an extensive resuscitation may be needed. The technique of endotracheal intubation will be described in Lesson 5.

## Key Points

1. Chest compressions are indicated when the heart rate remains below 60 beats per minute, despite 30 seconds of effective positive-pressure ventilation.

2. Once the heart rate is below 60 beats per minute, the oximeter may stop working. You should increase the oxygen to 100% until return of the oximeter reading to guide you in the appropriate adjustment of delivered oxygen.

3. Chest compressions
   - Compress the heart against the spine.
   - Increase intrathoracic pressure.
   - Circulate blood to the vital organs, including the brain.

4. There are 2 acceptable techniques for chest compressions—the thumb technique and the 2-finger technique—but the thumb technique is preferred.

## Key Points—*continued*

5. Locate the correct area for compressions by running your fingers along the lower edge of the rib cage until you locate the xiphoid. Then place your thumbs or fingers on the sternum, above the xiphoid and on a line connecting the nipples.

6. To ensure proper rate of chest compressions and ventilation, the compressor repeats "One-and-Two-and-Three-and-Breathe-and...."

7. During chest compressions, the breathing rate is 30 breaths per minute and the compression rate is 90 compressions per minute. This equals 120 "events" per minute. One cycle of 3 compressions and 1 breath takes 2 seconds.

8. If you anticipate that the baby will need medication by the umbilical route, you can continue chest compressions by moving to the head of the bed to continue giving compressions using the thumb technique. Performing chest compressions from the head of the bed is most easily accomplished if the trachea has been intubated.

9. During chest compressions, ensure that
   • Chest movement is adequate during ventilation.
   • Supplemental oxygen is being used.
   • Compression depth is one-third of the diameter of the chest.
   • Pressure is released fully to permit chest recoil during relaxation phase of chest compression.
   • Thumbs or fingers remain in contact with the chest at all times.
   • Duration of the downward stroke of the compression is shorter than duration of the release.
   • Chest compressions and ventilation are well coordinated.

10. After 45 to 60 seconds of chest compressions and ventilation, check the heart rate. If the heart rate is
   • Greater than 60 beats per minute, discontinue compressions and continue ventilation at 40 to 60 breaths per minute.
   • Greater than 100 beats per minute, discontinue compressions and gradually discontinue ventilation if the newborn is breathing spontaneously.
   • Less than 60 beats per minute, intubate the newborn (if not already done), and give epinephrine, preferably intravenously. Intubation provides a more reliable method of continuing ventilation.

## Lesson 4 Review

*(The answers follow.)*

1. A newborn is apneic and bradycardic. Her airway is cleared, and she is stimulated. At 30 seconds, positive-pressure ventilation is begun. At 60 seconds, her heart rate is 80 beats per minute. Chest compressions (should) (should not) be started. Positive-pressure ventilation (should) (should not) continue.

2. A newborn is apneic and bradycardic. She remains apneic, despite having her airway cleared, being stimulated, receiving 30 seconds of positive-pressure ventilation, and ensuring that all ventilation techniques are optimal. Nevertheless, her heart rate is only 40 beats per minute. Chest compressions (should) (should not) be started. Positive-pressure ventilation (should) (should not) continue.

3. The heart rate is 40 beats per minute as determined by auscultation, and the oximeter has stopped working. Chest compressions have begun, but the baby is still receiving room air oxygen. What should be done about oxygen delivery? (continue room air) (increase the oxygen concentration to 100%)

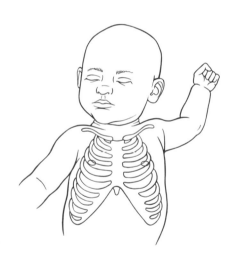

4. During the compression phase of chest compressions, the sternum compresses the heart, which causes blood to be pumped from the heart into the (veins) (arteries). In the release phase, blood enters the heart from the (veins) (arteries).

5. Mark the area on this baby (see illustration at left) where you would apply chest compressions.

6. The preferred method of delivering chest compressions is the (thumb) (2-finger) technique.

7. If you anticipate that the baby will need medication by the umbilical route, you can continue chest compressions by one of the following actions:

   _____ or _____

8. The correct depth of chest compressions is approximately
   A. One-fourth of the anterior-posterior diameter of the chest
   B. One-third of the anterior-posterior diameter of the chest
   C. One-half of the anterior-posterior diameter of the chest

## Lesson 4 Review—*continued*

**9.** Which drawing shows the correct release motion?

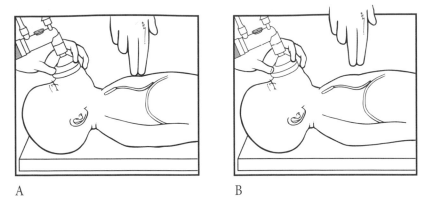

A                                    B

**10.** What phrase is used to time and coordinate chest compressions and ventilation? _____.

**11.** The ratio of chest compressions to ventilation is _____ to

_____.

**12** During positive-pressure ventilation without chest compressions, the rate of breaths per minute should be _____ to _____ breaths per minute.

**13.** During positive-pressure ventilation with chest compressions, the rate of "events" per minute should be _____ "events" per minute.

**14.** The count "One-and-Two-and-Three-and-Breathe-and" should take about _____ seconds.

**15.** A baby has required ventilation and chest compressions. After 30 seconds of chest compressions, you stop and count **8 heartbeats in 6 seconds.** The baby's heart rate is now _____ beats per minute. You should (continue) (stop) chest compressions.

**16.** A baby has required chest compressions and is being ventilated with bag and mask. The chest is not moving well. You stop and count **4 heartbeats in 6 seconds.** The baby's heart rate is now _____ beats per minute. You may want to consider

_____, _____,

and _____.

## Lesson 4 Review—*continued*

**17.** Complete the chart.

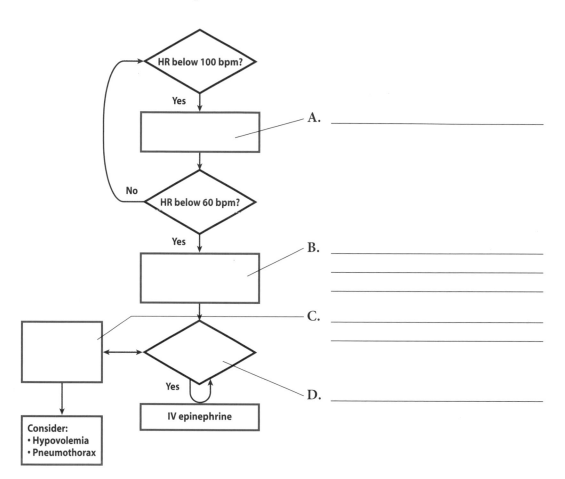

A. _____

B. _____
_____
_____

C. _____
_____

D. _____

## Answers to Questions

1. Chest compressions **should not** be started. Positive-pressure ventilation **should** continue.

2. Chest compressions **should** be started. Positive-pressure ventilation **should** continue.

3. **Oxygen concentration should be increased to 100%** until the oximeter begins to work again, at which time it should be adjusted to match the table in the flow diagram.

4. Blood is pumped into the **arteries** during the compression phase, and from the **veins** during the release phase.

## Answers to Questions—*continued*

**5.** Compression area.

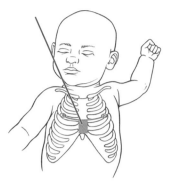

**6.** The preferred method of delivering chest compressions is the **thumb** technique.

**7.** You can continue chest compressions by **moving to the head of the bed to continue the thumb technique** or **changing to the 2-finger technique.**

**8.** The correct depth of chest compressions is approximately **one-third of the anterior-posterior diameter of the chest** (B).

**9.** Drawing **A** is correct (fingers remain in contact during release).

**10.** **"One-and-Two-and-Three-and-Breathe-and ..."**

**11.** The ratio is **3:1.**

**12.** The rate of ventilation without chest compressions should be **40 to 60** breaths per minute.

**13.** There should be **120** "events" per minute during chest compressions.

**14.** The count "One-and-Two-and-Three-and-Breathe-and" should take about **2** seconds.

**15.** Eight heartbeats in 6 seconds is **80** beats per minute. You should **stop** chest compressions.

**16.** Four heartbeats in 6 seconds is **40** beats per minute. You may want to consider **endotracheal intubation, insertion of an umbilical catheter,** and **administration of epinephrine.**

## Answers to Questions—*continued*

**17.** The missing text is shown below:

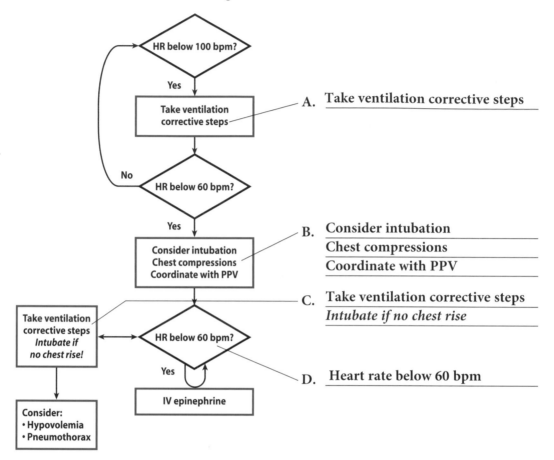

A.  Take ventilation corrective steps

B.  Consider intubation
    Chest compressions
    Coordinate with PPV

C.  Take ventilation corrective steps
    *Intubate if no chest rise*

D.  Heart rate below 60 bpm

# Lesson 4: Chest Compressions Performance Checklist

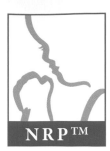

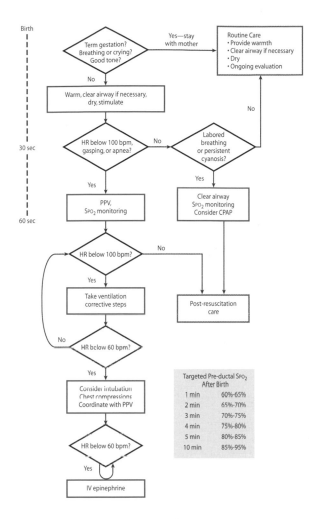

## The Performance Checklist Is a Learning Tool

The learner uses the checklist as a reference during independent practice or as a guide for discussion and practice with a Neonatal Resuscitation Program™ (NRP™) instructor. When the learner and instructor agree that the learner can perform the skills correctly and smoothly without coaching and within the context of a scenario, the learner may move on to the next lesson's Performance Checklist.

## Knowledge Check

• What are the indications for beginning chest compressions?

• Which method is preferred: 2-finger or thumb technique? Why?

• What is the indication for discontinuing chest compressions?

**Learning Objectives**

1. Identify the newborn who requires chest compressions.

2. Demonstrate correct technique for performing chest compressions.

3. Identify the sign that indicates chest compressions should be discontinued.

4. Demonstrate behavioral skills to ensure clear communication and teamwork during this critical component of newborn resuscitation.

**"You are called to attend an emergency cesarean birth due to fetal bradycardia. How would you prepare for the resuscitation of this baby? As you work, say your thoughts and actions aloud so your assistant and I will know what you are thinking and doing."**

Instructor should check boxes as the learner responds correctly.

Note: This scenario takes the learner from Lesson 1 through Lesson 4. The instructor who finds the "Details" column helpful for assessing performance may use this Performance Checklist as the Basic Integrated Skills Station Checklist (Lessons 1 through 4) instead of the more abbreviated Basic Integrated Skills Performance Checklist.

| Participant Name: | | |
|---|---|---|
| | ☐ Obtains relevant perinatal history | Gestational age? Fluid clear? How many babies? Other risk factors? |
| | ☐ Performs equipment check <br> ☐ Assembles resuscitation team (at least one other person) and discusses plan and roles <br> ☐ If obstetric provider indicates that meconium is present in amniotic fluid, prepares for intubation and suctioning meconium | Warm, Clear airway, Auscultate, Oxygenate, Ventilate, Intubate, Medicate, Thermoregulate |

| | **"The baby has just been born."** | |
|---|---|---|
| **Sample Vital Signs** | **Performance Steps** | **Details** |
| Gestational age as indicated <br> Apneic <br> Limp | ☐ Completes initial assessment <br> ☐ Receives baby at radiant warmer | Asks 3 questions: Term? Breathing or crying? Good tone? |

| Sample Vital Signs | Performance Steps | Details |
|---|---|---|
| | *Meconium management (optional)* | |
| | ☐ Performs initial steps | Warm, position airway, suction mouth and nose, dry, remove wet linen, stimulate. |
| Respiratory rate (RR)-apneic<br>Heart rate (HR)-40 beats per minute (bpm) | ☐ Evaluates respirations and heart rate | Auscultates apical pulse or palpates umbilicus. |
| | ☐ Initiates positive-pressure ventilation (PPV) | Begins with ___% oxygen per hospital protocol at about 20 cm $H_2O$ pressure. Rate = 40-60/min |
| | ☐ Calls for additional help if necessary | A minimum of 2 resuscitators are necessary if PPV required. Team should be assembled before birth. |
| | ☐ Requests pulse oximetry | Assistant places probe on right hand or wrist before plugging into monitor. |
| RR-apneic<br>HR-40 bpm<br>$S_{PO_2}$ — — - -<br>No breath sounds or chest movement | ☐ Requests assessment of heart rate, pulse oximetry<br><br>☐ If not rising, requests assessment of bilateral breath sounds and chest movement | Pulse oximetry not functioning at low HR. |
| | ☐ Takes ventilation corrective steps (MR SOPA) | **M**ask adjustment and **R**eposition airway (reattempt 5-10 breaths).<br>**S**uction mouth and nose and **o**pen mouth (reattempt 5-10 breaths).<br>Gradually increase the **p**ressure every few breaths until there are bilateral breath sounds and visible chest movement with each breath, up to a maximum of 40 cm $H_2O$ pressure, if necessary. |
| + chest movement<br>+ breath sounds | ☐ Requests evaluation of chest rise and breath sounds | If all corrective steps done but still no chest movement, breath sounds, or rising heart rate, learner indicates need for **a**lternative airway, such as intubation. |
| + chest movement<br>+ breath sounds | ☐ Performs 30 seconds of PPV; notes breath sounds and chest movement | Assistant notes bilateral breath sounds and chest movement. |
| HR-50 bpm<br>$S_{PO_2}$ — — — | ☐ Evaluates heart rate and $S_{PO_2}$ | Assistant auscultates or palpates HR (oximetry not yet functioning due to low heart rate). |
| | ☐ Calls for additional help<br>☐ Initiates chest compressions<br>☐ Increases oxygen to 100% | Team may already be present. Do not forget someone needs to document events on the code sheet.<br>Leader delegates PPV and other tasks as necessary. |
| | ☐ Locates appropriate position on lower third of sternum | |

| Sample Vital Signs | Performance Steps | Details |
|---|---|---|
| | ☐ 2-finger technique:<br>• Uses fingertips of middle and index or ring fingers<br>☐ Thumb technique:<br>• Uses distal portion of both thumbs (one thumb over the other if baby is small) | Thumb technique is preferred because you can control the depth of compression better than with 2-finger technique. Thumb technique generates superior peak systolic and coronary arterial perfusion pressure. |
| | ☐ Compresses sternum one-third of anterior-posterior diameter of chest, straight up and down.<br>☐ Keeps fingertips/thumbs on sternum during release. Allows chest expansion between compressions, but does not lift thumbs or fingers from chest. | Duration of downward stroke should be somewhat shorter than the duration of the release for generation of maximum cardiac output.<br><br>During thumb technique, beware of tight grip around thorax that impedes ventilation. |
| | ☐ Compressor counts cadence: "One-and-Two-and-Three-and-Breathe-and"<br>☐ Ventilates during pause at "Breathe-and" | One cycle of 3 compressions and 1 breath takes 2 seconds. |
| | ☐ Provides 45-60 seconds of chest compressions and coordinated ventilations<br>Assesses heart rate:<br>☐ Palpates umbilicus and continues ventilation<br>Or, if no pulsations felt,<br>☐ Auscultates apical pulse and pauses ventilation | Heart rate assessment is a good place to ask learner and assistant to change places so learner can demonstrate roles of compressor and ventilator.<br>Instructor chooses<br>**Option 1:** Recovery to free-flow oxygen.<br><br>**Option 2:** Indicate need to proceed to umbilical venous catheter (UVC) placement and administration of epinephrine. |
| **Option 1** | | |
| HR-70 bpm<br>$SpO_2$-67%<br><br>Apneic<br>+ breath sounds<br>+ chest movement | ☐ Discontinues compressions<br><br>☐ Continues ventilations<br><br>☐ Adjusts oxygen based on oximetry and newborn's age | Discontinue compressions when HR >60 bpm.<br><br><br>Continue to monitor HR and $SpO_2$. |

| Sample Vital Signs | Performance Steps | Details |
|---|---|---|
| HR-120 bpm<br>$SpO_2$-74%<br>RR-10 breaths per minute<br><br><br>HR-140 bpm<br>$SpO_2$-97%<br>RR-weak cry | ☐ Provides additional 30 seconds of effective ventilation *without* chest compressions.<br>☐ Assesses newborn's respiratory effort, HR, pulse oximetry.<br>☐ Slows PPV rate as newborn breathes spontaneously.<br>☐ Gradually withdraws PPV and adjusts free-flow oxygen based on oximetry. Eventually discontinues free-flow oxygen based on oximetry. | Team should be noting newborn's improving vital signs and discussing next steps together. |
|  | ☐ Updates family<br>☐ Directs appropriate post-resuscitation care |  |
| **Option 2** | | |
| HR-40 bpm<br>$SpO_2$ - - -<br>(Oximeter—no signal) | ☐ Provides additional 45-60 seconds of chest compressions and coordinated ventilations and considers reasons for poor response | Consider reasons for poor response:<br>• Ineffective ventilation?<br>• Dislodged endotracheal tube (or need to intubate now)?<br>• Supplemental oxygen being given?<br>• Appropriate compression technique (location, depth, rate)?<br>• Coordinated compressions and ventilations? |
| HR-50 bpm<br>$SpO_2$ - - -<br>(Oximeter—no signal) | ☐ Requests HR assessment after completing more than 45-60 seconds of coordinated compressions and PPV<br>☐ Communicates plan for next steps<br>• Intubate if not yet done<br>• Insert emergency UVC and give epinephrine | Team may need additional help to place emergency UVC and administer epinephrine and intubate newborn. |

Instructor asks the learner Reflective Questions to enable self-assessment, such as:

1 What went well during this resuscitation?

2 Who assumed the leadership role in this scenario?

3 Did you (leader) get what you needed from your assistant(s)? What behavioral skills did you use to ensure good teamwork? Give me an example of what you did or said that used that behavioral skill.

4 When the baby did not respond to chest compressions and coordinated, effective ventilation, what did team members do to support (or not support) each other?

5 What would you do differently when faced with this scenario again?

### Neonatal Resuscitation Program Key Behavioral Skills

| | |
|---|---|
| Know your environment. | Allocate attention wisely. |
| Anticipate and plan. | Use all available information. |
| Assume the leadership role. | Use all available resources. |
| Communicate effectively. | Call for help when needed. |
| Delegate workload optimally. | Maintain professional behavior. |

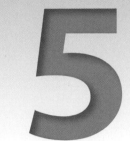
# Endotracheal Intubation and Laryngeal Mask Airway Insertion

## In Lesson 5 you will learn

- The indications for endotracheal intubation during resuscitation
- How to select and prepare the appropriate equipment for endotracheal intubation
- How to use the laryngoscope to insert an endotracheal tube
- How to determine if the endotracheal tube is in the trachea
- How to use the endotracheal tube to suction meconium from the trachea
- How to use the endotracheal tube to administer positive-pressure ventilation
- When to consider using a laryngeal mask airway for positive-pressure ventilation
- How to place a laryngeal mask airway

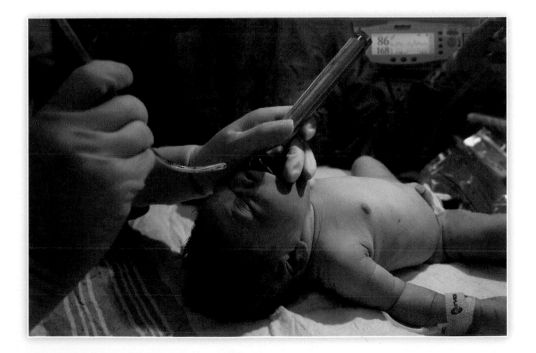

## When should endotracheal intubation be considered?

Endotracheal intubation may be performed at various points during resuscitation (as indicated by the asterisks [✳] in the flow diagram).

- If there is meconium and the baby has depressed respirations, muscle tone, or heart rate, you need to intubate the trachea as the very first step, before any other resuscitation measures are started.

- If positive-pressure ventilation (PPV) is not resulting in adequate clinical improvement and there is not good chest movement, you may decide to intubate to be able to provide adequate ventilation rather than to continue corrective efforts to optimize mask ventilation.

- If the need for PPV lasts beyond a few minutes, you may decide to intubate to improve the efficacy and ease of assisted ventilation.

- If chest compressions are necessary, intubating will facilitate coordination of chest compressions and ventilation and maximize the efficiency of each positive-pressure breath.

- When special indications occur, such as extreme prematurity, surfactant administration, or suspected diaphragmatic hernia. (See Lessons 7 and 8.)

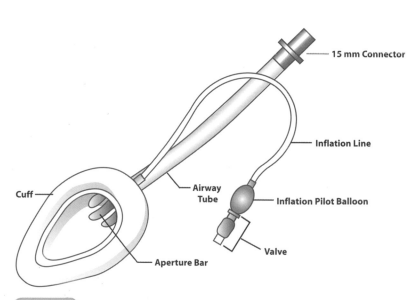

**Figure 5.1.** Laryngeal mask airway

## What alternatives are there to endotracheal intubation?

Masks that fit over the laryngeal inlet (laryngeal mask airways) have been shown to be an effective alternative for assisting ventilation when PPV by bag and mask or mask and T-piece resuscitator is ineffective and attempts at intubation are considered not feasible or are unsuccessful (Figure 5.1). However, laryngeal mask airways have not been studied for suctioning of meconium, and experience with their use in preterm newborns is limited. Placement of these devices will be covered at the end of this chapter.

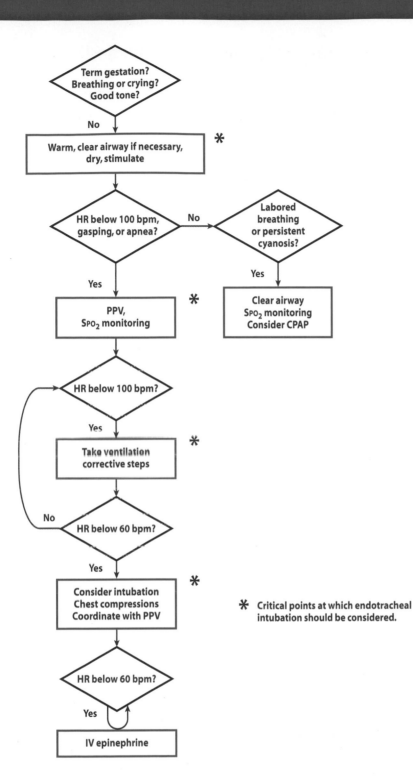

* Critical points at which endotracheal
  intubation should be considered.

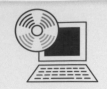

You are encouraged to view this video on the DVD that accompanies this textbook: *Endotracheal Intubation*

## What equipment and supplies are needed?

The supplies and equipment necessary to perform endotracheal intubation should be kept together and readily available. Each delivery room, nursery, and emergency department should have at least one complete set of the following items (Figure 5.2):

1. Laryngoscope with an extra set of batteries and extra bulbs.

2. Blades: No. 1 (term newborn), No. 0 (preterm newborn), No. 00 (optional for extremely preterm newborn). Straight rather than curved blades are preferred.

3. Endotracheal tubes with inside diameters of 2.5, 3.0, 3.5, and 4.0 mm.

4. Stylet (optional) that fits into the endotracheal tubes.

5. Carbon dioxide ($CO_2$) monitor or detector.

6. Suction setup with catheters of size 10F (for suctioning the pharynx), size 8F, and either size 5F or 6F (for suctioning endotracheal tubes of various sizes).

7. Roll of waterproof tape (1/2 or 3/4 inch), or endotracheal tube securing device.

8. Scissors.

9. Oral airway.

10. Meconium aspirator.

11. Stethoscope (with neonatal head).

12. Positive-pressure device (bag or T-piece resuscitator) and tubing for delivering air and/or supplemental oxygen. Self-inflating bag should have an oxygen reservoir and all types of devices should have a pressure manometer.

13. Pulse oximeter and neonatal probe.

14. Laryngeal mask airway (size 1) with 5-mL syringe.

This equipment should be stored together in a clearly marked container placed in a readily accessible location.

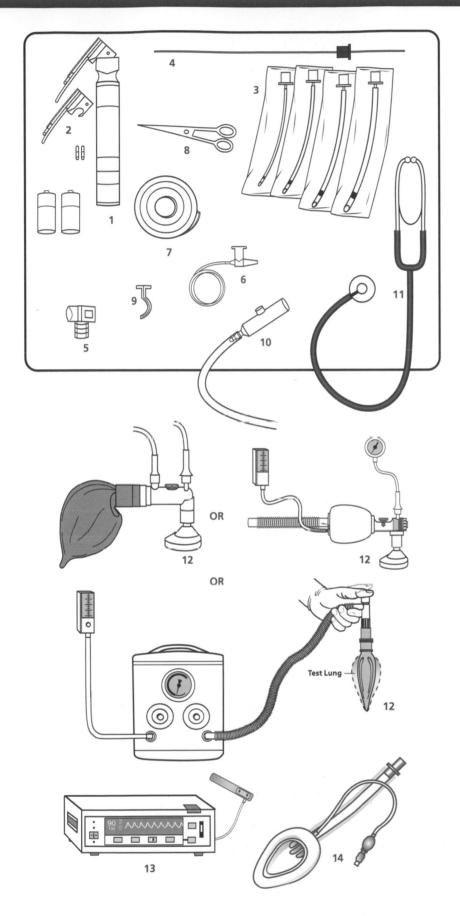

**Figure 5.2.** Neonatal resuscitation equipment and supplies

Intubation is best performed as a clean procedure. The endotracheal tubes and stylet should be clean and protected from contamination by being opened, assembled, and placed back in their packaging until just before insertion. The laryngoscope blades and handle should be cleaned after each use.

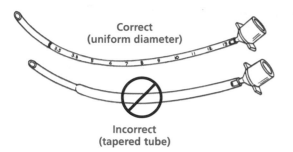

**Figure 5.3.** Endotracheal tubes with uniform diameter are preferred for newborns

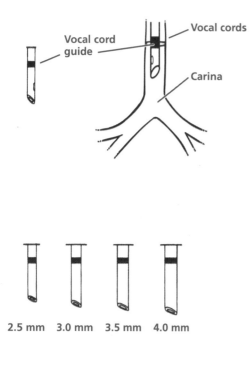

## What kind of endotracheal tubes are best to use?

Endotracheal tubes are supplied in sterile packages and should be handled with clean technique. They should be of uniform diameter throughout the length of the tube, not tapered near the tip (Figure 5.3). One disadvantage of the tapered tube is that, during intubation, your view of the tracheal opening is easily obstructed by the wide part of the tube. In addition, the shoulders created by changing diameter are more likely to obstruct the view and may cause trauma to the vocal cords.

Most endotracheal tubes for newborns have a black line near the tip of the tube, which is called a "vocal cord guide" (Figure 5.4). Such tubes are meant to be inserted so that the vocal cord guide is placed at the level of the vocal cords. This technique usually positions the tip of the tube above the bifurcation of the trachea (carina).

The length of the trachea in a low birthweight newborn is less than that of a term, appropriately grown newborn—3 cm versus 5 to 6 cm. Therefore, the smaller the tube, the closer the vocal cord guide is to the tip of the tube. However, there is some variability among tube manufacturers regarding the placement of the vocal cord guide.

Although tubes are available with cuffs at the level of the vocal cord guide, cuffed tubes are not recommended for neonatal resuscitation.

Most endotracheal tubes made for newborns come with centimeter markings along the side of the tube, identifying the distance from the tip of the tube. Later, you will learn to use these markings to identify the appropriate depth of insertion of the tube.

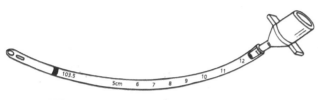

**Figure 5.4.** Characteristics of endotracheal tubes used for neonatal resuscitation

# How do you prepare the endotracheal tube for use?

Select the preferred tube size.

**Table 5-1.** Endotracheal tube size for babies of various weights and gestational ages

| Weight (g) | Gestational Age (wks) | Tube Size (mm) (inside diameter) |
|---|---|---|
| Below 1,000 | Below 28 | 2.5 |
| 1,000-2,000 | 28-34 | 3.0 |
| 2,000-3,000 | 34-38 | 3.5 |
| Above 3,000 | Above 38 | 3.5-4.0 |

> **Once resuscitation has started, delays in providing appropriate therapy, especially ventilation, may result in prolonged hypoxemia. Preparation of intubation equipment before an anticipated high-risk delivery is important.**

The appropriate size of the endotracheal tube to use is determined from the baby's weight. Table 5-1 gives the recommended tube size for various weight and gestational age categories. It may be helpful to post the table in each delivery room, on or near the radiant warmers. Sometimes it is necessary to use a smaller endotracheal tube than is recommended; however, this results in increased resistance to air flow. As a result, more pressure may be required to deliver the same tidal volumes. In addition, small diameter tubes become easily plugged.

**Consider cutting the tube to a shorter length.**

Many endotracheal tubes come from the manufacturer much longer than necessary for orotracheal use. The extra length will increase resistance to airflow. Some clinicians find it helpful to shorten the endotracheal tube before insertion (Figure 5.5). The endotracheal tube may be shortened to 13 to 15 cm to make it easier to handle during intubation and to lessen the chance of inserting the tube too far. A 13- to 15-cm tube will provide enough tube extending beyond the baby's lips for you to adjust the depth of insertion, if necessary, and to properly secure the tube to the face. Remove the connector (note that the connection to the tube may be tight), and then cut the tube diagonally to make it easier to reinsert the connector.

Replace the endotracheal tube connector. The fitting should be tight so that the connector does not inadvertently separate during insertion or use. Ensure that the connector and

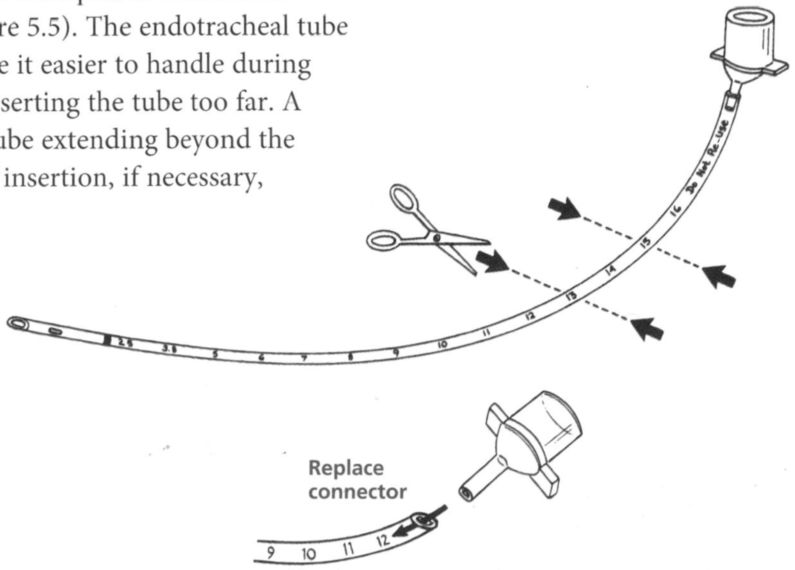

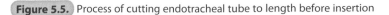

**Replace connector**

**Figure 5.5.** Process of cutting endotracheal tube to length before insertion

tube are properly aligned so that kinking of the tube is avoided. Connectors are made to fit a specific-sized tube. They cannot be interchanged among tubes of different sizes.

Some clinicians prefer to leave the tube long initially and then cut the tube to length after insertion if it is decided to leave it in place for longer than the immediate resuscitation. Note that the 15-cm length may be preferred to accommodate some types of endotracheal tube securing devices.

**Consider using a stylet (optional).**

Some people find it helpful to place a stylet through the endotracheal tube to provide rigidity and curvature to the tube, thus facilitating intubation (Figure 5.6). When inserting the stylet, it is essential that

- The tip does not protrude from the end or side hole of the endotracheal tube (to avoid trauma to the tissues).

- The stylet is secured so that it cannot advance farther into the tube during intubation.

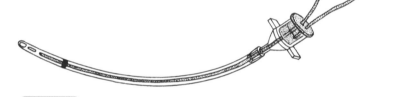

**Figure 5.6.** Optional stylet for increasing endotracheal tube stiffness and maintaining curvature during intubation

Although many find the stylet helpful, others find the stiffness of the tube alone adequate. Use of a stylet is optional and depends on the operator's preference and skill.

## How do you prepare the laryngoscope and additional supplies?

**Select blade and attach to handle.**

First, select the appropriate-sized blade and attach it to the laryngoscope handle.

- No. 0 for preterm newborns, or, for extremely preterm babies, No. 00

- No. 1 for term newborns

**Check light.**

Next, turn on the light by clicking the blade into the "open" position to verify that the batteries and bulb are working. Check to see that the bulb is screwed in tightly to ensure that it will not flicker or fall out during the procedure.

**Prepare suction equipment.**

- Adjust the suction source to 80 to 100 mm Hg by increasing or decreasing the level of suction while occluding the end of the suction tubing.

- Connect a 10F (or larger) suction catheter to the suction tubing so that it is available to suction secretions from the mouth and nose.

- Smaller suction catheters (5F, 6F, or 8F, depending on the size of the endotracheal tube) should be available for suctioning secretions from the tube if it becomes necessary to leave the endotracheal tube in place. Appropriate sizes are listed in Table 5-2.

**Prepare device for administering positive pressure.**

A resuscitation bag or T-piece resuscitator and mask should be on hand to ventilate the baby between intubation attempts, if intubation is unsuccessful, or to provide PPV, if required, after suctioning for meconium. The resuscitation device without the mask also can be used to check tube placement and, subsequently, to provide continued ventilation, if necessary. Check the operation of the device as described in Lesson 3.

**Put the end-tidal $CO_2$ detector within reach.**

It will be needed to help confirm endotracheal tube placement in the trachea.

**Turn on oxygen-air mixture from blender.**

The tubing should be connected to the blender and be available to deliver a variable amount of oxygen from 21% to 100% free-flow oxygen and to connect to the resuscitation device. The flow from the blender should be set at 5 to 10 L/min.

Make sure a **stethoscope** is on the resuscitation bed.

A stethoscope will be needed to check heart rate and breath sounds.

**Cut tape or prepare stabilizer.**

Cut several strips of adhesive tape to secure the tube to the face, or prepare an endotracheal tube holder, if used at your hospital.

**Table 5-2.** Suction catheter size for endotracheal tubes of various inner diameters

| Endotracheal Tube Size | Catheter Size |
| --- | --- |
| 2.5 | 5F or 6F |
| 3.0 | 6F or 8F |
| 3.5 | 8F |
| 4.0 | 8F or 10F |

 **When anticipating a resuscitation, such as for a baby with a known malformation or fetal distress, or for a premature baby, prepare to use a blender to provide a variable amount of oxygen. If there is insufficient time to fully prepare, you can begin resuscitation with room air until blended oxygen and oximetry are available.**

 **Review**

*(The answers are in the preceding section and at the end of the lesson.)*

1. A newborn with meconium and depressed respirations (will) (will not) require suctioning via an endotracheal tube before other resuscitation measures are started.

2. A newborn receiving ventilation by mask is not improving after 2 minutes of apparently good technique. Despite ventilation corrective steps, the heart rate is not rising and there is poor chest movement. Endotracheal intubation (should) (should not) be considered.

**3.** For babies weighing less than 1,000 g, the inside diameter of the endotracheal tube should be _____ mm.

**4.** The preferred blade size for use in term newborns is No. _____. The preferred laryngoscope blade size for use in preterm newborns is No. _____, or, for extremely preterm newborns, No. _____.

Note: When intubation is performed immediately following birth, as part of resuscitation, there is generally insufficient time or vascular access to administer a pre-medication. However, some clinicians will give a pre-medication (eg, a sedative and/or a narcotic and vagolytic) prior to an elective intubation, such as prior to surgery or before initiation of mechanical ventilation in the neonatal intensive care unit (NICU). This program focuses on resuscitation of the newly born baby. Therefore, the details of pre-medication will not be covered.

## How do you continue resuscitation while you intubate?

Unfortunately, you cannot continue most resuscitation actions during intubation.

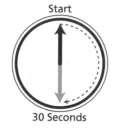

Start

30 Seconds

- Ventilation must be discontinued because the mask must be removed from the airway during the procedure.

- Chest compressions must be interrupted because the compressions cause movement and prevent you from seeing landmarks.

  - Make every effort to minimize the amount of hypoxemia imposed during intubation by limiting the time taken to complete the procedure. Do not try to intubate for longer than approximately 30 seconds. If you are unable to visualize the glottis and insert the tube within 30 seconds, remove the laryngoscope and attempt to ventilate the baby with mask ventilation, particularly if the intubation effort has resulted in bradycardia. Ensure that the baby is stable, and then try again.

## What anatomy do you need to know to insert the tube properly?

The anatomic landmarks that relate to intubation are labeled in Figures 5.7 through 5.9. Study the relative position of these landmarks, using all the figures, because each is important to your understanding of the procedure.

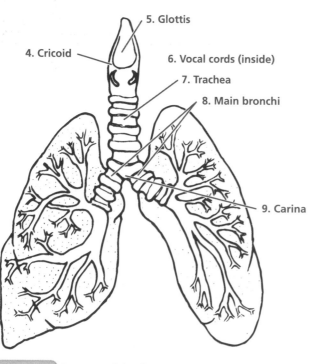

4. Cricoid
5. Glottis
6. Vocal cords (inside)
7. Trachea
8. Main bronchi
9. Carina

**Figure 5.7.** Anatomy of the airway

1. **Epiglottis**—The lidlike structure overhanging the entrance to the trachea

2. **Vallecula**—The pouch formed by the base of the tongue and the epiglottis

3. **Esophagus**—The passageway extending from the throat to the stomach

4. **Cricoid**—Lower portion of the cartilage of the larynx

5. **Glottis**—The opening of the larynx leading to the trachea, flanked by the vocal cords

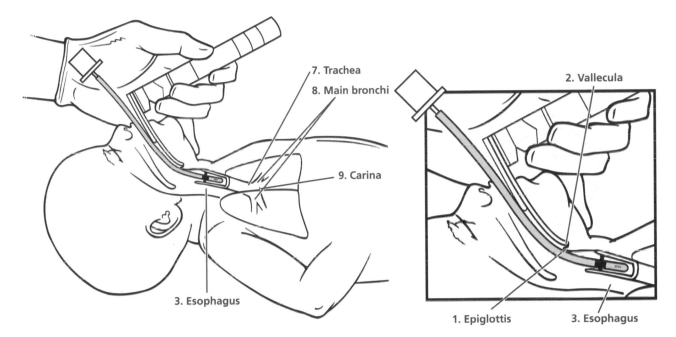

**Figure 5.8.** Sagittal section of the airway, with laryngoscope in place

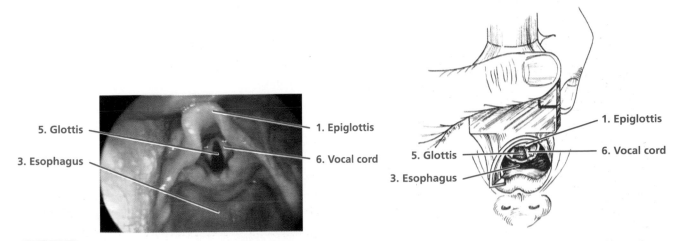

**Figure 5.9.** Photograph and drawing of laryngoscopic view of glottis and surrounding structures. (Drawing from Klaus M, Fanaroff A. *Care of the High Risk Neonate,* Philadelphia, PA: WB Saunders, 1996.)

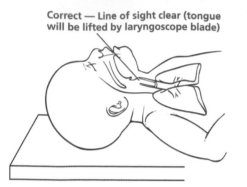

Correct — Line of sight clear (tongue will be lifted by laryngoscope blade)

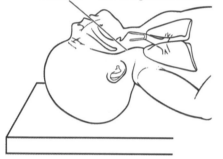

Incorrect — Line of sight obstructed

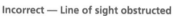

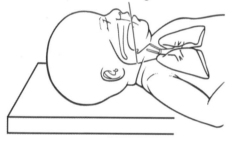

Incorrect — Line of sight obstructed

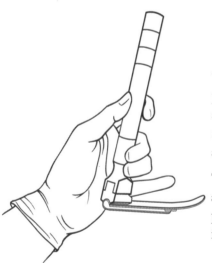

**Figure 5.10.** Correct (top) and incorrect (middle and bottom) positioning for intubation

**6** **Vocal cords**—Mucous membrane-covered ligaments on both sides of the glottis

**7** **Trachea**—The windpipe or air passageway, extending from the throat to the main bronchi

**8** **Main bronchi**—The 2 air passageways leading from the trachea to the lungs

**9** **Carina**—Where the trachea branches into the 2 main bronchi

## How should you position the newborn for intubation?

The correct position of the newborn for intubation is the same as for mask ventilation—on a flat surface with the head in a midline position and the neck slightly extended. It may be helpful to place a roll under the baby's shoulders to maintain slight extension of the neck. However, if the roll used is too large, the head may be overextended, obstructing the airway (see below).

This "sniffing" position aligns the trachea for optimal viewing by allowing a straight line of sight into the glottis once the laryngoscope has been properly placed (Figure 5.10).

It is important not to hyperextend the neck, because this will raise the glottis above your line of sight and narrow the trachea.

If there is too much flexion of the head toward the chest, you will be viewing the posterior pharynx and may not be able to directly visualize the glottis.

## How do you hold the laryngoscope?

Turn on the laryngoscope light by opening the blade until it clicks into place and hold the laryngoscope in your *left* hand, between your thumb and first 2 or 3 fingers, with the blade pointing away from you (Figure 5.11). For clinicians with small hands, thin laryngoscope handles are available that allow better control of this instrument.

The laryngoscope is designed to be held in the *left* hand—by both right- and left-handed persons. If held in the right hand, the closed curved part of the blade will block your view of the glottis, as well as make insertion of the endotracheal tube impossible.

**Figure 5.11.** Correct hand position when holding a laryngoscope for neonatal intubation

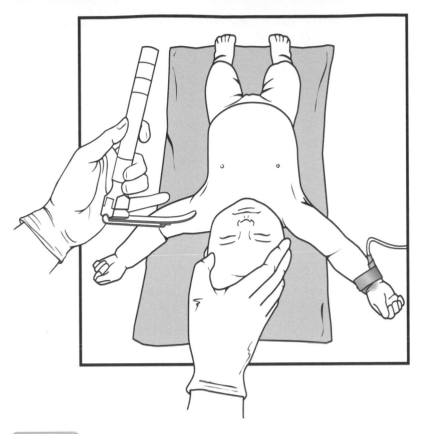

**Figure 5.12.** Preparing to insert the larynogoscope

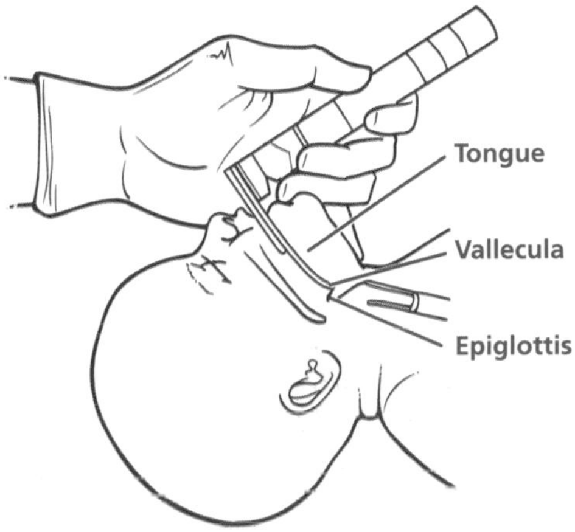

**Figure 5.13.** Landmarks for placement of the laryngoscope

Tongue

Vallecula

Epiglottis

## How do you visualize the glottis and insert the tube?

**First,** stabilize the baby's head with your right hand (Figure 5.12). It may be helpful to have a second person hold the head in the desired "sniffing" position.

**Second,** open the baby's mouth. You may need to use your right index finger to open the baby's mouth to make it easier to insert the laryngoscope. Slide the laryngoscope blade over the right side of the tongue and toward the midline, pushing the tongue to the left side of the mouth, then advance the blade until the tip lies in the vallecula, just beyond the base of the tongue (Figure 5.13).

Note: Although this lesson describes placing the tip of the blade in the vallecula, some prefer to place it directly on the epiglottis, *gently* compressing the epiglottis against the base of the tongue.

**Third,** lift the blade slightly, thus lifting the tongue out of the way to expose the pharyngeal area (Figure 5.14). When lifting the blade, raise the *entire* blade by pulling up in the direction the handle is pointing.

> ❗ **Do not elevate the tip of the blade by using a rocking motion and pulling the handle toward you.**

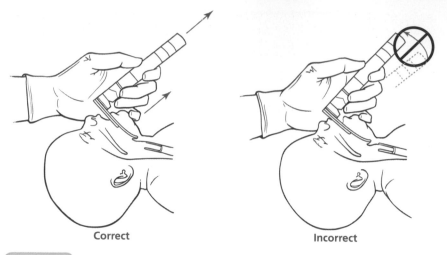

**Figure 5.14.** Correct (left) and incorrect (right) method for lifting the laryngoscope blade to expose the larynx

Rocking rather than elevating the tip of the blade will not produce the view of the glottis you desire and will put excessive pressure on the alveolar ridge. The motion to lift the blade should come from your shoulder, not your wrist.

**Fourth,** look for landmarks (Figure 5.15).

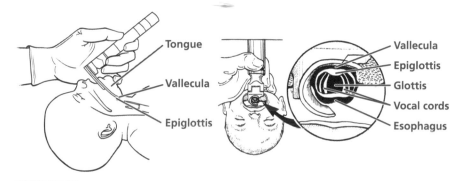

**Figure 5.15.** Identification of landmarks before placing endotracheal tube through glottis

If the tip of the blade is correctly positioned in the vallecula, you should see the epiglottis at the top, with the glottic opening below. You also should see the vocal cords appearing as vertical stripes on each side of the glottis or as an inverted letter "V" (Figures 5.15 and 5.16D).

If these structures are not immediately visible, quickly adjust the blade until the structures come into view. You may need to advance or withdraw the blade slowly to see the vocal cords. Applying downward pressure to the cricoid (the cartilage that covers the larynx) may help bring the glottis into view (Figure 5.17). The pressure may be applied by an assistant.

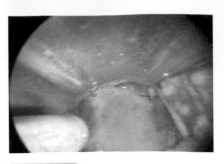

**Figure 5.16A.** View of posterior pharynx after first inserting laryngoscope

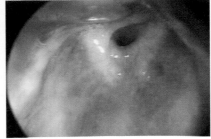

**Figure 5.16B.** View of esophagus after laryngoscope has been inserted too far

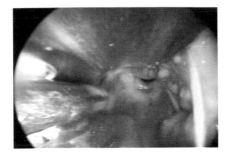

**Figure 5.16C.** View of arytenoids and posterior glottis as laryngoscope blade is withdrawn slightly

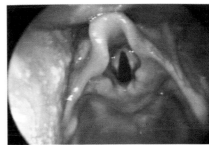

**Figure 5.16D.** View of glottis and vocal cords as laryngoscope is gently lifted

Suctioning of secretions may help to improve your view (Figure 5.18).

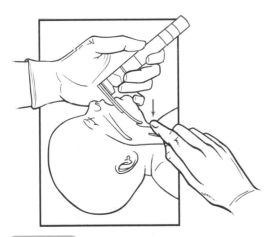

**Figure 5.17.** Improving visualization with pressure applied to larynx by an assistant

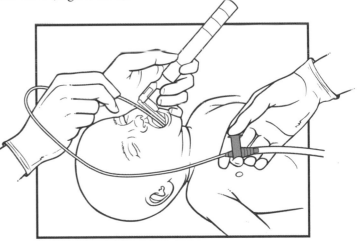

**Figure 5.18.** Suctioning of secretions

**Fifth,** insert the tube (Figure 5.19).

Holding the tube in your right hand, introduce it into the right side of the baby's mouth, with the curve of the tube lying in the horizontal plane so that the tube curves from left to right. This will prevent the tube from blocking your view of the glottis.

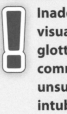

**Inadequate visualization of the glottis is the most common reason for unsuccessful intubation.**

**Figure 5.19.** Insertion of endotracheal tube between the vocal cords

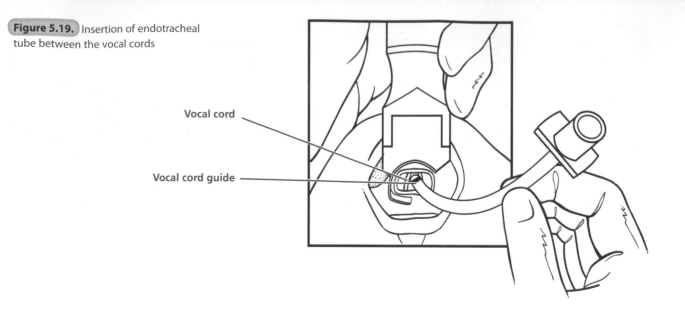

Vocal cord

Vocal cord guide

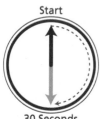

Start

30 Seconds

Keep the glottis in view and, when the vocal cords are apart, insert the tip of the endotracheal tube until the vocal cord guide is at the level of the cords.

If the cords are together, wait for them to open. Do not touch the closed cords with the tip of the tube because it may cause spasm of the cords. Never try to force the tube between closed cords. If the cords do not open within 30 seconds, stop and ventilate with a mask. After the heart rate and color have improved, you can try again.

Be careful to insert the tube only so far as to place the vocal cord guide at the level of the vocal cords (Figure 5.20). In most cases, this will position the tube in the trachea approximately halfway between the vocal cords and the carina.

Note the marking on the tube that aligns with the baby's lip.

**Sixth,** stabilize the tube with your right hand and *carefully* remove the laryngoscope without displacing the tube. Use your thumb and finger to hold the baby's head securely, which prevents accidental dislodgement of the tube. Hold the tube securely against the baby's hard palate (Figure 5.21).

If you are right-handed, you may want to transfer the endotracheal tube from your right hand to your left hand.

If a stylet was used, remove it from the endotracheal tube—again be careful to hold the tube in place while you do so (Figure 5.22).

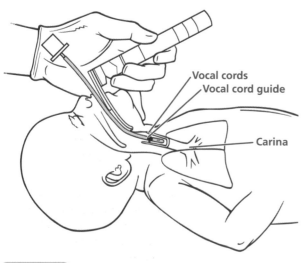

Vocal cords
Vocal cord guide

Carina

**Figure 5.20.** Correct depth of insertion of endotracheal tube

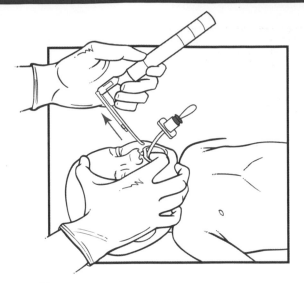

**Figure 5.21.** Stabilizing the tube while laryngoscope is withdrawn

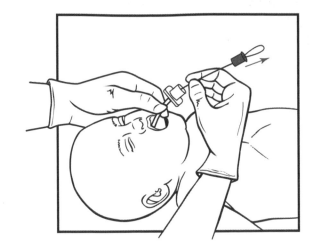

**Figure 5.22.** Removing stylet from endotracheal tube

You are now ready to use the tube for the reason you inserted it.

- If the purpose is to *suction meconium,* then use the tube as described on pages 176 through 178.

- If the purpose is to *ventilate the baby,* then quickly attach a ventilation bag or T-piece resuscitator to the tube, take steps to be certain the tube is in the trachea by attaching a $CO_2$ detector to the tube and observing for color change, and resume PPV (Figure 5.23). Ask another team member to secure the tube with tape or an endotracheal tube securing device. These steps will be described after the section on meconium suctioning.

**Although it is important to hold the tube firmly, be careful not to press or squeeze the tube so tightly that the stylet cannot be removed or the compressed tube obstructs airflow.**

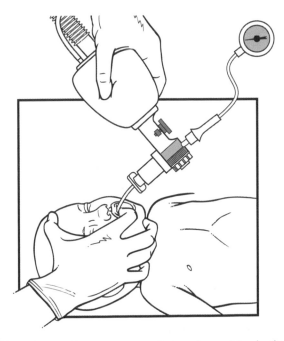

**Figure 5.23.** Resuming positive-pressure ventilation after endotracheal intubation

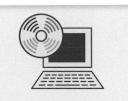

**You are encouraged to view the video in the accompanying DVD, as it shows the details of the complete intubation sequence.**

## For how long should you attempt intubation?

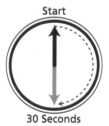

Start

30 Seconds

Although the steps of intubation are described in detail in the previous section, they need to be completed very quickly—within approximately **30** seconds—during an actual resuscitation. The baby will not be ventilated during this process, so quick action is essential. If the patient appears to be compromised (eg, severe decrease in heart rate or oxygen saturation [$Spo_2$] because of the length of time of the procedure), it is usually preferable to stop, resume PPV with a mask, and then try again. Assistance should be requested if initial attempts are unsuccessful (eg, by calling an anesthesiologist, emergency department physician, respiratory therapist, neonatal nurse practitioner, or other individual with intubation experience in your institution).

## What do you do next if the tube was inserted to suction meconium?

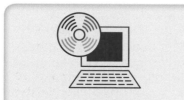

**You are encouraged to view this video on the DVD that accompanies this textbook:** *Using a Meconium Aspirator*

As described in Lesson 2, if there is meconium in the amniotic fluid and the baby has depressed muscle tone, depressed respirations, or a heart rate below 100 beats per minute (bpm) (ie, is not vigorous), the trachea should be intubated and suctioned.

As soon as the endotracheal tube has been inserted and the stylet, if used, has been removed,

• Connect the endotracheal tube to a meconium aspirator, which has been connected to a suction source. Several alternative types of meconium aspirators are commercially available, some of which include the endotracheal tube as part of the device.

• Occlude the suction-control port on the aspirator to apply suction to the endotracheal tube (Figure 5.24), and gradually withdraw the tube as you continue suctioning any meconium that may be in the trachea.

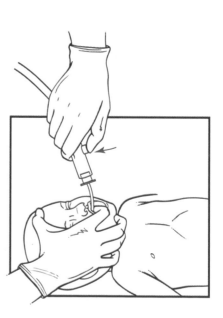

**Figure 5.24.** Suctioning meconium from trachea using an endotracheal tube, meconium aspiration device, and suction tubing connected to a suction source

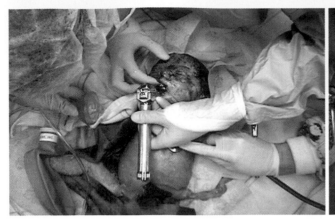

A

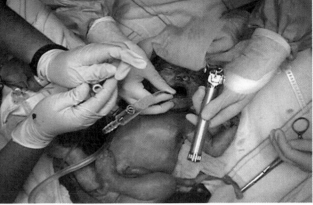

B

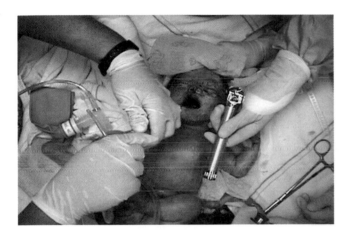

C

**Figure 5.25.** Sequence of intubation for meconium. **A.** Laryngoscope is inserted into mouth of flaccid baby covered in meconium. **B.** Endotracheal tube has been inserted and a meconium aspiration device has been attached to the tube. **C.** Suction tubing has been attached to the aspirator and the control port has been occluded to apply suction to the endotracheal tube as it is gradually withdrawn.

## For how long do you try to suction meconium?

Judgment is required when suctioning meconium. You have learned to suction the trachea only if the meconium-stained baby has depressed respirations or muscle tone, or has a heart rate below 100 bpm. Therefore, at the time you begin to suction the trachea, it is likely that the baby will already be significantly compromised and will eventually need resuscitation. You will need to delay resuscitation for a few seconds while you suction meconium, but you do not want to delay longer than absolutely necessary.

The following are a few guidelines:

• Do not apply suction to the endotracheal tube for longer than 3 to 5 seconds as you withdraw the tube.

• If no meconium is recovered, do not repeat the procedure; proceed with resuscitation.

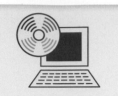

You are encouraged to view this video on the DVD that accompanies this textbook: *Using an End-tidal CO₂ Detector*

- If you recover meconium the first time you suction the trachea, you may want to consider intubating and suctioning a second time, as the presence of meconium in the airway may impede your ability to provide effective PPV. However, repeated intubations may delay further resuscitative efforts. Before intubating a second time, check the heart rate. If the baby does not have bradycardia, reintubate and suction again. If the heart rate is low, you may decide to administer positive pressure without repeating the procedure.

## If you intubated to ventilate the baby, how do you check to be sure that the tube is in the trachea?

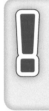

Be certain the tube is in the trachea. A misplaced tube is worse than having no tube at all.

Watching the tube pass between the cords, watching for chest movement following application of positive pressure, and listening for breath sounds are all helpful signs that the tube is in the trachea rather than the esophagus. However, these signs can be misleading. An increasing heart rate and evidence of exhaled $CO_2$ in the tube are the primary methods for confirming endotracheal tube placement (Figure 5.26).

There are 2 basic types of $CO_2$ detectors available.

- Colorimetric devices are connected to the endotracheal tube and change color in the presence of $CO_2$ (Figures 5.26 and 5.27).

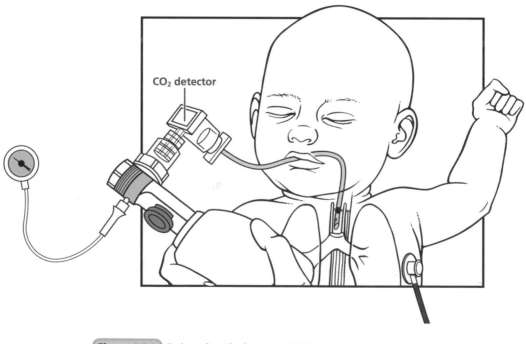

**CO₂ detector**

**Figure 5.26.** Carbon dioxide detector will change color during exhalation if endotracheal tube is in trachea

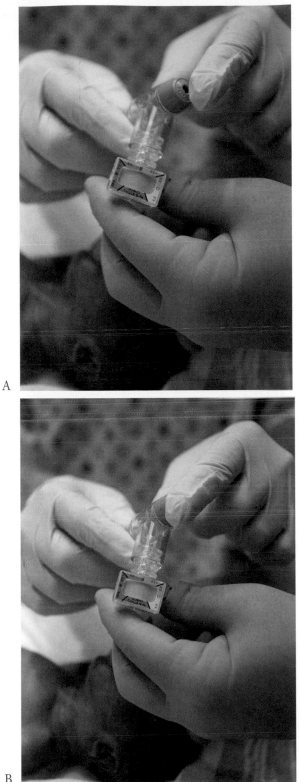

A

B

Figure 5.27. **A.** The colorimetric $CO_2$ detector is a purple or blue color before being connected to the endotracheal tube. **B.** It turns yellow when the tube is in the airway of a breathing or ventilated baby.

- Capnographs rely on placement of a special electrode at the endotracheal tube connector. The capnograph should display a waveform showing good oscillation with each breath if the tube is in the trachea.

The colorimetric device is the most commonly used method of $CO_2$ detection.

As soon as you have inserted the endotracheal tube, connect a $CO_2$ detector and note the presence or absence of $CO_2$ during exhalation. If $CO_2$ is not detected after several positive-pressure breaths, consider removing the tube, resuming ventilation, and repeating the intubation process as described on pages 170 through 177.

## Can the $CO_2$ detector be used to confirm adequate ventilation when providing positive-pressure ventilation via a mask or laryngeal mask airway?

The $CO_2$ detector also may be used to determine adequate ventilation during PPV being delivered via a mask or laryngeal mask airway. The device should be inserted between the PPV device (flow-inflating or self-inflating bag or T-piece resuscitator) and the mask or laryngeal mask airway. If $CO_2$ is not detected by a change in color of the device, PPV may not be adequate and standard corrective measures described in Lesson 3 should be considered, especially if the baby's heart rate is not increasing. However, there are limited studies to confirm the accuracy of using $CO_2$ detectors during ventilation via a mask.

- **Babies with very poor cardiac output may not exhale sufficient $CO_2$ to be detected reliably by $CO_2$ detectors.**
- **Any colorimetric $CO_2$ detection device that has already changed color in the package is defective and should not be used.**
- **If epinephrine is administered via the endotracheal tube and contaminates the colorimetric device, it may turn the screen yellow and give a false positive reading (indicating that the tube is in the trachea when it is not).**

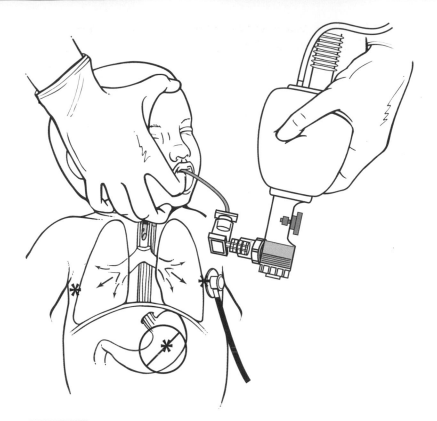

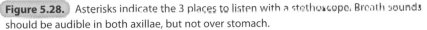

**Figure 5.28.** Asterisks indicate the 3 places to listen with a stethoscope. Breath sounds should be audible in both axillae, but not over stomach.

If the tube is positioned correctly, you also should observe the following:

- Improvement in heart rate and $SpO_2$

- Breath sounds audible over both lung fields but decreased or absent over the stomach (Figure 5.28)

- No gastric distention with ventilation

- Vapor condensing on the inside of the tube during exhalation

- Symmetrical movement of the chest with each breath

When listening to breath sounds, be sure to use a small stethoscope and place it laterally and high on the chest wall (in the axilla). A large stethoscope, or a stethoscope placed either too near the center or too low on the chest, may transmit sounds from the esophagus or stomach.

 **Be cautious when interpreting breath sounds in newborns. Because sounds are easily transmitted, those heard over the anterior portions of the chest may be coming from the stomach or esophagus. Breath sounds also can be transmitted to the abdomen.**

Observe for absence of gastric distension and movement of both sides of the chest with each ventilated breath.

Listening for bilateral breath sounds and observing symmetrical chest movement with PPV provide secondary confirmation of correct endotracheal tube placement in the airway with the tip of the tube positioned above the carina. A rapid, sustained increase in heart rate is the best indicator of *effective* PPV.

## What do you do if you suspect that the tube may not be in the trachea?

The tube is likely not in the trachea if one or more of the following occurs:

- The newborn remains bradycardic and the $Spo_2$ is not increasing despite PPV.

- The $CO_2$ detector does not indicate presence of $CO_2$.

- You do not hear good breath sounds over the lungs.

- The abdomen appears to become distended.

- You **_do_** hear air noises over the stomach.

- There is no mist in the tube.

- The chest is not moving symmetrically with each positive-pressure breath.

If you suspect the tube is not in the trachea, you should do the following:

- Use your right hand to hold the tube in place while you use your left hand to reinsert the laryngoscope so that you can visualize the glottis and see if the tube is passing between the vocal cords.

and/or

- Remove the tube, use a resuscitation device and mask to stabilize the heart rate and color, and then repeat the intubation procedure.

## How do you know if the tip of the tube is in the right location within the trachea?

You can use the tip-to-lip measurement to estimate if the tube has been inserted the correct distance (Table 5-3). Adding 6 to the baby's weight in kilograms will give you a rough estimate of the correct distance from

**Table 5-3.** Estimated distance from tip of tube to baby's lip, based on baby's weight

| Depth of insertion | |
| --- | --- |
| Weight (kg) | Depth of insertion (cm from upper lip) |
| 1* | 7 |
| 2 | 8 |
| 3 | 9 |
| 4 | 10 |

*Babies weighing less than 750 g may require only 6-cm insertion.

the tube tip to the vermilion border of the upper lip. It may help you to remember "Tip-to-lip: 1-2-3 7-8-9". (Note: This rule is less reliable in those babies who have congenital anomalies of the neck and mandible [eg, Robin syndrome].)

Remember that the tip-to-lip distance is only an estimate of correct tube position. Therefore, you should listen to breath sounds in both axillae after positioning the endotracheal tube. If the tube is correctly placed and the lungs are inflating, you will hear breath sounds of equal intensity on each side.

If the tube is in too far, you will hear breath sounds that are louder on one side than the other (usually the right). If that is the case, pull back the tube very slowly while listening to the left side of the chest. When the tube is pulled back and the tip reaches the carina, you should hear an increase in breath sounds on the obstructed side and equal breath sounds when comparing the 2 sides.

If the tube is going to be left in place beyond the initial resuscitation, you should obtain a chest x-ray as a final confirmation that the tube is in the proper position.

If the tube is correctly placed, the tip will be located in the trachea, midway between the vocal cords and the carina. On the x-ray, the tip should be visible at the level of the clavicles, or slightly below (Figure 5.29). If it is in too far, it generally will be down the right main bronchus, and you will be ventilating only the right lung (Figure 5.30).

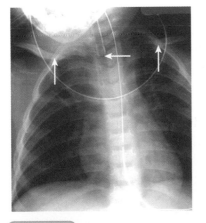

**Figure 5.29.** *Correct* placement of endotracheal tube with tip in midtrachea. The horizontal arrow points to the tip of tube. The vertical arrows point to the clavicles.

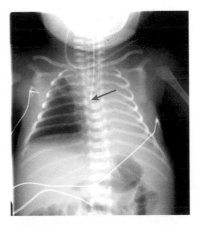

**Figure 5.30.** *Incorrect* placement of endotracheal tube with tip in right main bronchus. Note atelectasis of left lung.

# What can go wrong while you are trying to intubate?

*You may have trouble visualizing the glottis (Figure 5.31).*

| Problem | Landmarks | Corrective Action |
|---|---|---|
| 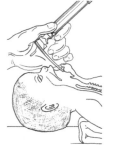 | 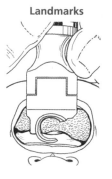 | 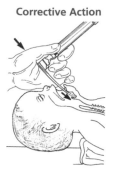 |
| Laryngoscope not inserted far enough. | You see the tongue surrounding the blade. | Advance the blade farther. |
| 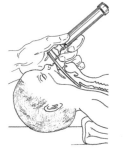 | 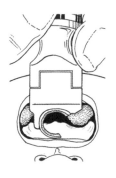 | 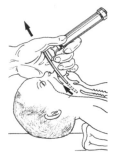 |
| Laryngoscope inserted too far. | You see the walls of the esophagus surrounding the blade. | Withdraw the blade slowly until the epiglottis and glottis are seen. |
| 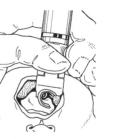 | | 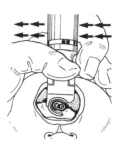 |
| Laryngoscope inserted off to one side. | You see part of the glottis off to one side of the blade. | Gently move the blade back to the midline. Then advance or retreat according to landmarks seen. |

**Figure 5.31.** Common problems associated with intubation

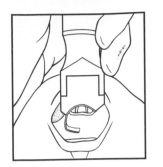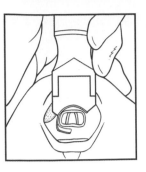

**Figure 5.32.** Poor visualization of the glottis (left) can be improved by elevating the tongue or depressing the larynx (right and Figure 5.31)

Poor visualization of the glottis also may be caused by not elevating the tongue high enough to bring the glottis into view (Figure 5.32).

Sometimes, pressure applied to the cricoid, which is the cartilage covering the larynx, helps to bring the glottis into view (Figure 5.33).

This is accomplished by using the fourth or fifth finger of the left hand or by asking an assistant to apply the pressure.

Practice intubating a manikin enough times so that you can quickly find the correct landmarks and insert the tube within 30 seconds.

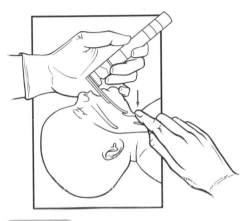

**Figure 5.33.** Improving visualization with pressure applied to the larynx by an assistant (right)

### You may inadvertently insert the tube into the esophagus instead of the trachea.

An endotracheal tube in the esophagus is worse than having no tube at all, because the tube will obstruct the baby's pharyngeal airway without providing a secure intratracheal airway. Therefore,

- Be certain that you visualize the glottis before inserting the tube. Watch the tube enter the glottis between the vocal cords.

- Look carefully for signs of inadvertent esophageal intubation after the tube has been inserted (eg, distention of the stomach and poor response to intubation). Use a $CO_2$ detector to verify endotracheal placement.

If you are concerned that the tube may be in the esophagus, visualize the glottis and tube with a laryngoscope and/or remove the tube, and reintubate quickly.

> ### Signs of an endotracheal tube in the esophagus instead of the trachea
>
> - Poor response to intubation (continued bradycardia, low $S_{PO_2}$, etc)
> - $CO_2$ detector fails to show presence of expired $CO_2$
> - No audible breath sounds
> - Air heard entering the stomach
> - Gastric distension
> - No mist in tube
> - Poor chest movement

***You may inadvertently insert the tube too far into the trachea, down the right main bronchus.***

If the tube is inserted too far, it usually will pass into the right main bronchus (Figure 5.34).

When you insert the tube, it is important to watch the vocal cord guide on the tube and stop advancing the tube as soon as the vocal cord guide reaches the cords.

Signs of the tube being in the right main bronchus include

- Baby's heart rate or $S_{PO_2}$ shows no improvement.

- Breath sounds are heard over the right side of the chest but not the left side.

- Breath sounds are louder on the right side of the chest than on the left side.

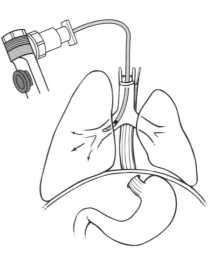

**Figure 5.34.** Endotracheal tube inserted too far (tip is down the right main bronchus). NOTE: Although a $CO_2$ detector will confirm that the tube is in the airway, it will likely not distinguish between it being in the trachea versus in a main bronchus.

In rare cases, unequal breath sounds also may be a sign of a unilateral pneumothorax or congenital diaphragmatic hernia. (See Lesson 7.)

If you think the tube may be down the right main bronchus, first check the tip-to-lip measurement to see if the number at the lip is higher than the estimated measurement (Table 5-3). Even if the measurement appears to be correct, if breath sounds remain asymmetric, you should withdraw the tube slightly while you listen over the left side of the chest to hear if the breath sounds on the left side become louder.

**You may encounter other complications (Table 5-4).**

**Table 5-4.** Some complications associated with endotracheal intubation

| Complication | Possible Causes | Prevention or Corrective Action to Be Considered |
|---|---|---|
| Hypoxia | Taking too long to intubate. Incorrect placement of tube. | Ventilate with mask if possible. Halt intubation attempt after 30 seconds. Reposition tube. |
| Bradycardia/apnea | Hypoxia. Vagal response from laryngoscope or suction catheter. | Ventilate with mask if possible. Oxygenate after intubation with bag or T-piece resuscitator and tube. Limit duration of intubation attempts. |
| Pneumothorax | Overventilation of one lung because of tube in right main bronchus, or from excessive ventilation pressures. | Place tube correctly. Use appropriate ventilating pressures. Consider transillumination and needle aspiration if pneumothorax is suspected (see Lesson 7). |
| Contusions or lacerations of tongue, gums, or airway | Rough handling of laryngoscope or tube; inappropriate "rocking" rather than lifting of laryngoscope. Laryngoscope blade too long or too short. | Obtain additional practice/skill. Be gentle when manipulating the laryngoscope. Select appropriate equipment. |
| Perforation of trachea or esophagus | Too vigorous insertion of tube. Stylet protrudes beyond end of tube. | Handle tube gently. Place stylet properly. |
| Obstructed endotracheal tube | Kink in tube or tube obstructed with secretions, meconium, or blood. | Try to suction tube with catheter. If unsuccessful, consider replacing tube. |
| Infection | Introduction of organisms via hands or equipment. | Pay careful attention to clean technique. |

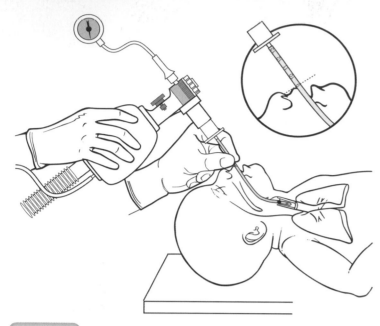

**Figure 5.35.** Measurement of endotracheal tube marking at the lip

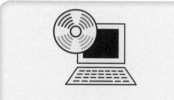

**You are encouraged to view this video on the DVD that accompanies this textbook:** *Endotracheal Tube: Emergency Tape Technique*

## If the tube is to be left in, how do you secure it in place?

After you have ensured that the tube is in the correct position, take note of the centimeter marking that appears at the upper lip. This can help you maintain the appropriate depth of insertion (Figure 5.35).

For PPV beyond a few minutes, the tube needs to be secured to the face. Specific methods of securing the tube vary among practitioners. Either water-resistant tape or a device specifically designed to secure an endotracheal tube can be used.

One method is to cut a piece of tape that is long enough to extend from one side of the baby's mouth, across the philtrum, and about 2 cm on the opposite cheek (Figure 5.36).

- Place a strip of clear adhesive dressing between the baby's nose and upper lip.

- Cut 2 pieces of one-half-inch tape approximately 4 inches long.

- Split each piece for half its length.

- Stick the unsplit section of the tape and one tab across the baby's upper lip.

- Wrap the other tab in a spiral around the endotracheal tube.

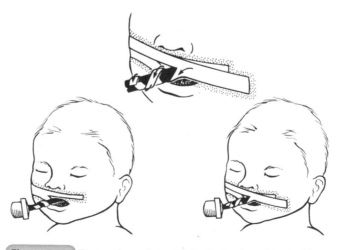

**Figure 5.36.** Taping the endotracheal tube in place. (Used with permission from Kattwinkel J, Cook LJ, Hurt H, Nowacek GA, Short JG, Crosby WM, eds. *Maternal and Fetal Evaluation and Immediate Newborn Care.* Elk Grove Village, IL: American Acadamy of Pediatrics; 2007:199. *PCEP Perinatal Continuing Education Program;* book 1.)

- Place second tape in reverse direction.

- Listen with a stethoscope over both sides of the chest to be sure the tube has not been displaced.

If you did not previously shorten the tube, it would be appropriate to do so now. However, be prepared to reinsert the connector quickly, as you will be unable to attach the resuscitation bag or T-piece resuscitator until you do so.

## What is a laryngeal mask airway, and when should you consider using it?

The laryngeal mask airway is an airway device that can be used to provide PPV. The neonatal device (Figure 5.37) is a soft elliptical mask with an inflatable cuff (rim) attached to a flexible airway tube. The device is inserted into the baby's mouth with your index finger and guided along the baby's hard palate until the tip nearly reaches the esophagus. No instruments are used. Once the mask is fully inserted, the cuff is inflated. The inflated mask covers the laryngeal opening and the cuff conforms to the contours of the hypopharynx, occluding the esophagus with a low-pressure seal. The airway tube has a standard 15-mm adaptor that is attached to a resuscitation bag, T-piece resuscitator, or ventilator. A pilot balloon attached to the cuff is used to monitor the mask's inflation. Both reusable and disposable versions are commercially available. Only the size-1 device is small enough for use in newborns.

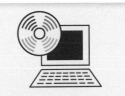

You are encouraged to view this video on the DVD that accompanies this textbook: *Laryngeal Mask Airway Placement*

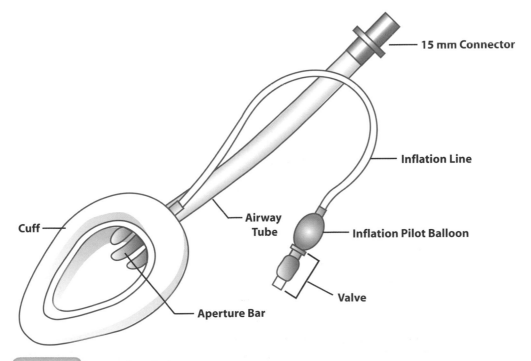

**Figure 5.37.** Laryngeal mask airway

The following case is an example of how a laryngeal mask airway can be used to provide PPV during neonatal resuscitation. As you read the case, imagine yourself as part of the resuscitation team.

## Case 5.
## Difficult intubation

A baby is delivered at term after a labor complicated by fetal decelerations. The fluid is clear, without meconium staining. The baby is brought to the radiant warmer limp, blue, and apneic. The initial steps of resuscitation are performed and positive-pressure ventilation (PPV) is initiated with a bag-and-mask device, but the team cannot achieve effective ventilation, despite appropriate adjustments. The resuscitation team unsuccessfully attempts to place an endotracheal tube using direct laryngoscopy. The team leader notes that the baby has a relatively small jaw. The baby remains limp and apneic.

One team member rapidly places a laryngeal mask airway, inflates the cuff, attaches a resuscitation bag, and achieves effective PPV, resulting in an increasing heart rate and good breath sounds. The baby's oxygen saturation (SPo2) improves, and he begins to show spontaneous respirations. Because of the apparent upper airway obstruction, the laryngeal mask airway is left in place and he is transferred to the neonatal intensive care unit for further evaluation and post-resuscitative care.

## How does a laryngeal mask airway work?

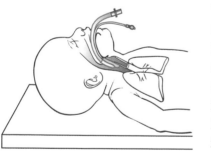

**Figure 5.38.** Laryngeal mask airway in place over the laryngeal opening

The larynx is a firm structure that forms the opening of the trachea into the anterior pharynx. The distal end of the device is a soft mask that functions like a cap that fits over the larynx. The mask has a donut-shaped cuff that can be inflated to make a seal over the larynx (Figure 5.38). The mask has bars across the middle that prevent the epiglottis from becoming trapped within the airway tube. (See "aperture bar" in Figure 5.37.) After the mask has been placed over the larynx, the cuff is inflated, thus providing a seal. When positive pressure is applied to the airway tube, the pressure is transmitted through the airway tube and the mask into the baby's trachea. As with an endotracheal tube, babies can breathe spontaneously through the device, but, without a tube between the vocal cords, you may hear crying or grunting.

## In what situations might a laryngeal mask airway be useful?

Laryngeal mask airways may be useful in situations when positive pressure with a face mask fails to achieve effective ventilation, and endotracheal intubation is either not feasible or unsuccessful. When you "can't ventilate and can't intubate," the device may provide a successful rescue airway.

For example, a laryngeal mask airway may be helpful when a newborn presents with the following:

- Congenital anomalies involving the mouth, lip, or palate, where achieving a good seal with a mask is difficult.

- Anomalies of the mouth, tongue, pharynx, or neck that result in difficulty visualizing the larynx with a laryngoscope.

- A very small mandible or relatively large tongue, such as with Robin syndrome and Trisomy 21.

- Positive-pressure ventilation provided by bag and mask or T-piece resuscitator is ineffective, and attempts at intubation are not feasible or are unsuccessful.

The laryngeal mask airway does not require a firm seal against the face. Furthermore, unlike a face mask, the flexible laryngeal mask bypasses the tongue, allowing more effective ventilation of the lungs than with a face mask. In addition, no instrument is needed to visualize the larynx to place the device. It is placed "blindly" by using the operator's finger to guide it into place. Although a laryngeal mask airway does not provide as tight a seal in the airway as an endotracheal tube, it can provide an acceptable alternative in many cases.

The laryngeal mask airway is used by anesthesiologists for ventilating patients with normal lungs during anesthesia in many hospital operating rooms.

## What are the limitations of the laryngeal mask airway?

- The device cannot be used to suction meconium from the airway.

- If you need to use high ventilation pressures, air may leak through the seal between the larynx and the mask, resulting in insufficient pressure to inflate the lungs and causing gastric distention.

- There is insufficient evidence to recommend using a laryngeal mask airway when chest compressions are required. However, if an endotracheal tube cannot be placed successfully and chest compressions are required after a laryngeal mask airway has been placed to allow provision of PPV, it is reasonable to attempt compressions with the device in place.

- There is insufficient evidence to recommend using the laryngeal mask airway to administer intratracheal medications. Intratracheal medications may leak between the mask and larynx into the esophagus and, therefore, not enter the lung.

- There is insufficient evidence to recommend the laryngeal mask airway for prolonged assisted ventilation in newborns.

- Laryngeal masks cannot be used in very small newborns. The smallest currently available laryngeal mask airway devices are intended for use in babies greater than approximately 2 kg. However, some providers have used the size-1 laryngeal masks successfully in babies as small as 1,500 g. Remember that, as soon as it becomes apparent that obtaining a secure airway in a small baby, or in a baby with an airway malformation, may be necessary, assistance should be requested from providers with expertise in airway management.

## How do you place the laryngeal mask airway?

The following instructions apply to the disposable device. If you are using the reusable laryngeal mask airway, refer to the manufacturer's instructions for proper cleaning and maintenance procedures.

Note: If you think that the stomach is distended in a baby in whom you have decided to place a laryngeal mask airway, an orogastric tube should be placed, and air in the stomach aspirated, before inserting the laryngeal mask airway. The orogastric tube should be removed before laryngeal mask airway placement, as its presence may prevent you from obtaining a proper seal with the laryngeal mask airway.

**Prepare the laryngeal mask airway.**

1. Wear gloves and follow standard precautions.

2. Remove the size-1 device from the sterile package and use clean technique.

3. Quickly inspect the device to ensure that the mask, midline aperture bars, airway tube, 15-mm connector, and pilot balloon are intact.

④ Attach the included syringe to the pilot balloon valve port and test the cuff by inflating it with 4 mL of air. Using the attached syringe, remove the air from the cuff.

⑤ Check to be sure that the cuff is deflated before insertion. Some clinicians believe that leaving a small amount of air in the cuff (enough to remove the wrinkles) makes insertion easier. However, this has not been systematically evaluated.

**Get ready to insert the laryngeal mask airway.**

⑥ Stand at the baby's head and position the head in the "sniffing" position as you would for endotracheal intubation.

⑦ Hold the device like a pen in either hand, with your index finger placed at the junction of the cuff and the tube (Figure 5.39). The bars in the middle of the mask opening must be facing forward, toward the baby's tongue. The flat part of the mask has no bars or openings, and it will be facing the baby's palate.

⑧ Some clinicians lubricate the back of the laryngeal mask with a water-soluble lubricant. If you choose to do so, be careful to keep the lubricant away from the apertures on the front side, inside the mask.

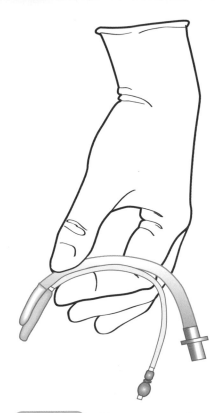

**Figure 5.39.** Holding the laryngeal mask airway prior to insertion. It may be held in the right or left hand.

**Insert the laryngeal mask airway.**

⑨ Gently open the baby's mouth and press the cuff end of the device, with the open side of the cuff facing anterior, against the baby's hard palate (Figure 5.40A).

⑩ Flatten the back side of the mask against the baby's palate with your index finger just above the cuff. Ensure that the tip of the mask remains flat and does not curl backward on itself.

⑪ Using your index finger, gently guide the device along the contours of the baby's hard palate toward the back of the throat (Figure 5.40B). **Do not use force.** Use a smooth movement to guide the mask past the tongue and into the hypopharynx until you feel resistance.

**Set and secure the laryngeal mask airway in place.**

⑫ Before removing your finger, grasp the airway tube with your other hand to hold it in place (Figure 5.40C). This prevents the device from being pulled out of position while you are moving your finger. At this point, the tip of the mask should be resting near the entrance to the esophagus (upper esophageal sphincter).

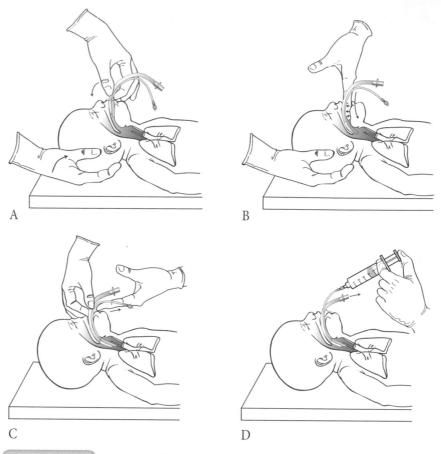

A                                 B

C                                 D

**Figure 5.40. A-D.** Inserting the laryngeal mask airway. The cuff should be inserted while deflated and then be inflated after insertion.

13 Inflate the cuff by injecting 2 to 4 mL of air via the inflation valve (Figure 5.40D). The cuff should be inflated with only enough air to achieve a seal. Do not hold the airway tube when you inflate the mask. You may note that the device moves slightly outward when it is inflated. This is normal. ***Never inflate the cuff of the size-1 laryngeal mask airway with more than 4 mL of air***.

**Ventilate through the laryngeal mask airway.**

14 Attach your resuscitation bag or T-piece resuscitator to the 15-mm adaptor on the device and begin PPV (Figure 5.41).

15 Confirm proper placement by the presence of rising heart rate, chest wall movement, and breath sounds audible with a stethoscope.

16 Secure the tube with tape, as you would an endotracheal tube.

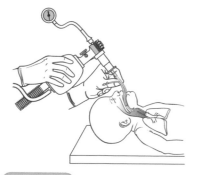

**Figure 5.41.** Providing positive-pressure ventilation using a laryngeal mask airway

## How do you know that the laryngeal mask airway is properly placed?

If the device is properly placed, you should notice a prompt increase in the baby's heart rate, equal breath sounds when you listen with a stethoscope, increasing $Spo_2$, and chest wall movement, similar to what you would expect with a properly placed endotracheal tube. If you place a colorimetric $CO_2$ monitor on the adaptor, you should note a rapid color change indicating expired $CO_2$. It is possible for the baby to breathe spontaneously through the laryngeal mask airway; therefore, you may hear grunting or crying through the device. You should not hear a large leak of air coming from the baby's mouth or see a growing bulge in the baby's neck.

## What are the possible complications that may occur with the laryngeal mask airway?

The device may cause soft-tissue trauma, laryngospasm, or gastric distension from air leaking around the mask. Prolonged use over hours or days has been infrequently associated with oropharyngeal nerve damage or lingual edema in adults; however, no information is available on the incidence of these complications in newborns.

## When should you remove the laryngeal mask airway?

The laryngeal mask airway can be removed when the baby establishes effective spontaneous respirations or when an endotracheal tube can be inserted successfully. Babies can breathe spontaneously through the device. If necessary, the laryngeal mask airway can be attached to a ventilator or continuous positive airway pressure (CPAP) device during transport to the neonatal intensive care unit, but long-term use for ventilation of newborns has not been investigated. When you decide to remove the device, suction secretions from the mouth and throat before you deflate the cuff and remove the device.

## Key Points

1. A person experienced in endotracheal intubation should be immediately available to assist at every delivery.

2. Indications for endotracheal intubation include the following:
   - To suction the trachea in the presence of meconium when the newborn is not vigorous
   - To improve efficacy of ventilation if mask ventilation is ineffective
   - To improve efficacy of ventilation if mask ventilation is required for more than a few minutes
   - To facilitate coordination of chest compressions and ventilation and to maximize the efficiency of each ventilation
   - To improve ventilation in special conditions, such as extreme prematurity, surfactant administration, or suspected diaphragmatic hernia (see Lessons 7 and 8)

3. The laryngoscope is always held in the operator's left hand.

4. The correct-sized laryngoscope blade for a term newborn is No. 1. The correct-sized blade for a preterm newborn is No. 0 or, in extremely preterm infants, No. 00.

5. Choice of the proper endotracheal tube size is based on weight.

| Weight (g) | Gestational Age (wks) | Tube Size (mm) (inside diameter) |
|---|---|---|
| Below 1,000 | Below 28 | 2.5 |
| 1,000-2,000 | 28-34 | 3.0 |
| 2,000-3,000 | 34-38 | 3.5 |
| Above 3,000 | Above 38 | 3.5-4.0 |

6. The intubation procedure ideally should be completed within 30 seconds.

7. The steps for intubating a newborn are as follows:
   - Stabilize the newborn's head in the "sniffing" position.
   - Slide the laryngoscope over the right side of the tongue, pushing the tongue to the left side of the mouth, and advancing the blade until the tip lies just beyond the base of the tongue.
   - Lift the blade slightly. Raise the entire blade, not just the tip.
   - Look for landmarks. Vocal cords should appear as vertical stripes on each side of the glottis or as an inverted letter "V". Suction with a large bore catheter, if necessary, for visualization.

- Insert the tube into the right side of the mouth with the curve of the tube lying in the horizontal plane so that the tube curves from left to right.
- If the cords are closed, wait for them to open. Insert the tip of the endotracheal tube until the vocal cord guide is at the level of the cords.
- Hold the tube firmly against the baby's palate while removing the laryngoscope. Hold the tube in place while removing the stylet if one was used.

8. Correct placement of the endotracheal tube is indicated by
   - Improved vital signs (heart rate, color/oximetry, activity)
   - Presence of exhaled $CO_2$ as determined by a $CO_2$ detector
   - Breath sounds over both lung fields but decreased or absent over the stomach
   - No gastric distention with ventilation
   - Vapor in the tube during exhalation
   - Chest movement with each breath
   - Tip-to-lip measurement: add 6 to newborn's estimated weight in kilograms
   - Direct visualization of the tube passing between the vocal cords
   - Chest x-ray confirmation if the tube is to remain in place past initial resuscitation

9. Placement of a laryngeal mask airway may be useful in the following situations:
   - When facial or upper airway malformations render ventilation by mask ineffective
   - When positive-pressure ventilation with a face mask fails to achieve effective ventilation and intubation is not possible

10. The limitations of a laryngeal mask airway are
    - Currently available devices are too large for small preterm babies (or babies less than approximately 32 weeks' gestational age).
    - The device cannot be used to suction meconium from the airway.
    - An air leak at the mask-larynx interface may result in delivery of insufficient pressure to the lungs.
    - Its use during chest compressions or to deliver medications to the lungs may not be as effective as with an endotracheal tube.
    - There is insufficient evidence to recommend the laryngeal mask airway for prolonged assisted ventilation in newborns.

## Lesson 5 Review

*(The answers follow.)*

1.  A newborn with meconium and depressed respirations (will) (will not) require suctioning via an endotracheal tube before other resuscitation measures are started.

2.  A newborn receiving ventilation by mask is not improving after 2 minutes of apparently good technique. Despite ventilation corrective steps, the heart rate is not rising and there is poor chest movement. Endotracheal intubation (should) (should not) be considered.

3.  For babies weighing less than 1,000 g, the inside diameter of the endotracheal tube should be _____ mm.

4.  The preferred blade size for use in term newborns is No. _____. The preferred laryngoscope blade size for use in preterm newborns is No. _____, or, for extremely preterm newborns, No. _____.

5.  Which illustration shows the view of the oral cavity that you should see if you have the laryngoscope correctly placed for intubation?

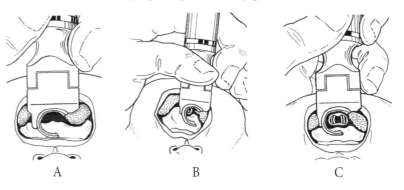

A          B          C

6.  Both right- and left-handed people should hold the laryngoscope in their _____ hand.

7.  You should try to take no longer than _____ seconds to complete endotracheal intubation.

8.  If you have not completed endotracheal intubation within the time limit in Question 7, what should you do? _____
    _____

## Lesson 5 Review—*continued*

9. Which illustration shows the correct way to lift the tongue out of the way to expose the pharyngeal area?

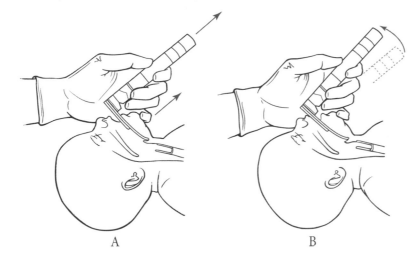

A                                  B

10. You have the glottis in view, but the vocal cords are closed. You (should) (should not) wait until they are open to insert the tube.

11. What 2 guidelines are helpful for determining the depth that the endotracheal tube be inserted into the baby's trachea?
   _____ and _____

12. You have inserted an endotracheal tube and are giving positive-pressure ventilation through it. When you check with a stethoscope, you hear breath sounds on both sides of the baby's chest, with equal intensity on each side and no air entering the stomach. The tube likely (is) (is not) correctly placed.

13. Which x-ray shows the correct placement of an endotracheal tube?

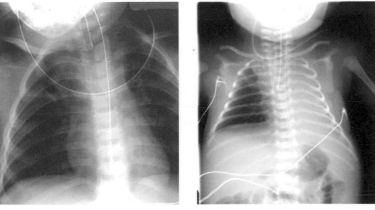

A                                  B

## Lesson 5 Review—*continued*

14. You have inserted an endotracheal tube and are giving positive-pressure ventilation through it. When you check with a stethoscope, you hear no breath sounds over either side of the chest and you hear air entering the stomach. The tube is placed in the (esophagus) (trachea).

15. You have inserted an endotracheal tube and are giving positive-pressure ventilation through it. When you check with a stethoscope, you hear breath sounds over the right side of the chest, but not the left. When you check the tip-to-lip measurement, the first number seen at the lip is higher than expected. You should (withdraw) (advance) the tube slightly and listen with the stethoscope again.

16. A baby is born at term following abruption of the placenta and is not improving despite positive-pressure ventilation by mask. You have tried to intubate the trachea but have been unsuccessful. Help has not yet arrived. A reasonable next step would be: _____ _____

17. A baby is born with bilateral cleft lip and palate and a very small mandible and requires positive-pressure ventilation. You are unable to achieve a seal with bag and mask. A reasonable next step would be: _____

18. An extremely low birthweight baby is born and requires assisted ventilation. Insertion of a laryngeal mask airway would be a reasonable alternative to intubation. (True, False)

## Answers to Questions

1. A newborn with meconium and depressed respirations **will** require suctioning by endotracheal intubation before other resuscitation measures are started.

2. Endotracheal intubation **should** be considered for a newborn who is not improving, despite good technique.

3. For babies weighing less than 1,000 g, the inside diameter of the endotracheal tube should be **2.5** mm.

## Answers to Questions—*continued*

4.  The blade of a laryngoscope should be No. **1** for term newborns, No. **0** for preterm newborns, and No. **00** for extremely preterm newborns.

5.  Illustration **C** shows the correct view for intubation.

6.  Both right- and left-handed people should hold the laryngoscope in their **left** hand.

7.  The goal should be to insert an endotracheal tube and connect it to a resuscitation device within **30 seconds.**

8.  If you have not completed endotracheal intubation within 30 seconds, you should **remove the laryngoscope, ventilate with positive-pressure ventilation by mask, and then try again.**

9.  Illustration **A** is correct.

10. You **should** wait until the vocal cords are open to insert the tube.

11. You should insert the tube **to the level of the vocal cord guide** and **"tip-to-lip 1-2-3 7-8-9".**

12. The tube **is** correctly placed.

13. X-ray **A** shows correct placement of an endotracheal tube. The tube is too low in B, and the left lung is airless, probably from the tube being down the right main bronchus.

14. The tube is placed in the **esophagus.**

15. You should **withdraw** the tube slightly and listen with the stethoscope again.

16. **Insert a laryngeal mask airway.**

17. **Insert a laryngeal mask airway.**

18. **False.** The laryngeal mask airway device is too large for an extremely low birthweight baby.

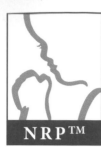

# Lesson 5: Endotracheal Intubation and Laryngeal Mask Airway Placement

# Performance Checklist

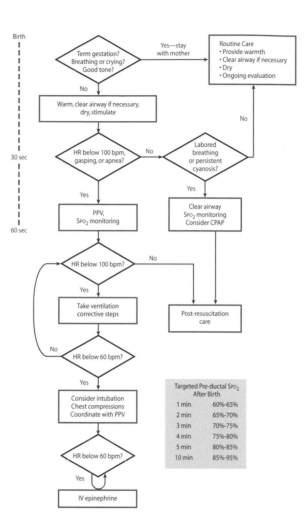

## The Performance Checklist Is a Learning Tool

The learner uses the checklist as a reference during independent practice, or as a guide for discussion and practice with a Neonatal Resuscitation Program™ (NRP™) instructor. When the learner and instructor agree that the learner can perform the skills correctly and smoothly without coaching and within the context of a scenario, the learner may move on to the next lesson's Performance Checklist.

**Knowledge Check**

- What are the indications for endotracheal intubation during resuscitation?

- How do you determine if a baby born with meconium-stained amniotic fluid requires tracheal suction?

- What are the signs of correct placement of the endotracheal tube in the trachea?

- What are the indications for placing a laryngeal mask airway?

- What are the limitations of a laryngeal mask airway?

**Learning Objectives**

1. Identify the newborn who requires endotracheal intubation during resuscitation.

2. Demonstrate correct technique for performing/assisting with endotracheal intubation and administering positive-pressure ventilation (PPV).

3. Demonstrate correct technique for suctioning meconium from the trachea of a non-vigorous newborn.

4. Identify when placement of a laryngeal mask airway is indicated.

5. List the limitations of a laryngeal mask airway.

6. Demonstrate correct technique in placing and removing a laryngeal mask airway.

7. Demonstrate behavioral skills to ensure clear communication and teamwork during this critical component of newborn resuscitation.

**"You are called to attend the birth of a full-term newborn because of meconium in the amniotic fluid. How would you prepare for the resuscitation of this baby? As you work, say your thoughts and actions aloud so your assistant and I will know what you are thinking and doing."**

Instructor should check boxes as the learner responds correctly.

| Participant Name: | | |
|---|---|---|
| | ☐ Obtains relevant perinatal history | Gestational age? (confirms information) Fluid clear? (confirms information) How many babies? Other risk factors? |
| | ☐ Performs equipment check<br>☐ Assembles resuscitation team (at least one other person) and discusses plan and roles | **Warm**er on, Towels to **dry**, **Clear airway** (bulb syringe, wall suction set at 80-100 mm Hg, meconium aspirator), **Auscultate** (stethoscope), **Oxygenate** (checks oxygen, blender, pulse oximeter, and probe), **Ventilate** (checks positive-pressure ventilation [PPV] device), **Intubate** (laryngoscope and blades, endotracheal tubes, stylets, end-tidal $CO_2$ detector) **Medicate** (code cart accessible), **Thermoregulate.** |
| | **Prepares for intubation**<br>• Selects correct-sized tube<br>• Inserts stylet correctly (stylet optional)<br>• Checks light on blade (size 1 for full-term newborn)<br>• Ensures that suction functions at 80-100 mm Hg and ensures connection to 10F or 12F catheter<br>• Obtains meconium aspiration device<br>• Obtains end-tidal $CO_2$ detector<br>• Prepares tape or obtains endotracheal tube securing device | The team prepares for a non-vigorous newborn who will require intubation and tracheal suction with a meconium aspiration device.<br><br><br><br><br><br><br><br><br>Due to the high-risk scenario, the team also prepares to intubate and ventilate with an endotracheal tube and PPV device. |
| | **"The baby has been born."** | |

| Sample Vital Signs | Performance Steps | Details |
|---|---|---|
| Appears term<br>Apneic<br>Limp | Completes initial assessment when baby is born.<br>☐ Asks 3 questions: Term? Breathing or crying? Good tone? | |
| | ☐ Indicates tracheal suctioning is required | Newborn is meconium stained and not vigorous (apneic, and poor muscle tone). |
| Respiratory Rate (RR)-apneic<br>Heart rate (HR)-<100 beats per minute (bpm)<br>Tone-limp | ☐ Receives baby at radiant warmer, does not dry or stimulate | Vigorous meconium-stained newborn may stay with his mother and receive routine care. |

During the intubation procedure, the role of the intubator is in the left column and the role of the assistant is in the right column. Some actions and decisions can be made by either or both the intubator and assistant (merged columns).

| Performing Intubation | Assisting With Intubation |
|---|---|
| ☐ Holds laryngoscope correctly in left hand | ☐ Positions newborn's head. |
| ☐ Inserts blade carefully to base of tongue | ☐ Monitors 30-second time frame for intubation. |
| ☐ Requests suction if needed for visualization | ☐ Places suction catheter in intubator's hand and provides suction if needed. Intubator should not have to look away from landmarks. |
| ☐ Lifts using correct motion (no rocking back) | ☐ Taps out heart rate (HR) (if no audio HR from pulse oximeter) where intubator can view with peripheral vision. |
| ☐ Requests cricoid pressure if needed | ☐ Applies cricoid pressure if requested. |
| ☐ Identifies landmarks seen | |
| ☐ Takes corrective action to visualize glottis if needed | |
| ☐ Inserts tube from right side, does not insert tube down center of laryngoscope blade | |
| ☐ Aligns vocal cord guide with vocal cords | ☐ Attaches meconium aspiration device to suction tubing. |
| ☐ Removes laryngoscope (and stylet) while firmly holding tube against baby's palate | ☐ Attaches meconium aspiration device to endotracheal tube. |
| ☐ Holds endotracheal tube in place and applies suction to meconium aspiration device; slowly withdraws endotracheal tube from trachea | |

☐ Assesses the need to repeat procedure with a clean endotracheal tube (decision is based on amount of meconium recovered and baby's status)

**OR**

☐ Proceeds with Initial Steps

| | Proceeds With Initial Steps | |
|---|---|---|
| **Sample Vital Signs** | **Performance Steps** | **Details** |
| | ☐ Performs initial steps | Position airway, dry, stimulate, remove wet linen. |
| RR-apneic<br>HR-40 bpm | ☐ Evaluates respirations and heart rate | Auscultates apical pulse or palpates umbilicus. |
| | ☐ Initiates PPV | Begins with ___% oxygen per hospital protocol at about 20 cm $H_2O$ pressure. Rate = 40-60/min |
| | ☐ Calls for additional help if necessary | A minimum of 2 resuscitators are necessary if PPV required. Team should already be assembled. |
| | ☐ Requests pulse oximetry | Places probe on right hand or wrist before plugging into monitor. |
| RR-apneic<br>HR-40 bpm<br>$SPO_2$ - - -<br><br>No breath sounds or chest movement | ☐ Requests assessment of heart rate, pulse oximetry<br><br>☐ If not rising, requests assessment of bilateral breath sounds and chest movement | Pulse oximetry not functioning at low HR. |
| | ☐ Takes ventilation corrective steps (MR SOPA) | **M**ask adjustment, **R**eposition airway (re-attempt PPV). **S**uction mouth and nose and **o**pen mouth (re-attempt PPV). If no breath sounds or chest movement, gradually increase **p**ressure every few breaths until there are bilateral breath sounds and chest movement with each breath. Move to next step if reaching 40 cm $H_2O$. |
| No chest movement<br>No breath sounds<br><br>HR-50 bpm<br>$SPO_2$ - - - | ☐ Requests evaluation of chest movement and breath sounds<br><br>☐ Evaluates heart rate and pulse oximetry | If all corrective steps are done but there still is no chest movement, breath sounds, or rising heart rate, learner indicates need for intubation. |
| | ☐ Indicates need for intubation | Ventilation of the newborn is the highest priority; chest compressions will be ineffective until ventilation is established by mask or endotracheal tube. |
| | ☐ Directs assistant to continue monitoring HR and oxygen saturation ($SPO_2$)<br>☐ Turns up oxygen to 100% in preparation for chest compressions<br>☐ Assistant may continue to try corrective steps to improve PPV | Assistant monitors HR and $SPO_2$ (if possible) throughout procedure. |

| Performing Intubation | Assisting With Intubation |
|---|---|
| □ **Prepares for intubation** (Most of these steps were done in preparation for the birth.) • Selects correct-sized tube • Inserts stylet correctly (stylet optional) • Checks light on blade (size 1 for full-term newborn) • Ensures that suction functions at 80-100 mm Hg and ensures connection to 10F or 12F catheter • Obtains end-tidal $CO_2$ detector • Prepares tape or obtains endotracheal tube securing device | |
| □ Holds laryngoscope correctly in left hand | □ Positions newborn's head. |
| □ Inserts blade carefully to base of tongue | □ Monitors 30-second time frame for intubation. |
| □ Requests suction if needed for visualization | □ Places suction catheter in intubator's hand and provides suction if needed. Intubator should not have to look away from landmarks. |
| □ Lifts using correct motion (no rocking back) | □ Taps out heart rate (HR) (if no audio HR from pulse oximeter) where intubator can view with peripheral vision. |
| □ Requests cricoid pressure if needed | □ Applies cricoid pressure if requested. |
| □ Identifies landmarks seen | |
| □ Takes corrective action to visualize glottis if needed | |
| □ Inserts tube from right side, does not insert tube down center of laryngoscope blade | |
| □ Aligns vocal cord guide with vocal cords | |
| □ Removes laryngoscope (and stylet) while firmly holding tube against baby's palate | □ Removes mask from positive-pressure ventilation (PPV) device. Attaches $CO_2$ detector to endotracheal tube and attaches PPV device to $CO_2$ detector. |
| □ Holds tube against baby's palate with one hand and PPV device with other hand and resumes ventilation | □ Assistant hands off PPV device to intubator so that intubator is holding both the endotracheal tube and the PPV device. |

□ Ensures correct depth of insertion:
Estimate weight of newborn in kg + 6
Example: 3 kg + 6 = 9 cm marking at upper lip
□ Looks and listens for signs to confirm correct tube placement.
• Mist in tube during exhalation
• $CO_2$ detector confirmation (may not function if newborn has very poor cardiac perfusion)
• Rising heart rate
• Rising oxygen saturation
• Bilateral breath sounds
• Symmetrical chest movement (do not over inflate)

If correct placement cannot be confirmed, assistant and intubator discuss and take necessary corrective action.
□ Repeat confirmation steps.
□ Reassess correct tip-to-lip measurement.
□ Reinsert laryngoscope and visualize placement of stripe at vocal cords.
and/or
□ Remove endotracheal tube, ventilate with mask and PPV device, and repeat intubation.
Or
□ Consider rescue airway (laryngeal mask airway). GO TO ALTERNATIVE AIRWAY.

Chest compressions resume after successful intubation

| Sample Vital Signs | Performance Steps | Details |
|---|---|---|
| HR-50 bpm | ☐ Assesses respiratory effort, HR, and $SpO_2$ as PPV resumes | |
| | ☐ Chest compressions resume | Assistant resumes chest compressions and calls out cadence. Now that baby is intubated, compressor may move to head of bed to allow access to umbilicus, if needed. |
| HR-70 bpm<br>$SpO_2$-67% | ☐ Checks heart rate after 45-60 seconds of chest compressions<br>☐ Discontinues compressions<br>☐ Continues ventilations<br>☐ Adjusts oxygen based on oximetry and newborn's age | |
| RR-apneic<br>HR-120 bpm<br>$SpO_2$-74% | ☐ After 30 seconds of PPV with endotracheal tube, checks respiratory effort, HR, and $SpO_2$<br>☐ Adjusts oxygen based on oximetry and newborn's age | |
| RR-occasional gasp<br>HR-140 bpm<br>$SpO_2$-97% | ☐ May continue PPV for 30 additional seconds. Adjust oxygen based on oximetry and newborn's age.<br>Or<br>☐ Make a team decision to<br>• Update family.<br>• Secure endotracheal tube.<br>• Move to post-resuscitation care. | |
| **ALTERNATIVE AIRWAY: Placement of a laryngeal mask airway**<br>**"You have been unable to ventilate or intubate the baby. You decide to insert a laryngeal mask airway."** | | |
| Sample Vital Signs | Performance Steps | Details |
| HR-50 bpm<br>$SpO_2$ - - - | ☐ Directs chest compressions to begin while preparing rescue airway | Newborn requires continued efforts at ventilation and chest compressions. Oxygen concentration should be at 100% during chest compressions. |
| | ☐ Obtains size-1 laryngeal mask airway and 5-mL syringe | May consider placing orogastric tube to relieve gastric distention prior to placing laryngeal mask airway. |
| | ☐ Using the 5-mL syringe, quickly inflates the cuff with no more than 4 mL of air to check for leaks or tears | Learner should be moving quickly to insert the rescue airway. |
| | ☐ Withdraws air; however, leaves just enough air in cuff to remove the wrinkles | We have little experience using the laryngeal mask airway. This technique may keep the airway from folding over on itself during insertion. |

| Sample Vital Signs | Performance Steps | Details |
|---|---|---|
| | ☐ Requests pause in chest compressions while placing airway | |
| | ☐ Places baby's head in sniffing position<br>☐ Holding laryngeal mask airway like a pen, gently opens baby's mouth and inserts airway smoothly and quickly along the hard palate until resistance is met, just past the base of the tongue | Unlike placement of an adult laryngeal mask airway, the airway is inserted directly into the baby's hypopharynx in its intended position. It is not "flipped" into position at the back of the throat. |
| | ☐ Holds airway in place with other hand and removes index finger without dislodging airway | |
| | ☐ Ensures that airway stays in place by holding it against the hard palate; however, holds it gently enough so airway may rise and seat as cuff is inflated<br>☐ Inflates cuff with 5-mL syringe to total of no more than 4 mL of air | Airway may not rise and seat in the manikin. It also may be possible to insert the airway too far into the manikin, resulting in ineffective ventilation. |
| | ☐ Connects airway to end-tidal $CO_2$ detector and PPV device<br>☐ Holds airway against baby's hard palate to protect from dislodgement | The provider holds the airway in place just as the endotracheal tube is held in place—with one finger against the baby's hard palate. The other hand holds the PPV device. |
| + breath sounds<br>+ chest movement | ☐ Begins PPV at 40-60 breaths/minute<br>☐ Confirms correct placement<br>• Bilateral breath sounds<br>• Chest movement<br>• Color change on $CO_2$ detector | |
| HR-70 bpm<br>$SPO_2$-67% | ☐ Discontinues chest compressions<br>☐ Continues ventilations for 30 seconds | |
| HR-120 bpm<br>Occasional respirations<br>$SPO_2$-74% | ☐ Slows PPV rate and stimulates baby to breathe<br>☐ Monitors pulse oximetry and decreases 100% oxygen to meet saturation target for baby's age | |

| Sample Vital Signs | Performance Steps | Details |
|---|---|---|
| HR-140 bpm<br>Spontaneous respirations<br>$SpO_2$-97% | ☐ Suctions baby's mouth and throat with suction catheter<br>☐ Withdraws air from airway and removes laryngeal mask airway | Laryngeal mask airway could remain in place if desired. The baby can breathe spontaneously with the airway in place. The airway may be taped in place using the emergency endotracheal tube taping technique. |
| | ☐ Monitors baby's respiratory efforts, heart rate, oximetry, and muscle tone<br>☐ Monitors pulse oximetry and adjusts oxygen if needed | |
| | ☐ Indicates need for post-resuscitation care<br>☐ Updates family | |

**Instructor asks the learner Reflective Questions to enable self-assessment, such as**

1. What went well during this resuscitation?

2. What was your main objective?

3. Who assumed the leadership role in this scenario? What skills did you use to ensure that your assistant understood what you needed? Give me an example of what you did or said that used that behavioral skill.

4. As the assistant, what suggestions might you make, if any, to help the team leader communicate clearly with team members?

5. Would you do anything differently when faced with this scenario again?

### Neonatal Resuscitation Program Key Behavioral Skills

Know your environment.
Anticipate and plan.
Assume the leadership role.
Communicate effectively.
Delegate workload optimally.

Allocate attention wisely.
Use all available information.
Use all available resources.
Call for help when needed.
Maintain professional behavior.

# Medications

## In Lesson 6 you will learn

- When to give medications during resuscitation

- What medications to give during resuscitation

- Where to give medications during resuscitation

- How to insert an emergency umbilical venous catheter

- How to administer epinephrine

- When and how to administer fluids intravenously to restore intravascular volume during a resuscitation

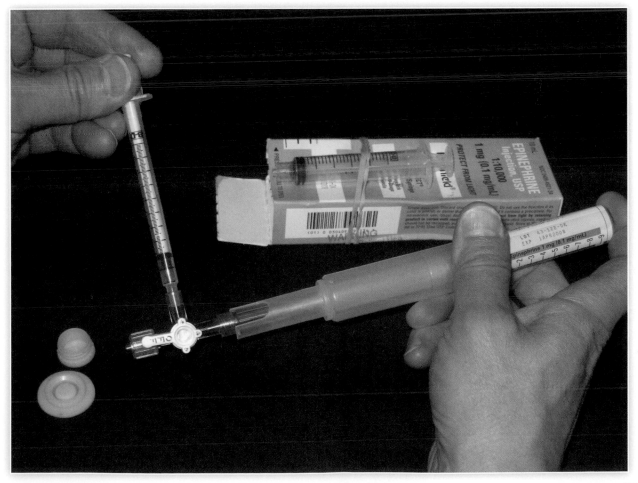

The following case is an example of how medications may be used during an extensive resuscitation. As you read the case, imagine yourself as part of the resuscitation team. The details of medication administration are described in the lesson.

## Case 6.
## Resuscitation with positive-pressure ventilation, chest compressions, and medications

A pregnant woman near term enters the emergency department in early labor with profuse vaginal bleeding.

A diagnosis of vasa previa is made, and repetitive late decelerations are noted on the fetal heart rate tracing. Additional skilled personnel are called to the delivery room, the radiant warmer is turned on, and resuscitation equipment is prepared. An umbilical catheter is primed with 0.9% saline, since the need for advanced resuscitation is anticipated. An emergency cesarean section is performed, and a limp, pale baby, appearing to weigh approximately 3 kg, is handed to the neonatal team.

A team member positions her head, suctions her mouth and nose, and stimulates her with drying. However, the baby remains limp, cyanotic, and without spontaneous respirations.

Positive-pressure ventilation (PPV) with a bag and mask and 21% oxygen is initiated and a pulse oximetry probe is placed on her right hand to monitor oxygenation. However, the baby remains apneic and cyanotic and PPV is ineffective, even after corrective measures are performed; therefore, the baby is intubated. After 30 seconds of effective ventilation, she remains cyanotic and limp and has a very low heart rate (20 to 30 beats per minute [bpm]). No signal can be detected using the pulse oximeter.

Chest compressions are provided and coordinated with PPV using 100% oxygen. A team member listens with a stethoscope to ensure that there are equal breath sounds and ventilation is adequately moving the chest. Nevertheless, after 60 seconds, the heart rate has not increased.

A team member cleans the cord stump and begins to insert the previously prepared umbilical venous line. The heart rate is now undetectable, so 1.5 mL of 1:10,000 epinephrine is instilled into the endotracheal tube while umbilical venous access is being secured. The heart rate is checked as coordinated chest compressions and PPV continue. The heart rate remains undetectable.

After the umbilical venous catheter is in place and a team member confirms that there is free flow of blood on aspiration with a syringe, a dose of 0.6 mL of 1:10,000 epinephrine is given into the catheter, followed by a normal saline flush. The heart rate is now audible with a stethoscope, but remains below 60 bpm. Because the baby has persistent bradycardia and a history of possible blood loss, 30 mL of normal saline

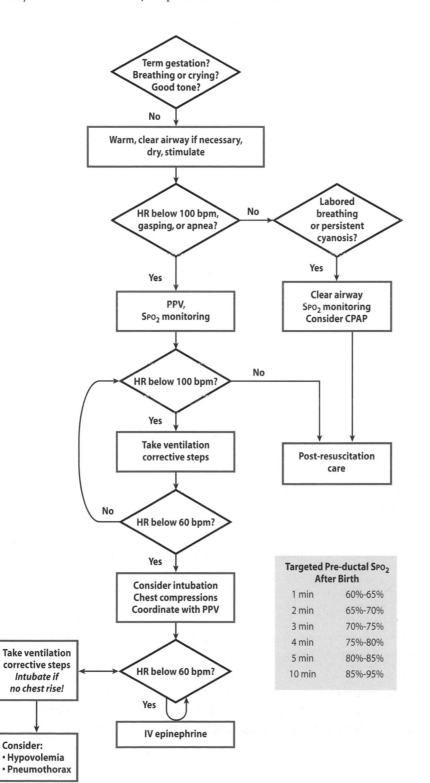

is given via the umbilical catheter. The heart rate gradually increases and the oximeter becomes consistent with the audible heart rate and shows an $SpO_2$ in the low 80s and rising.

By 8 minutes after birth, the baby makes an initial gasp. Chest compressions are stopped when the heart rate rises above 60 bpm. Assisted ventilation continues, the heart rate rises above 100 bpm, and the oxygen concentration is gradually reduced as the $SpO_2$ approaches 90%. The baby's color begins to improve, and she begins to have spontaneous respirations.

She is transferred to the nursery for post-resuscitation care with continued PPV.

---

If resuscitation steps (particularly, effective PPV) are implemented in a skillful and timely manner, more than 99% of newborns requiring resuscitation will improve without the need for medications. Before administering medications in an intensive resuscitation, you should check the effectiveness of ventilation several times, ensuring good chest movement and audible bilateral breath sounds with each breath, chest compressions should be started and coordinated with ventilations, and the oxygen concentration should be increased to 100%. With such poor cardiac output, the pulse oximeter usually will not give a reading. In most cases, you will choose to insert an endotracheal tube to ensure a stable airway and effective coordination of chest compressions and PPV if effective ventilation alone has not resulted in an increase in the baby's heart rate.

> ⚠ **If the heart rate remains below 60 bpm despite ongoing ventilation and chest compressions, your first action is to ensure that ventilation and compressions are being given optimally.**

Despite good ventilation of the lungs with PPV and augmented cardiac output from chest compressions, a small number of newborns (fewer than 7 per 10,000 births) will still have a heart rate below 60 bpm.

During asphyxia, the baby's blood pressure falls, resulting in poor coronary artery perfusion and decreased oxygen delivery to the heart. As a result, the heart muscle of these babies may not contract effectively, despite being perfused with oxygenated blood during resuscitation. These babies may benefit from receiving epinephrine to stimulate the heart and increase heart rate. Epinephrine also increases diastolic blood pressure, thus improving perfusion of coronary arteries. Newly born babies who have depressed respiratory and cardiac function because of acute blood loss also may benefit from volume replacement.

## What will this lesson cover?

This lesson will teach you when and why to give *epinephrine,* how to establish a route by which to give it, and how to determine dosage. The lesson also will discuss *volume expansion* for babies in shock from acute blood loss.

Administration of naloxone, a narcotic antagonist given to babies who have depressed respirations from maternal narcotics, is not necessary during the acute phases of resuscitation and will be discussed in Lesson 7. Sodium bicarbonate may be used to treat metabolic acidosis, and vasopressors, such as dopamine, may be used for hypotension or poor cardiac output, but these are administered more often in the post-resuscitative period and also are discussed in Lesson 7. Other drugs, such as atropine and calcium, are sometimes used during special resuscitation circumstances, but are not indicated during the acute phase of neonatal resuscitation.

The most reliable route of administration of medications is the intravenous route. Therefore, in this lesson, you will learn how to prepare the medications and how to prepare and insert an umbilical venous catheter. While a minimum of 2 people are required to administer coordinated PPV and chest compressions, a third and perhaps fourth person will be required to obtain intravenous access and administer intravenous medications.

You are encouraged to view these videos on the DVD that accompanies this textbook: *Preparing the Emergency UVC for Insertion*
and
*Placing an Emergency UVC*

## How do you establish intravenous access during resuscitation of a newborn?

### The umbilical vein

The umbilical vein is the most quickly accessible direct intravenous route in the newborn. If the use of epinephrine is anticipated because of unresponsiveness of the baby to the earlier steps of resuscitation, one member of the resuscitation team should begin work to place an umbilical venous catheter, while others continue to provide PPV and chest compressions.

- Put on sterile gloves and quickly set up a sterile field. Although you should use sterile technique, it is often difficult to perform this procedure in a truly sterile manner while working quickly so as not to delay resuscitation. If an ongoing need for the catheter is identified after resuscitation and stabilization, the catheter should be removed and a new one placed, using full sterile technique.

- Clean the cord with an antiseptic solution. Place a loose tie of umbilical tape around the base of the cord. This tie can be tightened if there is excessive bleeding after you cut the cord.

- Fill a 3.5F or 5F umbilical catheter with normal saline using a 3-mL syringe connected to a stopcock. The catheter should have a single end-hole. Close the stopcock to the catheter to prevent fluid loss and air entry.

- Cut the cord with a scalpel below the clamp that had been placed at birth and about 1 to 2 cm from the skin line (Figure 6.1). Make the cut perpendicular to the umbilical cord, rather than at an angle.

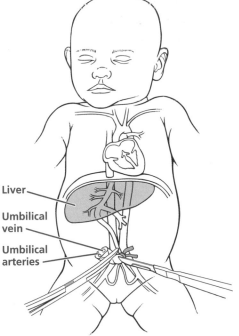

**Figure 6.1.** Cutting the umbilical stump in preparation for inserting umbilical catheter

*Liver*

*Umbilical vein*

*Umbilical arteries*

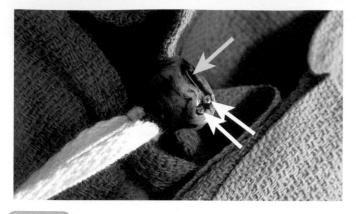

**Figure 6.2.** Cut umbilical cord, before placement of catheter. Note the umbilical arteries (shown by the white arrows) and the umbilical vein (shown by the yellow arrow).

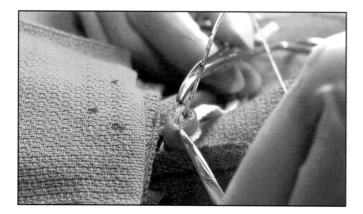

**Figure 6.3.** Saline-filled catheter has been placed 2 to 4 cm into the umbilical vein (note black centimeter marks on the catheter). Medications should not be administered until blood can be aspirated easily from the catheter.

- The umbilical vein will be seen as a large, thin-walled structure, usually at the 11- to 12-o'clock position. The 2 umbilical arteries have thicker walls and usually lie close together somewhere in the 4- and 8-o'clock positions (Figure 6.2). However, the arteries coil within the cord. Therefore, the longer the cord stump below your cut, the greater the likelihood that the vessels will not lie in the positions described.

- Insert the catheter into the umbilical vein (Figure 6.3). The course of the vein will be up, toward the heart, so this is the direction you should point the catheter. Continue inserting the catheter 2 to 4 cm (less in preterm babies) until you get free flow of blood when you open the stopcock to the syringe and gently aspirate. For emergency use during resuscitation, the tip of the catheter should be located only a short distance into the vein—only to the point at which blood is first able to be aspirated. If the catheter is inserted farther, there is risk of infusing medications directly into the liver, which may cause hepatic injury. (See Figure 6.4, right drawing.)

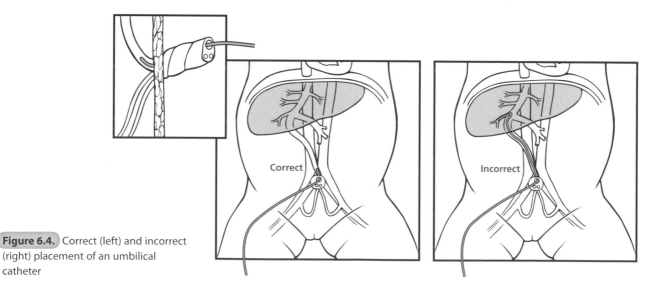

**Figure 6.4.** Correct (left) and incorrect (right) placement of an umbilical catheter

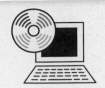

- While one person holds the catheter in place, another can administer the appropriate dose of epinephrine or volume expander (see pages 220 and 223), followed by 0.5 to 1 mL of normal saline to flush the drug through the catheter into the baby.

- After medications have been administered, either remove the catheter or secure it in place for continued IV access as the baby is transported to the nursery. Do not advance the catheter once the sterile field has been contaminated.

**You are encouraged to view this video on the DVD that accompanies this textbook:** *Securing and Safeguarding the Emergency UVC*

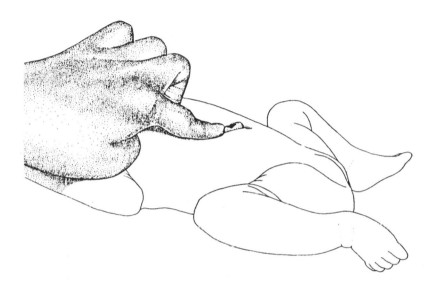

**Figure 6.5.** Stopping bleeding from the umbilical vein. (Used with permission from Kattwinkel J, Cook LJ, Hurt H, Nowacek GA, Short JG, Crosby WM, eds. *Neonatal Care*. Elk Grove Village, IL: American Academy of Pediatrics; 2007:151,221,228. *PCEP Perinatal Continuing Education Program*; book 2.)

If you remove the catheter, do it slowly and be prepared to control bleeding by tightening the cord tie. Because the umbilical vein runs just below the skin, superior to the umbilicus, umbilical venous bleeding usually can be stopped by applying pressure above the umbilicus (Figure 6.5).

If you decide to leave the catheter in place during continued stabilization or transport, it should be secured (Figure 6.6).

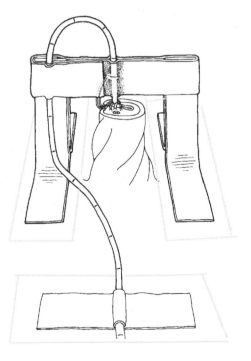

**Figure 6.6.** Taping in an umbilical catheter that has been sutured to the cord. The goal-post method of suturing and taping is an effective method for securing the umbilical line in the neonatal intensive care unit or nursery for prolonged use, but it takes time and may not be the best choice during resuscitation. Another technique is to use a clear adhesive dressing to temporarily secure the line to the newborn's abdomen. (Used with permission from Kattwinkel J, Cook LJ, Hurt H, Nowacek GA, Short JG, Crosby WM, eds. *Neonatal Care*. Elk Grove Village, IL: American Academy of Pediatrics; 2007:151,221,228. *PCEP Perinatal Continuing Education Program*; book 2.)

# Are there alternatives to intravenous access for administration of medications during resuscitation of a newborn?

## The endotracheal tube

Epinephrine given into the endotracheal tube may be absorbed by the lungs and enter blood that drains directly into the heart. Although this may be the fastest way to give epinephrine in an intubated baby, the process of absorption by the lungs makes the response time slower and more unpredictable than if epinephrine is given directly into the blood. There are many factors that make it particularly difficult for a newborn to achieve adequate lung absorption of epinephrine, including the presence of fluid-filled alveoli that may dilute endotracheal epinephrine and possible continued shunting of blood through fetal pathways (especially in the situation of acidemia and hypoxia), such that perfusion bypasses the lung, preventing absorption and distribution of endotracheally administered epinephrine. Data from both animal models and clinical studies suggest that the standard intravenous dose is ineffective if given via the endotracheal tube. There is some evidence in animal models that giving a higher dose can compensate for the delayed absorption from the lungs; however, no studies have confirmed the efficacy or safety of this practice in newly born babies. Nevertheless, since the endotracheal route is the most readily accessible, administration of a dose of epinephrine via an endotracheal tube may be considered *while the intravenous route is being established*. If endotracheal epinephrine is given, a larger dose will be needed and, therefore, a larger syringe will be necessary. The large syringe should be clearly labeled "For Endotracheal Use Only," to avoid inadvertently giving the higher dose intravenously. While this program includes an explanation of the endotracheal technique, the intravascular route is recommended as the best and most effective choice.

## Intraosseous access

When resuscitating a newborn in the hospital setting, the umbilical vein is clearly the most readily available vascular access. In the outpatient setting, where umbilical venous catheters may not be readily available, the intraosseous approach may be a reasonable alternative route for vascular access for those who have been trained in the technique. However, there are limited data regarding the delivery of medications via intraosseous lines in newborns, particularly newborns born preterm. In the delivery room, the umbilical venous route is the preferred route of drug administration.

## What is epinephrine and when should you give it?

Epinephrine hydrochloride (sometimes referred to as adrenaline chloride) is a stimulant. Epinephrine increases the strength and rate of cardiac contractions, but most importantly causes peripheral vasoconstriction, which increases blood flow to the brain and the coronary arteries so that the heart receives oxygen and substrate to provide energy for myocardial function. Administration of epinephrine can help re-establish normal myocardial and cerebral blood flow.

Epinephrine is not indicated before you have established adequate ventilation because

- Time spent administering epinephrine is better spent on establishing effective ventilation and oxygenation.

- Epinephrine will increase workload and oxygen consumption of the heart muscle, which, in the absence of available oxygen, may cause myocardial damage.

## How should you prepare epinephrine and how much should you give?

Although epinephrine comes in 2 concentrations, only the 1:10,000 preparation should be used in neonatal resuscitation.

Epinephrine should be given intravenously. However, since administration may be delayed by the time required to establish intravenous access, some clinicians may choose to give a dose of endotracheal epinephrine while the umbilical venous line is being placed. The endotracheal route may be faster to establish, but this route results in lower and less predictable blood levels that are often not effective. If the need for medications is anticipated, preparation of an umbilical venous catheter before delivery will allow rapid administration of intravenous epinephrine if it is indicated during the resuscitation.

The recommended intravenous dose in newborns is 0.1 to 0.3 mL/kg of a 1:10,000 solution (equal to 0.01 to 0.03 mg/kg). You will need to estimate the baby's weight after birth.

In the past, higher intravenous doses have been suggested for adults and older children when they did not respond to a lower dose. However, there is no evidence that this results in a better outcome, and there is some evidence that higher doses in babies may result in brain and heart damage.

Epinephrine is indicated when the heart rate remains below 60 beats per minute after you have given 30 seconds of *effective* assisted ventilation (preferably after endotracheal intubation) and at least another 45 to 60 seconds of coordinated chest compressions and effective ventilation.

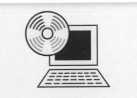

You are encouraged to view this video on the DVD that accompanies this textbook: *Drawing Up and Administering Epinephrine*

**Recommended concentration =**

1:10,000

**Recommended route =**

Intravenously (consider endotracheal route ONLY while intravenous access is being obtained)

**Recommended dose =**

0.1 to 0.3 mL/kg of 1:10,000 solution (consider 0.5 to 1 mL/kg, but only if giving endotracheally)

**Recommended preparation =**

1:10,000 solution in 1-mL syringe (or 3-6 mL syringe if giving endotracheally)

**Recommended rate of administration =**

*Rapidly*—as quickly as possible

Studies in animals and in both adults and newborn babies all demonstrate that, when given via the trachea, doses of epinephrine that are significantly higher than the intravenous dose are required to show a positive effect. If you decide to give a dose endotracheally while intravenous access is being obtained, consider giving a higher dose (0.5 to 1 mL/kg, or 0.05 to 0.1 mg/kg) by the endotracheal route *only*. However, the safety of these higher endotracheal doses has not been studied. *Do not give doses higher than 0.1 to 0.3 mL/kg intravenously.*

Epinephrine should be given quickly, whether by the intravenous or intratracheal route. When giving epinephrine via the endotracheal tube, be sure to give the drug directly into the tube, being careful not to leave it deposited in the endotracheal tube connector or along the walls of the tube. Some people prefer to use a catheter to give the drug deeply into the tube, but this has not been shown to be more effective. Because you will need to give a higher dose intratracheally, you will be giving a relatively large volume of fluid into the endotracheal tube (up to 1 mL/kg). You should follow the drug with several positive-pressure breaths to distribute the drug throughout the lungs for absorption. When the drug is given intravenously through a catheter, you should follow the drug with a 0.5- to 1-mL flush of normal saline to be sure that the drug has reached the blood.

# Review

*(The answers are in the preceding section and at the end of the lesson.)*

1. Fewer than _____% of babies requiring resuscitation will need epinephrine to stimulate their hearts.

2. As soon as you suspect that medications may be needed during a resuscitation, one member of the team should begin to insert a(n) _____ to deliver the drug(s).

3. Effective ventilation and coordinated chest compressions have been performed for 45 to 60 seconds, the trachea has been intubated, and the baby's heart rate is below 60 beats per minute. You should now give _____ while continuing chest compressions and _____.

4. What is the potential problem with administering epinephrine through an endotracheal tube? _____.

5. You should follow an intravenous dose of epinephrine with a flush of _____ to ensure that most of the drug is delivered to the baby and not left in the catheter.

6. Epinephrine (increases) (decreases) the blood pressure and strength of cardiac contractions and (increases) (decreases) the rate of cardiac contractions.

7. The recommended concentration of epinephrine for newborns is (1:1,000) (1:10,000).

8. The recommended dose of epinephrine for newborns is _____ to _____ mL/kg, if given intravenously, and _____ to _____ mL/kg, if given intratracheally, of a 1:10,000 solution.

9. Epinephrine should be given (slowly) (as quickly as possible).

## What should you expect to happen after giving epinephrine?

Check the baby's heart rate about 1 minute after administering epinephrine (longer if given endotracheally). As you continue PPV with 100% oxygen and chest compressions, the heart rate should increase to more than 60 bpm within approximately 1 minute after you give epinephrine intravenously; the increase in heart rate may take longer (or may not occur) if you give epinephrine via the endotracheal tube. The primary mechanism for epinephrine's effect is that it increases vascular resistance and, therefore, systemic blood pressure, thus improving blood flow to the coronary arteries, resulting in improved contractility of heart muscle.

If the heart rate does not increase to above 60 bpm after the first dose of epinephrine, you can repeat the dose every 3 to 5 minutes. If you started at the lower end of the dosage range, you should consider increasing subsequent doses to the maximum dose. Any repeat doses should be given intravenously if possible. In addition, ensure that

**Minimize interruption of chest compressions to assess the heart rate, as every interruption will cause a fall in diastolic pressure, which will take significant time to recover following resumption of compressions.**

- There is good air exchange as evidenced by adequate chest movement and presence of bilateral breath sounds. Endotracheal intubation should be strongly considered if not already done.

- The endotracheal tube has not been dislodged from the trachea during resuscitation.

- Chest compressions are being given to a depth of one-third of the diameter of the chest and are well coordinated with ventilations.

If there is a poor response to resuscitation, and the baby is pale or there is evidence of blood loss, you will want to consider the possibility of hypovolemia.

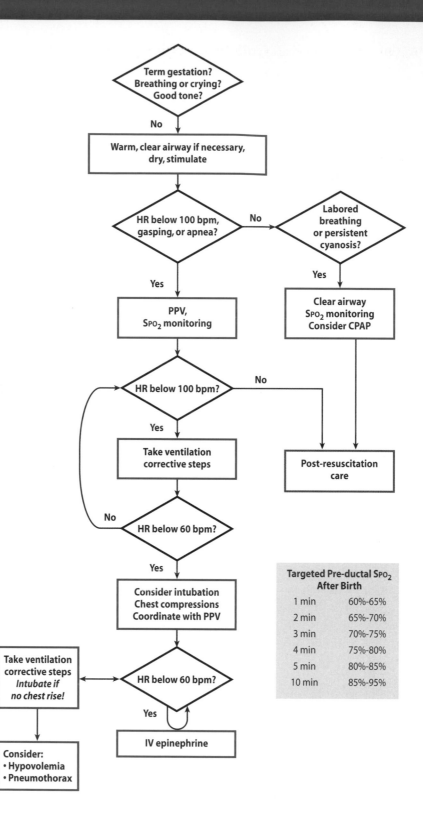

Term gestation?
Breathing or crying?
Good tone?

No

Warm, clear airway if necessary, dry, stimulate

HR below 100 bpm, gasping, or apnea?

No → Labored breathing or persistent cyanosis?

Yes

PPV, SPO₂ monitoring

Yes → Clear airway SPO₂ monitoring Consider CPAP

HR below 100 bpm?

No

Yes

Take ventilation corrective steps

Post-resuscitation care

HR below 60 bpm?

No

Yes

Consider intubation
Chest compressions
Coordinate with PPV

HR below 60 bpm?

Take ventilation corrective steps
*Intubate if no chest rise!*

Yes

IV epinephrine

Consider:
• Hypovolemia
• Pneumothorax

**Targeted Pre-ductal SPO₂ After Birth**

| | |
|---|---|
| 1 min | 60%-65% |
| 2 min | 65%-70% |
| 3 min | 70%-75% |
| 4 min | 75%-80% |
| 5 min | 80%-85% |
| 10 min | 85%-95% |

## What should you do if the baby remains bradycardic after epinephrine administration, and there is strong suspicion of acute blood loss?

If there has been a placenta previa, or blood loss from the umbilical cord, the baby may be in hypovolemic shock. In some cases, the baby may have lost blood into the maternal circulation and there will be signs of shock with no obvious evidence of blood loss. Babies who are hypovolemic may appear pale, have delayed capillary refill, and/or have weak pulses. They may have a persistently low heart rate, and circulatory status often does not improve in response to effective ventilation, chest compressions, and epinephrine.

> **!** If the baby appears to be in shock and is not responding to resuscitation, administration of a volume expander may be indicated.

## What can you give to expand blood volume? How much should you give? How can you give it?

The recommended solution for acutely treating hypovolemia is an isotonic crystalloid solution. Acceptable solutions include

- 0.9% NaCl (normal saline)

- Ringer's lactate

O Rh-negative packed red blood cells should be considered as part of the volume replacement when severe fetal anemia is documented or expected. If timely diagnosis permits, the donor unit can be cross-matched to the mother, who would be the source of any problematic antibody. Otherwise, it may be necessary to request emergency release of non–cross-matched O Rh-negative packed cells from your blood bank. However, volume should be administered cautiously in babies who are known to have chronic in utero anemia, as the baby's intravascular volume may be normal even though the hemoglobin level is low, and rapid administration of packed red blood cells could precipitate heart failure.

Volume expanders should not be routinely given during resuscitation in the absence of a history or indirect evidence of acute blood loss. Giving a large volume load to a baby whose myocardial function is already compromised by hypoxia can decrease cardiac output and further compromise the newborn.

> **Recommended solution =**
>
> Normal saline

The initial dose of the selected volume expander is 10 mL/kg. However, if the baby does not improve significantly after the first dose, you may need to give another aliquot of 10 mL/kg. In unusual cases of documented large blood loss, administration of additional volume might be considered.

> **Recommended dose =**
>
> 10 mL/kg

**Recommended route =**

**Umbilical vein**

**Recommended rate of administration =**

**Over 5-10 minutes**

If hypovolemia is suspected, fill a large syringe with normal saline or other volume expander while others on the team continue resuscitation. A volume expander must be given into the vascular system. The umbilical vein is usually the most accessible vein in a newborn. Other routes (eg, intraosseous) may be used, although this is more likely in a setting outside the nursery or delivery room. (See page 218.)

Acute hypovolemia, resulting in a need for resuscitation, should be corrected fairly quickly in most cases. Some evidence suggests that rapid administration of a volume expander in a newborn may result in intracranial hemorrhage, particularly in preterm babies; thus, it may be advisable to give the volume over a longer duration during resuscitation of a newborn of less than 30 weeks' gestational age. No clinical trials have been conducted to define an optimum infusion rate, but a steady infusion over 5 to 10 minutes is reasonable.

## Review

*(The answers are in the preceding section and at the end of the lesson.)*

10. What should you do approximately 1 minute after giving epinephrine? _____

11. If the baby's heart rate remains below 60 beats per minute, you can repeat the dose of epinephrine every _____ to _____ minutes.

12. If the baby's heart rate remains below 60 beats per minute after you have given epinephrine, you also should check to make sure that ventilation is producing adequate lung inflation, and that _____ are being done correctly.

13. If the baby appears to be in shock, or there is evidence of blood loss, and resuscitation is not resulting in improvement, you should consider giving _____ mL/kg of _____ by what route? _____

## How much time should you take to reach this point, and what should you do if there is still no improvement?

If the baby has been severely compromised, but all resuscitation efforts have gone smoothly, you should have reached the point of giving epinephrine relatively quickly. Carrying out each of the first 3 basic steps of resuscitation in sequence may take as little as 30 seconds each, with somewhat longer intervals of interruptions for evaluation once chest compressions have started. Also, additional time may be required

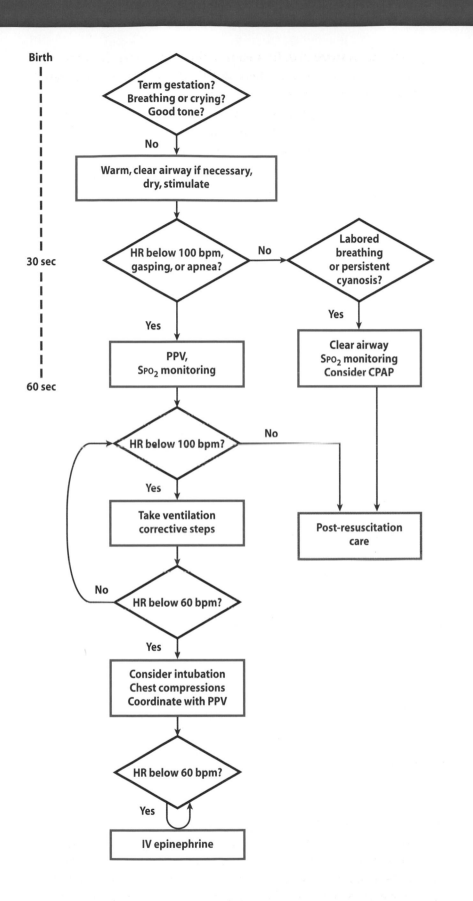

Birth

30 sec

60 sec

if corrective actions are needed to ensure that each step is being performed optimally before the next step is considered.

- Assessment and initial steps
- Positive-pressure ventilation
- Positive-pressure ventilation and chest compressions
- Positive-pressure ventilation, chest compressions, and epinephrine

Endotracheal intubation is often performed when resuscitation progresses to this point. You will have checked the efficacy of each of the steps, and considered the possibility of hypovolemia. If the heart rate is detectable but remains below 60 bpm, it is still possible that the baby will eventually respond to resuscitation, unless the baby is either extremely immature or has a severe congenital malformation. If you are certain that effective ventilation, chest compressions, and medications are being provided, you might then consider mechanical causes of poor response, such as an airway malformation, pneumothorax, diaphragmatic hernia, or congenital heart disease (discussed in Lesson 7).

If the heart rate is absent, or no progress is being made in certain conditions, such as extreme prematurity, it may be appropriate to consider discontinuing resuscitative efforts. How long to continue resuscitation efforts and the ethical considerations involved in deciding whether to discontinue resuscitation will be discussed in Lesson 9.

## Key Points

1. Epinephrine is a cardiac stimulant that also increases blood pressure. Preferably, it should be given by umbilical venous catheter. Its administration is indicated when the heart rate remains below 60 beats per minute despite 30 seconds of effective assisted ventilation, and administration should be followed by another 45 to 60 seconds of coordinated chest compressions and ventilations.

2. Recommended epinephrine
   - Concentration: 1:10,000 (0.1 mg/mL)
   - Route: Intravenously. Endotracheal administration may be considered while intravenous access is being established.
   - Dose: 0.1 to 0.3 mL/kg of a 1:10,000 concentration solution (consider higher dose, 0.5 to 1 mL/kg, for endotracheal route only)
   - Rate: *Rapidly*—as quickly as possible

3. Epinephrine should be given by umbilical vein. Administration via the endotracheal route is often faster and more accessible than placing an umbilical catheter, but is associated with unreliable absorption and is very likely not to be effective.

**4.** Indications for volume expansion during resuscitation include
* Baby is not responding to resuscitation.

AND
* Baby appears in shock (pale color, weak pulses, persistently low heart rate, no improvement in circulatory status despite resuscitation efforts).

OR
* There is a history of a condition associated with fetal blood loss (eg, extensive vaginal bleeding, placenta previa, twin-to-twin transfusion, etc).

**5.** Recommended volume expander
* Solution: Normal saline, Ringer's lactate, or O Rh-negative blood
* Dose: 10 mL/kg
* Route: Umbilical vein
* Preparation: Correct volume drawn into a large syringe
* Rate: Over 5 to 10 minutes

## Lesson 6 Review

*(The answers follow.)*

**1.** Fewer than _____% of babies requiring resuscitation will need epinephrine to stimulate their hearts.

**2.** As soon as you suspect that medications may be needed during a resuscitation, one member of the team should begin to insert a(n) _____ _____ to deliver the drug(s).

**3.** Effective ventilation and coordinated chest compressions have been performed for 45 to 60 seconds, the trachea has been intubated, and the baby's heart rate is below 60 beats per minute. You should now give _____ while continuing chest compressions and _____.

**4.** What is the potential problem with administering epinephrine through an endotracheal tube? _____

**5.** You should follow an intravenous dose of epinephrine with a flush of _____ to ensure that most of the drug is delivered to the baby and not left in the catheter.

## Lesson 6 Review—*continued*

6. Epinephrine (increases) (decreases) the blood pressure and strength of cardiac contractions and (increases) (decreases) the rate of cardiac contractions.

7. The recommended concentration of epinephrine for newborns is (1:1,000) (1:10,000).

8. The recommended dose of epinephrine for newborns is _____ to _____ mL/kg, if given intravenously, and _____ to _____ mL/kg, if given endotracheally, of a 1:10,000 solution.

9. Epinephrine should be given (slowly) (as quickly as possible).

10. What should you do approximately 1 minute after giving epinephrine? _____

11. If the baby's heart rate remains below 60 beats per minute, you can repeat the dose of epinephrine every _____ to _____ minutes.

12. If the baby's heart rate remains below 60 beats per minute after you have given epinephrine, you also should check to make sure that ventilation is producing adequate lung inflation, and that _____ are being done correctly.

13. If the baby appears to be in shock, there is evidence of blood loss, and resuscitation is not resulting in improvement, you should consider giving _____ mL/kg of _____ by what route? _____

## Answers to Questions

1. Fewer than **1**% of babies requiring resuscitation will need epinephrine to stimulate their hearts.

2. One member of the team should begin to insert an **umbilical venous catheter** when you anticipate that drugs will be needed.

## Answers to Questions—*continued*

3. You should give **epinephrine** while continuing chest compressions and **ventilation.**

4. **Epinephrine is not reliably absorbed in the lungs when given by the endotracheal route. A higher dose (0.5 to 1 mL/kg) should be considered if epinephrine is given via the endotracheal tube while umbilical venous access is being established.**

5. You should follow an intravenous injection of epinephrine with a flush of **normal saline.**

6. Epinephrine **increases** the blood pressure and strength of cardiac contractions and **increases** the strength and rate of cardiac contractions.

7. The recommended concentration of epinephrine for newborns is **1:10,000.**

8. The recommended dose of epinephrine for newborns is **0.1** to **0.3** mL/kg, if given intravenously, of a 1:10,000 solution. The recommended dose of epinephrine, if given endotracheally, is **0.5** to **1** mL/kg of a 1:10,000 solution.

9. Epinephrine should be given **as quickly as possible.**

10. You should **check the heart rate** approximately 60 seconds after giving epinephrine.

11. If the baby's heart rate remains below 60 beats per minute, you can repeat the dose of epinephrine every **3** to **5** minutes.

12. Check to make sure that ventilation is producing adequate lung inflation, and that **chest compressions** are being done correctly.

13. Consider giving **10** mL/kg of **volume expander** by **umbilical vein.**

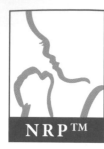

NRP™

# Lesson 6: Medication Administration via Endotracheal Tube and Emergency Umbilical Venous Catheter

# Performance Checklist

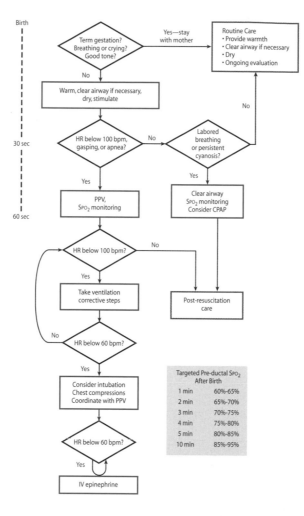

| Targeted Pre-ductal SPO₂ After Birth | |
|---|---|
| 1 min | 60%-65% |
| 2 min | 65%-70% |
| 3 min | 70%-75% |
| 4 min | 75%-80% |
| 5 min | 80%-85% |
| 10 min | 85%-95% |

**The Performance Checklist Is a Learning Tool**

The learner uses the checklist as a reference during independent practice or as a guide for discussion and practice with a Neonatal Resuscitation Program™ (NRP™) instructor. When the learner and instructor agree that the learner can perform the skills correctly and smoothly without coaching and within the context of a scenario, the learner may move on to the next lesson's Performance Checklist.

**Knowledge Check**

- What are the indications for epinephrine?

- What are the 2 routes? What are the 2 doses? Which route is preferred?

- What are indications for volume administration? What is used and what is the dose?

- How far is the emergency umbilical venous catheter (UVC) inserted into the vein?

**Learning Objectives**

1. Identify the newborn who requires epinephrine and/or volume during resuscitation.

2. Demonstrate correct technique for drawing up epinephrine.

3. Demonstrate correct technique for preparing/inserting an emergency UVC.

4. Demonstrate correct technique for administering epinephrine via endotracheal tube and UVC.

5. Demonstrate behavioral skills to ensure clear communication and teamwork during this critical component of newborn resuscitation.

**"You are called to attend the emergency cesarean birth of a baby whose mother has sustained injuries in an automobile crash. Paramedics report intermittent detection of a "low fetal heart rate." How would you prepare for the resuscitation of this baby? As you work, say your thoughts and actions aloud so your assistant and I will know what you are thinking and doing."**

This is a complex resuscitation. The learner and instructor decide how best to meet the learner's objectives. All learners taking Lesson 6 should know the correct concentration and dosage of epinephrine for both intratracheal and intravenous epinephrine. The learner and instructor may decide which additional skills are learning objectives: drawing up epinephrine, administering the medication, preparing and assisting with UVC insertion, and placing the UVC. Scope of practice may limit who may insert an umbilical catheter and order medication in the actual birth setting. The learner who is practicing medication administration and/or the leader of this resuscitation is not expected to perform all tasks, but may delegate tasks as required.

| Participant Name: | | |
|---|---|---|
| **Sample Vital Signs** | **Performance Steps** | **Details** |
| | ☐ Obtains relevant perinatal history | Gestational age? Fluid clear? How many babies? Other risk factors? |
| | ☐ Performs equipment check<br>☐ Assembles resuscitation team (preferably 2-3 other people) and discusses plan and roles<br>☐ Based on risk factors, team may prepare items needs for complex resuscitation | **Warm, Clear airway, Auscultate, Oxygenate, Ventilate, Intubate, Medicate, Thermoregulate.**<br><br>If there is time, team may prepare for intubation, umbilical venous catheter (UVC) placement, and medication/volume. |
| | **"The baby has just been born."** | |
| Term, Limp Apneic, Pale | Completes initial assessment when baby is born<br>☐ Asks 3 questions:<br>Term? Tone? Crying or breathing? | |
| | ☐ Receives baby at radiant warmer | |
| | ☐ Performs initial steps | Warm, position airway, dry, remove wet linen, stimulate. |
| Respiratory Rate (RR)-apneic<br>Heart Rate (HR)-30 beats per minute (bpm) | ☐ Evaluates respirations and heart rate | Auscultate pulse or palpates umbilicus. |
| | ☐ Initiates positive-pressure ventilation (PPV) at 40-60 breaths per minute<br>☐ Calls for additional help if necessary<br>☐ Requests pulse oximetry | Begins with ___% oxygen per hospital protocol at about 20 cm $H_2O$ pressure. |
| RR-apneic<br>HR-40 bpm<br>$SPO_2$ - - - -<br>No breath sounds or chest movement | ☐ Requests assessment of heart rate, pulse oximetry<br>☐ If not rising, requests assessment of bilateral breath sounds and chest movement | Pulse oximetry not functioning at low HR. Assistant must auscultate or palpate heart rate. |
| | ☐ Takes ventilation corrective steps | **MR SOPA** |

| Sample Vital Signs | Performance Steps | Details |
|---|---|---|
| + chest movement<br>+ breath sounds<br>HR-30 bpm<br>$SPO_2$ - - - - | ☐ Requests evaluation of chest movement and breath sounds<br>☐ Evaluates heart rate and pulse oximetry | Ventilation corrective steps may result in chest movement and bilateral breath sounds at any point in the sequence. |
| | ☐ Administers PPV by mask for 30 seconds | |
| HR-40 bpm<br>$SPO_2$ - - - -<br>+ chest movement<br>+ breath sounds | ☐ Evaluates heart rate and pulse oximetry | HR remains <60 bpm despite 30 seconds of effective ventilation. |
| | ☐ Requests chest compressions<br>☐ Increases oxygen to 100%<br>☐ Indicates need for intubation<br>☐ Directs assistant to continue monitoring HR and $SPO_2$ (when $SPO_2$ functioning) | Chest compressions begin as intubator prepares equipment. |
| | ☐ Requests pause in chest compressions (CC) while intubation occurs<br>☐ Takes corrective actions if signs of correct placement are not evident | If correct placement of endotracheal (ET) tube not evident: Repeat confirmation steps;<br>Check tip-to-lip measurement;<br>Reinsert laryngoscope and visualize placement;<br>Remove ET tube and ventilate with mask;<br>Repeat intubation or consider laryngeal mask airway. |
| | ☐ CC resume after tube placement is confirmed<br>☐ CC and ventilations continue for at least 45-60 seconds | Compressor may move to head of bed after intubation to increase access to umbilicus for UVC placement. |
| HR-40 bpm<br>$SPO_2$-63% | ☐ Evaluates HR and pulse oximetry | Assistant monitors HR and $SPO_2$ (if possible) throughout procedure. |
| | ☐ Requests epinephrine via ET tube while UVC is being placed<br>☐ Estimates baby's weight<br>☐ Orders dose of medication and route<br>☐ Asks medication person to repeat medication order (if necessary)<br>☐ Confirms that order was correctly received | Example: Leader states,<br>"The baby weighs about 3 kg. Let's give 3 mL of 1:10,000 epinephrine down the endotracheal tube."<br>Medication person repeats, "3 mL of 1:10,000 epinephrine down the ET tube."<br>Leader: "That's right." |
| | ☐ Draws up 1:10,000 epinephrine:<br>• Checks medication label<br>• Opens box<br>• Flips off yellow caps<br>• Twists 2 pieces together<br>• Removes needle guard cap<br>• Attaches 3-way stopcock or Luer lock syringe connector<br>• Attaches proper-size syringe to connector<br>• Draws up correct volume<br>• Labels syringe correctly | Use a 5- or 6-mL syringe for intratracheal dose. |

| Sample Vital Signs | Performance Steps | Details |
|---|---|---|
| | ☐ Administers intratracheal epinephrine<br>• Verbalizes medication, dose, and intended route<br>• Receives medication order confirmation<br>• Removes PPV device from ET tube<br>• Quickly gives drug directly into the tube<br>• Re-attaches PPV device to ET tube<br>• Announces that medication is in and may document dose, route, time, and response on code sheet | Example:<br>"I have 3 mL of 1:10,000 epinephrine for the ET tube."<br><br>If $CO_2$ detector gets wet, it is no longer reliable.<br><br>May repeat epinephrine every 3-5 minutes. |
| | ☐ Prepares emergency UVC<br>• Obtains syringe with normal saline<br>• Attaches 3-way stopcock to UVC<br>• Flushes UVC and stopcock with saline<br>• Closes stopcock to catheter | (if not already done with equipment check) |
| | ☐ Inserts emergency UVC<br>• Preps the base and lower 2 cm of the cord with antiseptic solution<br>• Ties umbilical tape loosely on skin around base of cord<br>• Cuts cord straight across not more than 2 cm above abdomen<br>• Inserts catheter into vein 2-4 cm<br>• Opens stopcock between baby and syringe and gently aspirates syringe to detect blood return<br>• Advances catheter until blood return is detected<br>• Clears any air from catheter and stopcock | Assistant may need to hold umbilicus up off abdomen with forceps or other instrument to allow cleaning, tying, and cutting of the umbilical cord.<br><br>Ensure that team is aware when scalpel enters the field.<br><br>Use sterile technique to the best of your ability under emergency circumstances. |
| HR-40 bpm<br>$SpO_2$-63%<br>+ breath sounds<br>+ chest movement | ☐ Evaluates HR and pulse oximetry<br>☐ May also re-evaluate effectiveness of ventilation | Re-evaluate heart rate and effectiveness of ventilation before each dose of epinephrine every 3 to 5 minutes. |
| | ☐ Requests epinephrine via UVC<br>☐ Estimates baby's weight<br>☐ States medication, desired dose, and route<br>☐ Asks medication person to repeat medication order (if necessary)<br>☐ Confirms that order was correctly received | Example:<br>Leader states,<br>"The baby is about 3 kg. Let's give 0.9 mL of 1:10,000 epinephrine through the UVC."<br>Medication person repeats, "0.9 mL of 1:10,000 epinephrine through the UVC."<br>Leader: "That's right." |
| | ☐ Administers epinephrine via UVC<br>• Attaches proper-sized syringe (1-mL syringe) to connector<br>• Draws up correct volume of medication<br>• Labels syringe correctly | |

| Sample Vital Signs | Performance Steps | Details |
|---|---|---|
| | ☐ Administers epinephrine via UVC<br>• Verbalizes medication, dose, and intended route<br>• Receives confirmation<br>• Ensures that catheter is being held in place; attaches syringe to stopcock and gives rapidly without air bubbles<br>• Flushes with .5 to 1 mL of normal saline<br>Announces, "epinephrine is in" and may document dose, route, time, and response on code sheet | |
| | ☐ Monitors HR and pulse oximetry (if functioning)<br>☐ Continues PPV and CC for at least 45-60 seconds after giving epinephrine | |
| HR-70 bpm<br>SpO$_2$-67%<br>RR-first gasps<br>Pale, poor perfusion | ☐ Evaluates HR and pulse oximetry in relation to baby's age<br>☐ Discontinues CC | |
| | ☐ Requests volume expander<br>• Reiterates estimated weight<br>• Orders 10 mL/kg of normal saline per UVC over 5-10 minutes<br>• Receives medication order confirmation<br>• Confirms that order was correctly received | Example:<br>Leader states,<br>"The baby is about 3 kg. Let's give 30 mL of normal saline through the UVC over 5-10 minutes."<br>Medication person repeats, "30 mL of normal saline through the UVC over 5-10 minutes."<br>Leader: "That's right." |
| | ☐ Administers normal saline per UVC<br>• Draws up correct volume normal saline or uses prefilled syringes. Numbers more than one syringe (#1, #2)<br>• Verbalizes medication, dose, and route<br>• Receives confirmation<br>• Ensures that catheter is being held in place; attaches syringe #1 to stopcock; gives entire dose in constant slow infusion over 5-10 minutes with no bubbles<br>• Announces that medication is in, and may document dose, route, time, and response on code sheet | |
| Respirations-occasional gasp<br>HR-120 bpm<br>SpO$_2$-74% | ☐ After 30 seconds of PPV with ET tube, checks respiratory effort, HR, and SpO$_2$<br>☐ Adjusts oxygen based on oximetry and newborn's age | |

| Sample Vital Signs | Performance Steps | Details |
|---|---|---|
| RR-occasional gasp<br>HR-140 bpm<br>$SpO_2$-97% | ☐ May continue PPV for 30 additional seconds to help ensure stability prior to transport to nursery<br>☐ Adjust oxygen based on oximetry and newborn's age<br>☐ Make a team decision to<br>• Update family<br>• Secure ET tube<br>• Secure or remove UVC<br>• Move to post-resuscitation care | |

**Instructor asks the learner Reflective Questions to enable self-assessment, such as the following:**

**1** What went well during this resuscitation?

**2** Who assumed the leadership role in this scenario? What skills did you use to ensure that your assistants understood what you needed? Give me an example of what you did or said that used that behavioral skill.

**3** As the assistant(s), what suggestions might you make (to the leader) to improve communication during a stressful resuscitation?

**4** Would you do anything differently when faced with this scenario again?

### Neonatal Resuscitation Program Key Behavioral Skills

| | |
|---|---|
| Know your environment. | Allocate attention wisely. |
| Anticipate and plan. | Use all available information. |
| Assume the leadership role. | Use all available resources. |
| Communicate effectively. | Call for help when needed. |
| Delegate workload optimally. | Maintain professional behavior. |

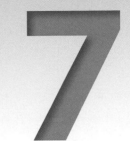

# Special Considerations

## In Lesson 7 you will learn about

- Special situations that may complicate resuscitation and cause ongoing problems

- Subsequent management of the baby who has required resuscitation

- How the principles in this program can be applied to babies who require resuscitation beyond the immediate newborn period or outside the hospital delivery room

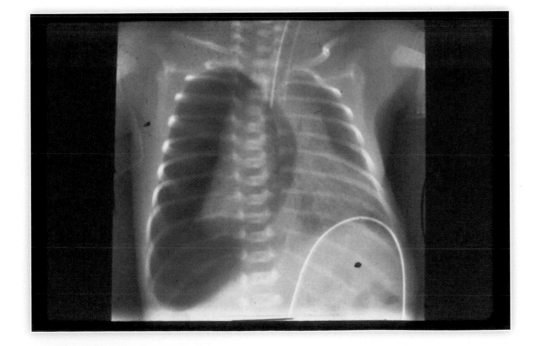

## What complications should you consider if the baby still is not doing well after initial attempts at resuscitation?

You have learned that nearly all compromised newborns will respond to appropriate stimulation and measures to improve ventilation. A few may require chest compressions and medications to improve, and a very small number will die, despite all appropriate resuscitation measures.

However, another small group of newborns will respond initially to resuscitation, but then remain compromised. These babies may have been born very preterm, may have a congenital malformation or infection, or may have experienced a complication of birth or resuscitation. Sometimes, you will know about the problem before birth because of an antepartum ultrasound or some other method of antenatal diagnosis.

The continuing difficulty you encounter will be different for every baby, depending on the underlying problem.

The most effective approach for babies who do not continue to improve after resuscitation will depend on their specific clinical presentation.

- Does positive-pressure ventilation (PPV) fail to result in adequate ventilation of the lungs?

- Does the baby remain bradycardic or hypoxemic, despite effective ventilation?

- Does the baby fail to begin spontaneous respirations?

Each of these 3 questions will be addressed separately.

## What if positive-pressure ventilation with a mask fails to result in adequate ventilation of the lungs?

Recall the MR SOPA acronym to ensure adequate ventilation (see page 95). If you have ensured a tight seal between the mask and the baby's face (M), repositioned the baby's head correctly in the "sniffing" position (R), cleared the airway by suctioning (S), opened the mouth slightly (O), and used sufficient pressure (P) to provide PPV, the heart rate, color, and oximetry reading should improve. If the baby is still bradycardic, you should assure yourself that there is perceptible chest movement with each positive-pressure breath and, when you listen to the lungs with a stethoscope, you should hear good airflow in and out of the baby's lungs. A carbon dioxide ($CO_2$) detector placed between the mask and the PPV device may be helpful in confirming that ventilation is being provided.

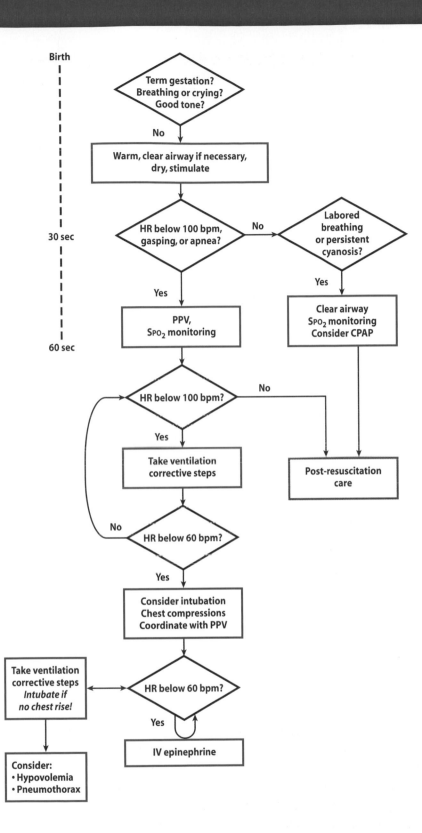

If you fail to see chest movement and do not hear good airflow, or a $CO_2$ detector does not confirm the presence of $CO_2$ with each exhalation, you should be doing all you can to establish an alternative airway (A) by intubating the trachea or inserting a laryngeal mask airway to establish good air movement by direct ventilation of the lungs. If you have taken all the steps of MR SOPA (Mask adjustment,

Reposition airway, Suction mouth and nose, Open mouth, Pressure increase, Airway alternative) and still are unable to detect good air movement, there may be other factors present that are interfering with establishing effective ventilation. While these factors are not commonly seen, you should be aware of the possibilities.

### Blockage of the airway

*Choanal atresia*

The anatomy of a baby's airway requires the nasal passages to be patent for air to reach the lungs during spontaneous breathing. Babies cannot breathe easily through their mouths unless they are actively crying. Therefore, if the nasal airway is filled with mucus or meconium, or if the nasal airway did not form properly (eg, choanal atresia), the baby will have severe respiratory distress (Figure 7.1). Although choanal atresia generally will not prevent you from ventilating the baby with positive pressure through the oropharynx, the baby may not be able to move air spontaneously through the blocked nasopharynx.

Test for choanal atresia by passing a small-caliber suction catheter into the posterior pharynx through one, and then the other, naris. Direct the catheter perpendicular to the baby's face so that it will travel along the floor of the nasal passageway. If the catheter will not pass when directed correctly, choanal atresia may be present. You will need to insert a plastic oral airway to allow air to pass through the mouth (Figure 7.2), or you may use an endotracheal tube as the oral airway, passing it through the mouth so that the tip of the tube reaches the posterior pharynx, without inserting it all the way into the trachea.

Congenital obstruction
of posterior nasopharynx

oral airway

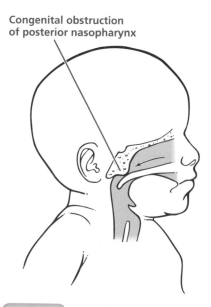

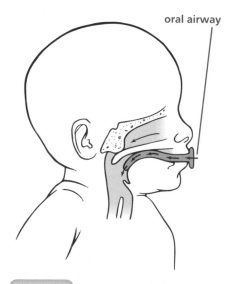

**Figure 7.1.** Choanal atresia with congenital blockage of the nasal airway

**Figure 7.2.** Temporary relief of nasal blockage by placement of an oral airway

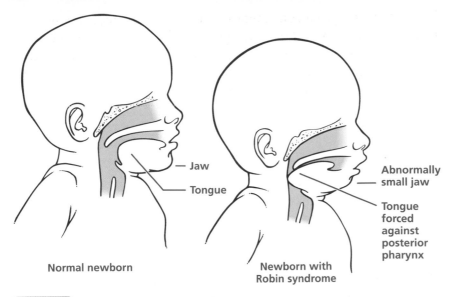

**Figure 7.3.** Newborn with normal anatomy (left) and newborn with Robin syndrome (right)

*Jaw*

*Tongue*

*Abnormally small jaw*

*Tongue forced against posterior pharynx*

**Normal newborn**

**Newborn with Robin syndrome**

### *Pharyngeal airway malformation (Robin syndrome)*

Some babies are born with a very small mandible, which results in a critical narrowing of the pharyngeal airway (Figure 7.3). During the first few months following birth, the mandible usually will grow to produce an adequate airway, but the baby may have considerable difficulty breathing immediately after birth. The main problem is that the posteriorly placed tongue falls far back into the pharynx and obstructs the airway just above the larynx.

If you suspect that the baby has this problem, your first action should be to turn the baby onto his stomach (prone). In this position, the tongue usually falls forward, thus opening the airway. If positioning is not successful, the next most effective means of achieving an airway for a baby with Robin syndrome is to insert a large catheter (12F) or small endotracheal tube (2.5 mm) through the nose, with the tip located deep in the posterior pharynx, past the base of the tongue, but not into the trachea; a laryngoscope is not required to do this (Figure 7.4). These 2 procedures (turning the baby prone and inserting a nasopharyngeal tube) usually permit the baby to move air well on his own without the need for endotracheal intubation, which may be quite difficult in this condition.

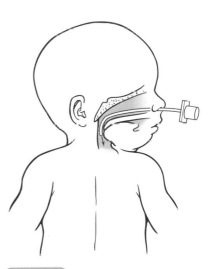

**Figure 7.4.** Relief of airway obstruction in a newborn with Robin syndrome by placement of a nasopharyngeal tube and placing the baby prone

> **!** It usually is very difficult to place an endotracheal tube into the trachea of a baby with Robin syndrome. Prone positioning and a nasopharyngeal tube are often sufficient to maintain the airway until more definitive treatment can be instituted.

If none of these procedures results in adequate air movement, and attempts at endotracheal intubation are unsuccessful, some clinicians have found placement of a laryngeal mask airway to be effective. (See Lesson 5.)

### Other rare conditions

Congenital malformations, such as laryngeal webs, cystic hygroma, or congenital goiter, have been reported as rare causes of airway compromise in the newborn. Most, but not all, of these malformations will be evident by external examination of the baby, and special expertise may be required for placement of an endotracheal tube or an emergency tracheostomy. If such problems are identified antenatally, the baby should be born in a facility where appropriate management of the airway is available in the delivery room.

## Impaired lung function

Lung function can be impaired because of intrinsic lung disease or because lung function is decreased due to extrinsic factors. Various abnormalities, such as intrathoracic air or fluid collections or masses, may prevent the lung from expanding within the chest. This causes respiratory distress and the baby may be persistently cyanotic and bradycardic despite adequate PPV.

### Pneumothorax

It is not uncommon for small air leaks to develop as the lung of the newborn fills with air. The likelihood is increased significantly if PPV is provided, particularly in the presence of meconium or a lung malformation, such as congenital diaphragmatic hernia. (See page 245.) Air that leaks from inside the lung and collects in the pleural space is called a pneumothorax (Figure 7.5). If the pneumothorax becomes large enough, the trapped air under tension can prevent the lung from expanding. It also can restrict blood flow to the lung, resulting in respiratory distress, oxygen desaturation, and bradycardia.

Breath sounds will be diminished on the side of the pneumothorax. Definitive diagnosis can be made with an x-ray. Transillumination of the chest may be helpful as a screening procedure. This involves holding a bright transillumination light against the chest wall on one side and comparing the transmission of light through the tissues with that on the other side (Figure 7.6). During transillumination, the side of the baby's chest that has the pneumothorax will appear brighter than the contralateral side. Be careful when interpreting the

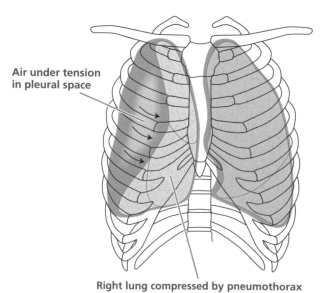

Air under tension in pleural space

Right lung compressed by pneumothorax

**Figure 7.5.** Pneumothorax compromising lung function

results of transillumination in very premature babies, because their thin skin may cause the chest to appear bright bilaterally even in the absence of a pneumothorax.

If a pneumothorax causes significant respiratory distress, it should be relieved by placing a percutaneous catheter or needle into the pleural space and evacuating the air. (See the following section.) A small pneumothorax usually will resolve spontaneously and often does not require treatment. In the case of a large pneumothorax, or if the baby has ongoing respiratory distress and/or low oxygen saturation (SpO$_2$), even after evacuation of the pneumothorax as described, placement of a tube to continually drain the air by suction (thoracostomy tube) by someone with appropriate training may be required.

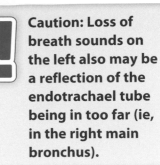

> **Caution: Loss of breath sounds on the left also may be a reflection of the endotrachael tube being in too far (ie, in the right main bronchus).**

> **If a baby has worsening bradycardia and decreasing SpO$_2$, and has asymmetric breath sounds after initial resuscitation, you may decide to emergently insert a percutaneous catheter or needle into the chest on the side of the decreased breath sounds and apply gentle suction to see if air can be evacuated while waiting for results of a chest x-ray.**

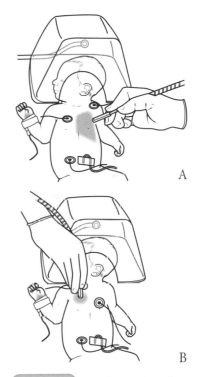

### Pleural effusions

In rare circumstances, edema fluid, chyle (lymph fluid), or blood collects in the pleural space of a newborn and prevents the lungs from adequately expanding. Collections of fluid within the pleural space cause the same symptoms as a pneumothorax. Often, other signs of problems, such as generalized edema (hydrops fetalis), are present in such newborns.

Confirmation of the presence of air or fluid in the pleural space can be made by x-ray. If respiratory distress is significant, you may need to insert a percutaneous catheter or needle into the pleural space to drain the air or fluid, as described for evacuating a pneumothorax.

### How do you evacuate a pneumothorax or pleural effusion?

The air may be aspirated by inserting a needle into either the fourth intercostal space at the anterior axillary line or the second intercostal space at the mid-clavicular line on the suspected side. (See "X" positions in Figure 7.7.) First, the baby should be turned with the aspiration site superior, to allow the air to rise.

**Figure 7.6.** Transillumination of a pneumothorax. Positive transillumination on the baby's left side (A), negative transillumination on the right (B). (Used with permission from Kattwinkel J, Cook LJ, Hurt H, Nowacek GA, Short JG, Crosby WM, eds. *Neonatal Care*. Elk Grove Village, IL: American Academy of Pediatrics; 2007:151, 221, 228. *PCEP Perinatal Continuing Education Program*; book 2.)

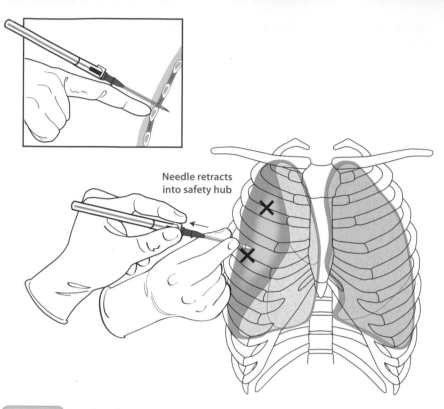

Figure 7.7.
Note that the needle enters just above the rib, so as to avoid the artery lying just under the rib above.

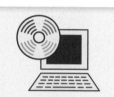

**You are encouraged to view this video on the DVD that accompanies this textbook:**
*Needle Thoracentesis*

An 18- or 20-gauge percutaneous catheter-over-needle device is inserted perpendicular to the chest wall and just over the top of the rib. The needle is placed just over the lower rib, rather than just below the upper rib, to avoid puncturing one of the intercostal arteries (Figure 7.7).

The needle is then removed from the catheter, and a 3-way stopcock connected to a 20-mL syringe is connected to the catheter (Figure 7.8). The stopcock is then opened between the syringe and the catheter, and the syringe is used to aspirate air or fluid. When the syringe is full, the stopcock may be closed to the chest while the syringe is emptied. The stopcock then may be reopened to the chest and more fluid or air may be aspirated until the baby's condition has improved. To avoid accidental reinjection of air or fluid into the chest cavity, care should be taken when manipulating the stopcock. An x-ray

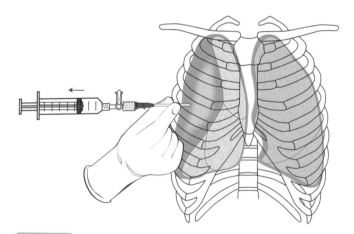

Figure 7.8. Insertion of a percutaneous catheter for drainage of a pneumothorax or pleural fluid (see text). The needle may be placed at either of the "X" marks shown in Figure 7.7, but should always be perpendicular to the chest surface. Note that the needle present in Figure 7.7 has been removed and only the catheter remains in the pleural space.

should be obtained to document the presence or absence of residual pneumothorax or effusion.

If an appropriate-gauge percutaneous catheter is not available, a 19- or 21-gauge butterfly needle may be used. In this case, the stopcock can be connected directly to the tubing of the butterfly needle. However, there is a small possibility of puncturing the lung with the butterfly needle as fluid or air is being aspirated.

### Congenital diaphragmatic hernia

The diaphragm normally separates the abdominal contents from the thoracic contents. When the diaphragm does not form completely, some of the abdominal contents (usually the intestines and the stomach, and sometimes the liver) enter the chest and prevent the lungs and its associated microvasculature from developing normally (Figure 7.9). A diaphragmatic hernia often can be diagnosed by ultrasound before birth. Without antenatal diagnosis, the baby with a diaphragmatic hernia may present at birth with completely unanticipated respiratory distress.

A baby with a diaphragmatic hernia typically presents with severe respiratory distress and often has an unusually flat-appearing (scaphoid) abdomen, because the abdomen has less contents than normal. Breath sounds may be diminished on the side of the hernia, or you may actually hear bowel sounds in the baby's chest. These babies often have pulmonary hypertension because of congenital abnormalities of the pulmonary blood vessels and, therefore, may remain persistently cyanotic from poor pulmonary blood flow. Abnormal lung structure also may contribute to hypoxemia in these babies.

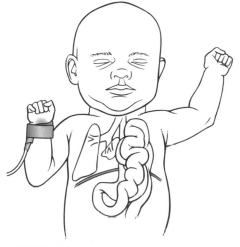

**Figure 7.9.** Compromised lung function from presence of a congenital diaphragmatic hernia

When the baby is born, the abnormal lungs cannot expand normally. If positive pressure is delivered by mask during resuscitation, some of the positive-pressure gas enters the stomach and intestines. Because the intestines are in the chest, lung inflation is increasingly inhibited. In addition, positive pressure may result in a pneumothorax because of the structural lung abnormalities.

 **Babies with known or suspected diaphragmatic hernia should not receive prolonged resuscitation with positive pressure by mask, or air will inflate the intestines in the chest. Intubate the trachea expeditiously and place a large orogastric catheter (10F) to evacuate the stomach contents (Figure 7.10). A double-lumen sump tube (Replogle tube) is most effective.**

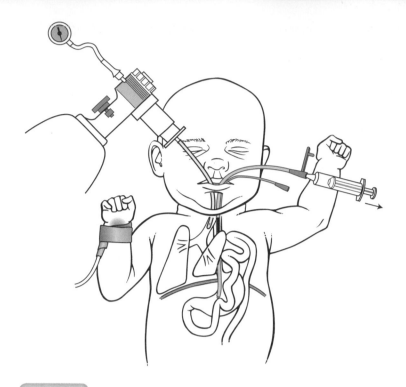

**Figure 7.10.** Stabilizing treatment for a baby with diaphragmatic hernia (endotracheal tube in trachea and Replogle tube in stomach). Replogle tube should be aspirated intermittently with a syringe or connected to vacuum. Both tubes should be secured to the face, but taping is not shown in this figure so as not to obscure other details in the figure.

### Pulmonary hypoplasia

Normal lung development requires the presence of amniotic fluid. Any condition that causes severe oligohydramnios (decreased amniotic fluid), such as renal agenesis, may result in poorly developed lungs (ie, pulmonary hypoplasia). High inflation pressures will be required to provide adequate ventilation in babies with this problem, and pneumothoraces are common. Severe pulmonary hypoplasia usually is incompatible with survival.

### Extreme immaturity

Extremely preterm babies may be very difficult to ventilate, because of structurally immature lungs and absence of pulmonary surfactant. High inflation pressures initially may be required to inflate the lungs during PPV, although continued high pressures should be avoided in immature lungs. (See Lesson 8.)

### Congenital pneumonia

Although congenital pneumonia usually presents as worsening lung disease after birth, some overwhelming infections (such as group B streptococcal disease) may present as respiratory failure immediately after delivery. Also, aspiration of amniotic fluid, particularly if contaminated with meconium, can cause severe respiratory compromise.

## What if the baby remains cyanotic or bradycardic despite good ventilation?

If a baby remains bradycardic or cyanotic, with $SpO_2$ confirming low oxygen saturation in the blood, first ensure that the baby's chest is moving adequately and that you can hear good equal breath sounds on both sides of the chest. If you have not already done so, increase the concentration of oxygen to 100%. If the baby still is bradycardic and/or has low $SpO_2$, she may have congenital heart disease, although this diagnosis usually cannot be established in the delivery room unless it was made prenatally. Remember that congenital heart block or even cyanotic congenital heart disease are rare conditions, while inadequate ventilation following birth is a much more common cause of persistent oxygen desaturation and bradycardia.

 **Babies with congenital heart disease are seldom critically ill immediately following birth. Lack of response to resuscitation is almost always because of failure to ventilate the baby effectively.**

## What if the baby fails to begin spontaneous respirations?

If PPV has resulted in normal heart rate and $SpO_2$, but the baby does not breathe spontaneously, the baby may have depressed respiratory drive or muscle activity due to

- Brain injury (hypoxic-ischemic encephalopathy [HIE]), severe acidosis, or a congenital defect such as a structural abnormality of the brain or neuromuscular disorder

or

- Sedation due to drugs received by the mother and passed to the baby across the placenta

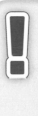 **Giving a narcotic antagonist is not the correct initial therapy for a baby who is not breathing. The first corrective action is to provide effective PPV.**

Narcotics given to the laboring mother to relieve pain may inhibit respiratory drive and activity in the newborn. In such cases, administration of naloxone (a narcotic antagonist) to the newborn will transiently reverse the effect of narcotics on the baby.

Administration of naloxone is not necessary as long as the baby can be adequately ventilated; however, improvement in respiratory effort after naloxone administration will confirm that the baby's respiratory depression was due to narcotic effects. Administration of naloxone may be considered in a baby with continued respiratory depression when there is a history of maternal narcotic administration within the past 4 hours.

After naloxone administration, continue to administer PPV until the baby is breathing normally. The duration of action of the narcotic often exceeds that of naloxone. Therefore, observe the baby closely for recurrent respiratory depression, which may necessitate ongoing respiratory support.

**Naloxone Hydrochloride**

**Recommended concentration =**

1.0-mg/mL solution

**Recommended route =**

Intravenous preferred; intramuscular acceptable, but delayed onset of action. There are no studies reporting the efficacy of endotracheal naloxone.

**Recommended dose =**

0.1 mg/kg

**Caution: Do not give naloxone to the newborn of a mother who is suspected of using narcotics or is on methadone maintenance. This may induce withdrawal seizures in the newborn.**

Other drugs given to the mother, such as magnesium sulfate or nonnarcotic analgesics or general anesthetics, also can depress respirations in the newborn; the effects of these drugs are not reversed by naloxone. If narcotics were not given to the mother or if naloxone does not result in restoring spontaneous respirations, transport the baby to the nursery for further evaluation and management while continuing to administer PPV and monitoring heart rate and pulse oximetry.

## Review

*(The answers are in the preceding section and at the end of the lesson.)*

1. Choanal atresia can be ruled out by what procedure? _____
_____

2. Babies with Robin syndrome and airway obstruction may be helped by placing a _____ and positioning the babies _____.
Endotracheal intubation of such babies is usually (easy) (difficult).

3. A pneumothorax or congenital diaphragmatic hernia should be considered if breath sounds are (equal) (unequal) on the 2 sides of the chest.

4. You should suspect a congenital diaphragmatic hernia if the abdomen is _____. Such babies should not be resuscitated with _____.

5. Persistent bradycardia and low SPo₂ during neonatal resuscitation most likely are caused by (heart problems) (inadequate ventilation).

6. Babies who do not have spontaneous respirations and whose mothers have been given narcotic drugs within 4 hours of delivery should first receive _____, and then, if spontaneous respirations do not begin, may be given _____ to confirm the cause of their respiratory depression.

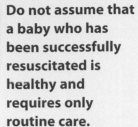

## What should you do after a baby has been successfully resuscitated?

Babies who required prolonged PPV, intubation, and/or chest compressions are likely to have been severely stressed and are at risk for multi-organ dysfunction that may not be immediately apparent.

Following resuscitation, some babies will breathe normally, some will have ongoing respiratory distress, and some will require continued assisted ventilation. All babies should have a heart rate above 100 beats per minute (bpm) and normal $SPO_2$.

If prolonged resuscitation was required, the baby needs to be kept in an environment where ongoing care can be provided. As described in Lesson 1, post-resuscitation care includes temperature control, close monitoring of vital signs (eg, heart rate, $SPO_2$, and blood pressure), and awareness of potential complications.

Laboratory studies, such as hematocrit and blood glucose levels, may need to be obtained to further assess the baby's status. Blood gas analysis also may be indicated. The extent of monitoring required and the location where monitoring is provided will depend on the specific details of the baby's presentation and availability of resources in your institution.

The likelihood of developing post-resuscitation complications increases with the length and extent of resuscitation required. The pH and base deficit determined from cord blood or from blood drawn from the baby soon after resuscitation may be helpful in estimating the extent of compromise.

> Do not assume that a baby who has been successfully resuscitated is healthy and requires only routine care.

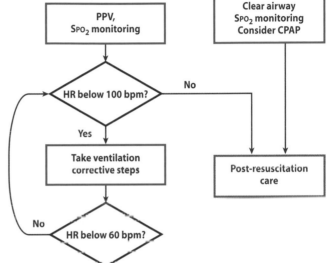

## What are common complications in babies who require prolonged/substantial resuscitation?

### Pulmonary hypertension

As explained in Lesson 1, the blood vessels in the lungs are tightly constricted in the fetus. Ventilation increases oxygen levels in the alveoli and causes the blood vessels to relax, thus increasing blood flow to the lungs and allowing the blood to pick up more oxygen.

The pulmonary blood vessels in babies who were hypoxemic and/or acidemic around the time of birth may remain constricted. This condition is called persistent pulmonary hypertension of the newborn (PPHN) and is most often seen in babies ≥34 weeks' gestational age, although, occasionally, it may occur in very low birthweight babies. Persistent pulmonary hypertension of the newborn usually is managed with supplemental oxygen therapy and, in most cases, mechanical ventilation to relax the pulmonary blood vessels and increase the baby's blood oxygen level. Severe pulmonary hypertension results in persistent, severe hypoxemia and may require therapies, such as inhaled nitric oxide and extracorporeal membrane oxygenation (ECMO), which can be provided only in tertiary care centers.

Exacerbation of pulmonary vasoconstriction may be prevented by avoiding episodes of hypoxemia after a baby has been resuscitated.

### Pneumonia and other lung complications

Babies who require resuscitation are at higher risk for developing pneumonia, either from aspiration syndrome or from a congenital infection that may have been responsible for the perinatal compromise. Neonatal pneumonia also is associated with pulmonary hypertension.

If a baby who required resuscitation continues to show signs of respiratory distress, or has a requirement for supplemental oxygen, consider evaluating the baby for pneumonia or sepsis and consider beginning parenteral antibiotics.

If acute respiratory deterioration occurs during or after resuscitation, consider the possibility that the baby may have developed a pneumothorax; or, if the baby has remained intubated after resuscitation, consider the possibility of a misplaced or obstructed endotracheal tube.

### Metabolic acidosis

The use of sodium bicarbonate during neonatal resuscitation is controversial. Its use may be helpful to correct metabolic acidosis that results from a buildup of lactic acid that may occur while the baby has hypoxemia and poor cardiac output. Lactic acid forms when tissues have insufficient oxygen. Severe acidosis causes the myocardium to contract poorly and causes the blood vessels of the lungs to constrict, thus decreasing pulmonary blood flow and preventing the lungs from adequately oxygenating the blood.

However, sodium bicarbonate can be harmful, particularly if given too early in a resuscitation. Use of sodium bicarbonate may increase the serum pH but can worsen intracellular acidosis. You must be certain that ventilation of the lungs is adequate before administering sodium bicarbonate. When sodium bicarbonate mixes with acid, $CO_2$ is formed. The lungs must be adequately ventilated to remove the $CO_2$.

**Use an oximeter and/or arterial blood gas determinations to be certain that a baby who required resuscitation remains adequately oxygenated.**

**Do not give sodium bicarbonate unless the lungs are being adequately ventilated.**

If you decide to give sodium bicarbonate, remember that it is very hypertonic and irritating to blood vessels and, therefore, must be given into a large vein, from which there is good blood return. The usual dose during resuscitation is 2 mEq/kg, given as a 4.2% solution (0.5 mEq/mL) at a rate no faster than 1 mEq/kg/min. Rapid administration of sodium bicarbonate has been implicated as a cause of intraventricular hemorrhage in preterm newborns; therefore, special care must be taken to administer it slowly in this population. (See Lesson 8.)

> ! Sodium bicarbonate is very caustic and is NEVER given through the endotracheal tube during resuscitation.

### Hypotension

Perinatal compromise can result in an insult to the heart muscle and/or result in decreased vascular tone, leading to hypotension. Heart murmurs often are audible from transient tricuspid insufficiency, which may be associated with decreased right ventricular output. If sepsis or blood loss is the reason that the baby required resuscitation, the effective circulating blood volume may be low, which also can contribute to hypotension.

Babies who require significant resuscitation should have heart rate and blood pressure monitoring until blood pressure and peripheral perfusion are normal and stable. Blood transfusion or other volume expansion may be indicated, as described in Lesson 6, and some babies may require an infusion of an inotropic agent, such as dopamine, to assist cardiac output and vascular tone if administration of an initial volume bolus does not result in normalization of blood pressure.

### Fluid management

After severe perinatal compromise, urine output, body weight, and serum electrolyte levels should be checked frequently for the first few days after birth. Perinatal compromise can result in renal dysfunction (eg, acute tubular necrosis [ATN]), which is usually transient, but can cause severe electrolyte abnormalities and fluid shifts. Consider checking the urine for signs of ATN, such as blood and/or protein in the urine, to rule out acute tubular necrosis. Electrolyte abnormalities also may increase the risk of cardiac arrhythmias.

Fluid and electrolyte intakes should be adjusted based on the baby's vital signs, urine output, and laboratory results. Because hypocalcemia may occur after perinatal asphyxia, supplemental calcium also may be required in these babies.

### Seizures or apnea

Newborns who have perinatal compromise and have required resuscitation may later manifest signs of HIE. Initially, the baby may have depressed muscle tone, but seizures may appear after several hours. Apnea or hypoventilation also may be a reflection of HIE. These same symptoms also may be a manifestation of metabolic abnormalities or electrolyte disturbances.

Babies who have required extensive resuscitation should be monitored closely for seizures and other neurologic abnormalities. For seizures thought to be associated with HIE, anticonvulsant therapy (such as phenobarbital) may be required.

### Hypoglycemia

Metabolism under conditions of oxygen deprivation, which may occur during perinatal compromise, consumes much more glucose than the same metabolism occurring in the presence of adequate oxygen. Although, initially, catecholamine secretion causes elevated serum glucose levels, glucose stores (glycogen) are depleted rapidly during perinatal stress, and hypoglycemia may result. Because glucose is an essential fuel for brain function in newborns, prolonged hypoglycemia may contribute to neurologic dysfunction after resuscitation.

Babies who require resuscitation need their blood glucose levels checked soon after resuscitation and then at regular intervals until several values are within normal limits and adequate glucose intake is ensured. Intravenous glucose is often necessary to maintain normal blood glucose levels, especially in babies who are not able to take oral feedings.

### Feeding problems

The gastrointestinal tract of a newborn is very sensitive to hypoxia-ischemia. Ileus, gastrointestinal bleeding, and even necrotizing enterocolitis can result. Also, because of neurologic dysfunction after resuscitation, sucking patterns and coordination of sucking, swallowing, and breathing may take several days to become normal. Intravenous fluids and nutrition will be required during this time.

### Temperature management

**!** Hyperthermia (overheating) can be very injurious to a baby. Be careful not to overheat the baby during or following resuscitation.

Babies who have been resuscitated can become cold for a variety of reasons. Special techniques for maintaining normal body temperature in premature babies are addressed in Lesson 8. Other babies (in particular, those born to mothers with chorioamnionitis) may have an elevated temperature in the delivery room. Since hyperthermia is associated with adverse outcomes in newborns, it is important not to overheat the baby during and following resuscitation. Babies' temperatures should be maintained in the normal range.

**Therapeutic hypothermia**

Recent studies have demonstrated that therapeutic hypothermia (body temperature of 33.5°C-34.5°C), instituted after resuscitation, improves neurologic outcomes in some late preterm and term babies with moderate to severe hypoxic-ischemic encephalopathy (HIE). Implementation of therapeutic post-asphyxial hypothermia must be guided by the degree of asphyxial insult and the time elapsed since the insult occurred. Based on published clinical trials, the following criteria should be applied when considering whether a baby is a candidate for therapeutic hypothermia post-resuscitation:

1. Gestational age ≥36 weeks

2. Evidence of an acute perinatal hypoxic-ischemic event

3. Ability to initiate hypothermia within 6 hours after birth

Use of therapeutic hypothermia in babies with HIE requires access to specialized equipment for inducing and maintaining hypothermia, and the ability to diagnose and treat seizures and other complications of asphyxia. A well-defined protocol for inducing and maintaining hypothermia is essential for avoiding hypothermia-related complications. If your hospital does not have an established program to provide therapeutic hypothermia in newborns, you should contact the closest center that provides this therapy as soon as you suspect that a baby born in your hospital may be a candidate for this therapy. Delaying the initial inquiry could mean that therapeutic hypothermia could not be initiated within the currently established therapeutic window.

If the decision is made to transport the baby to another center for this treatment, you should take steps to avoid unintentional hyperthermia while waiting for transport, including unwrapping the baby and uncovering her head. If the baby is under a radiant warmer, the warmer should be set to the servo control setting and slightly below the norm of 36.5°C, or the regional center may suggest that you turn off the radiant heat while you discuss the plan for stabilization pending transport.

Anticipated problems and management options post-resuscitation are summarized in Table 7-1.

> **!** Current evidence suggests that therapeutic hypothermia must be initiated within 6 hours of birth to be effective.

**Table 7-1.** Possible organ system injury following resuscitation and therapeutic measures

| Organ System | Potential Complication | Post-resuscitation Action |
|---|---|---|
| Brain | Apnea<br>Seizures<br>Change in neurologic examination | Monitor for apnea.<br>Support ventilation as needed.<br>Monitor glucose and electrolytes.<br>Avoid hyperthermia.<br>Consider anticonvulsant therapy.<br>Consider therapeutic hypothermia. |
| Lungs | Pulmonary hypertension<br>Pneumonia<br>Pneumothorax<br>Transient tachypnea<br>Meconium aspiration syndrome<br>Surfactant deficiency | Maintain adequate oxygenation and ventilation.<br>Consider antibiotics.<br>Obtain x-ray and blood gas.<br>Consider surfactant therapy.<br>Delay feedings if respiratory distress present. |
| Cardiovascular | Hypotension | Monitor blood pressure and heart rate.<br>Consider volume replacement followed by inotrope administration if hypotensive. |
| Kidneys | Acute tubular necrosis | Monitor urine output.<br>Monitor serum electrolytes.<br>Restrict fluids if baby is oliguric and vascular volume is adequate. |
| Gastrointestinal | Ileus<br>Necrotizing enterocolitis | Delay initiation of feedings.<br>Give intravenous fluids.<br>Consider parenteral nutrition. |
| Metabolic/<br>Hematologic | Hypoglycemia<br>Hypocalcemia; hyponatremia<br>Anemia if history of acute blood loss<br>Thrombocytopenia | Monitor blood glucose.<br>Monitor electrolytes.<br>Monitor hematocrit.<br>Monitor platelets. |

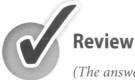 **Review**

*(The answers are in the preceding section and at the end of the lesson.)*

7. After resuscitation of a term or near-term newborn, vascular resistance in the pulmonary circuit is more likely to be (high) (low). Adequate oxygenation is likely to cause the pulmonary blood flow to (increase) (decrease).

8. If a meconium-stained baby has been resuscitated and then develops acute respiratory deterioration, a _____ should be suspected.

9. A baby who required resuscitation still has low blood pressure and poor perfusion after having been given a blood transfusion for suspected perinatal blood loss. He may require an infusion of _____ to improve his cardiac output and vascular tone.

10. Babies who have been resuscitated may have kidney damage and are likely to need (more) (less) fluids after the resuscitation.

11. Because energy stores are consumed faster in the absence of oxygen, blood _____ levels may be low following resuscitation.

12. List 3 causes of seizures following resuscitation.

    1. _____

    2. _____

    3. _____

13. A baby has a seizure 10 hours after being resuscitated. A blood glucose screen and serum electrolytes are normal. What class of drug should be used to treat her seizure? _____
    _____

## Are resuscitation techniques different for babies born outside the hospital or beyond the immediate newborn period?

Throughout this program, you have learned about resuscitating newly born babies who were born in the hospital and were having difficulty making the transition from intrauterine to extrauterine life. In addition, some babies may encounter difficulty and require resuscitation after being born, whether inside or outside the hospital, and other babies will require resuscitation after the immediate newborn period.

Some examples of babies who may require resuscitation under different circumstances include

- A baby who is delivered precipitously at home or in a motor vehicle, where resources are limited

- A baby who develops apnea in the nursery

- A 2-day-old baby with sepsis who presents in shock

- An intubated baby in the neonatal intensive care unit who deteriorates acutely

Although scenarios encountered outside the delivery room may be different from the events in the immediate post-delivery period, the physiologic principles and the steps you take to restore vital signs remain the same throughout the neonatal period (ie, the first month after birth).

- Warm and position the baby, clear the airway, and stimulate the baby to breathe.

- Establish effective ventilation, and provide supplemental oxygen if necessary.

- Perform chest compressions.

- Administer medications.

Once adequate ventilation is ensured, obtain further information about the baby's history to guide further resuscitation efforts.

Although this program is not designed to teach neonatal resuscitation in these other venues, some strategies for applying the principles of the Neonatal Resuscitation Program™ (NRP™) outside the delivery room are presented in the next few pages. More details are available through other programs, such as the Pediatric Advanced Life Support (PALS) program of the American Heart Association and the Pediatric Education for Prehospital Professionals (PEPP) program of the American Academy of Pediatrics. In general, where differences exist between the NRP and the recommendations presented in these other courses, you should apply the NRP recommendations during the time the newborn is still an inpatient following birth. In addition, you should consider the likely etiology of the arrest. For example, if the etiology is likely to be respiratory, as it usually is in very young babies, the lower compression-to-ventilation ratio (3:1) recommended by the NRP will be appropriate, while rescuers should consider using higher ratios, as recommended by PALS (eg, 15:2), if the arrest is believed to be of cardiac origin.

 **The priority for resuscitating babies at any time during the neonatal period, regardless of location, should be to restore adequate ventilation.**

## Case 7.
## Resuscitation of an apparently healthy newborn

A baby weighing 3,400 g is born in the hospital at term after an uncomplicated pregnancy, labor, and delivery. The transitional period is uneventful; he remains with his mother and begins breastfeeding soon after birth.

At approximately 20 hours of age, his mother notices that he is not breathing and is unresponsive in his bassinet. She activates the emergency alarm, and a perinatal nurse on the floor responds immediately.

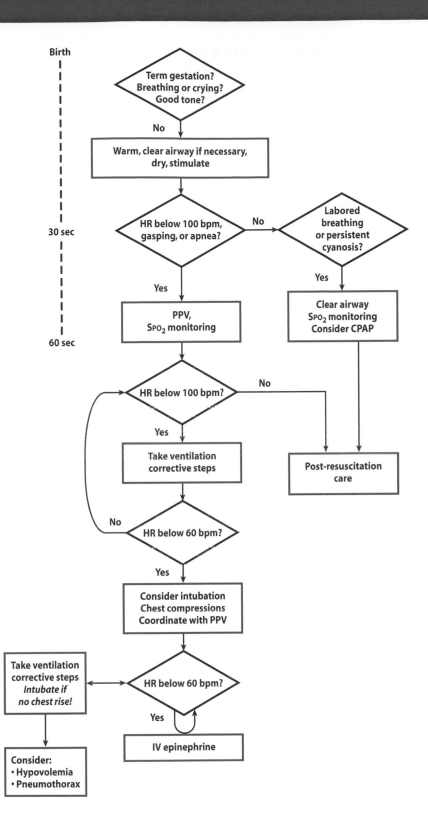

Birth

Term gestation?
Breathing or crying?
Good tone?

No

Warm, clear airway if necessary,
dry, stimulate

30 sec

HR below 100 bpm,
gasping, or apnea?

No

Labored
breathing
or persistent
cyanosis?

Yes

Yes

60 sec

PPV,
SpO₂ monitoring

Clear airway
SpO₂ monitoring
Consider CPAP

HR below 100 bpm?

No

Yes

Take ventilation
corrective steps

Post-resuscitation
care

No

HR below 60 bpm?

Yes

Consider intubation
Chest compressions
Coordinate with PPV

Take ventilation
corrective steps
*Intubate if
no chest rise!*

HR below 60 bpm?

Yes

Consider:
• Hypovolemia
• Pneumothorax

IV epinephrine

The nurse finds the baby apneic, limp, and blue. She places him on the
neonatal resuscitation table already in the LDRP room, and opens his
airway by placing his head in the "sniffing" position. She quickly
suctions his mouth and nose with a bulb syringe. She rubs his back and
flicks the soles of his feet, but he still does not resume breathing. The
nurse calls for help.

Using the self-inflating resuscitation bag and mask that is readily available in the mother's room, the nurse provides positive-pressure ventilation (PPV) with 21% oxygen. A second nurse arrives to help, bringing an emergency cart, and places a pulse oximetry probe on the baby's right hand. The SpO$_2$ is 70%, so she attaches the bag to the wall oxygen source. After approximately 30 seconds of effective PPV, the second nurse uses a stethoscope to confirm the oximeter's heart rate reading of 40 bpm.

Chest compressions are started and coordinated with PPV. After 45 to 60 seconds, the heart rate is checked again and found to be 50 bpm. A third clinician arrives and inserts an endotracheal tube. The umbilical cord is still sufficiently fresh to permit insertion of an umbilical venous catheter, and 1 mL of 1:10,000 epinephrine is administered into the line. After another 45 to 60 seconds, the heart rate is found to be 80 bpm.

Chest compressions are discontinued, and PPV continues. After another minute, the heart rate increases to more than 100 bpm, and the baby begins breathing spontaneously.

The oxygen is weaned as the pulse oximeter now reads 90% to 95%, and PPV is weaned as the baby begins to breathe spontaneously. A nurse provides support and information to the anxious mother as the baby is moved to the special care nursery in a transport incubator for evaluation of the cause of his respiratory arrest.

## What are some of the different strategies needed to resuscitate babies outside the hospital or beyond the immediate newborn period?

### Temperature control

When babies are born outside the delivery or birthing room environment, maintaining body temperature may become a major challenge because you likely will not have a radiant warmer readily available. Some suggestions for minimizing heat loss are as follows:

- Turn up the heat source in the room or vehicle, if applicable.

- Dry the baby well with bath towels, a blanket, or clean clothing.

- Use the mother's body as a heat source. Consider placing the baby skin-to-skin on the mother's chest and covering both baby and mother with a blanket.

- Rescue squads should consider having plastic wraps or chemical warmers on board emergency vehicles to help maintain the temperature of babies born extremely prematurely.

Maintaining normal body temperature is less difficult if the baby is not newly born, because the baby's body is generally not wet, so heat loss is decreased compared to a newborn. However, efforts should be made to prevent cooling, especially during the winter months, such as placing the baby on warm blankets, and using a hat, if one is available.

### Clearing the airway

If resuscitation is required outside a delivery room or nursery, vacuum suction will often not be readily available. Following are suggestions for methods of clearing the airway:

- Use a bulb syringe.
- Wipe the mouth and nose with a clean handkerchief or other cloth wrapped around your index finger.

### Ventilation

Most babies breathe spontaneously after birth. Drying the newborn, rubbing his back, and flicking the soles of the feet are acceptable methods of stimulation. However, some babies born outside the hospital may require PPV to ventilate the lungs. If a resuscitation bag-and-mask device is unavailable, PPV can be delivered by mouth-to-mouth-and-nose resuscitation. The baby is placed in the "sniffing" position, and the resuscitator's mouth is placed over the baby's mouth and nose, forming a tight seal. If the baby is very large, or the resuscitator has a small mouth, it may be necessary to cover only the baby's mouth with the resuscitator's mouth while the baby's nose is pinched to seal the airway. This technique poses a risk of transmission of infectious diseases.

### Chest compressions

Current recommendations for older infants, children, and adults call for chest compressions to be administered at a ratio of 30:2 with ventilations, or even continuously with no ventilations if there is only a single rescuer available. This change was made because, beyond the neonatal and pediatric age group, the etiology of an arrest is more often cardiac. During the first few weeks following birth, the cause of nearly all arrests will still be respiratory, and the NRP recommendation of a 3:1 compression-to-ventilation ratio should be employed. However, if there is a reason to suspect a cardiac etiology, use of the higher ratio should be considered.

### Vascular access

Catheterization of the umbilical vessels generally is not an option outside the hospital or beyond the first several days after birth. In such cases, prompt cannulation of a peripheral vein or insertion of an intraosseous needle into the tibia are reasonable alternatives. A detailed description of these techniques is beyond the scope of this program.

### Medications

Epinephrine should still be the primary drug used for resuscitation of babies who do not respond to PPV and chest compressions. However, other medications (such as calcium) also may be necessary, depending on the cause of the arrest. The diagnostic steps required and the details of using these drugs are beyond the scope of this program.

## Review

*(The answers are in the preceding section and at the end of the lesson.)*

14. You are likely to have (more) (less) (about the same) difficulty controlling body temperature of babies requiring resuscitation beyond the immediate newborn period.

15. The priority for resuscitating babies beyond the immediate newborn period should be to

    A. Defibrillate the heart.
    B. Expand blood volume.
    C. Establish effective ventilation.
    D. Administer epinephrine.
    E. Deliver chest compressions.

16. If vacuum suction is not available to clear the airway, 2 alternative methods are _____ and _____.

17. If a 15-day-old baby requiring resuscitation had blood loss, vascular access routes include _____ and _____.

18. A baby was delivered at term by emergency cesarean section for persistent fetal bradycardia lasting 30 minutes. He required chest compressions and now is profoundly obtunded, with absent deep tendon reflexes. What procedure may decrease the subsequent severity of hypoxic-ischemic encephalopathy, if instituted before 6 hours following birth? _____
_____

## Key Points

1. The appropriate action for a baby who fails to respond to resuscitation will depend on the presentation—failure to ventilate, persistent oxygen desaturation or bradycardia, or failure to initiate spontaneous breathing.

2. Respiratory distress due to choanal atresia can be helped by placing an oral airway.

3. Airway obstruction from Robin syndrome can be helped by inserting a nasopharyngeal tube and placing the baby prone.

4. In an emergency, a pneumothorax can be detected by transillumination and treated by aspirating air with a syringe attached to a needle inserted into the chest.

5. If diaphragmatic hernia is suspected, avoid positive-pressure ventilation by mask. Immediately intubate the trachea in the delivery room and insert an orogastric tube to decompress the stomach and intestines.

6. Persistent oxygen desaturation and/or bradycardia are rarely caused by congenital heart disease in a newborn. More commonly, the persistent desaturation and bradycardia are caused by inadequate ventilation.

7. A baby who has required resuscitation must have close monitoring and management of oxygenation, blood pressure, fluid status, respiratory effort, blood glucose, nutritional issues, and temperature.

8. Be careful not to overheat the baby during or following resuscitation.

9. If a mother has recently received narcotics and her baby fails to breathe, first provide effective positive-pressure ventilation to maintain a heart rate above 100 bpm, then you might consider giving naloxone to the baby.

10. Restoring adequate ventilation is the priority when resuscitating babies at birth in the delivery room or later in the nursery or other location.

11. Management steps for babies requiring resuscitation outside the delivery room include the following:
    • Maintain temperature by placing the baby skin-to-skin with the mother and raising the environmental temperature.
    • Clear airway with a bulb syringe or a cloth on your finger.
    • Use mouth-to-mouth-and-nose breathing for providing positive-pressure ventilation.
    • Obtain vascular access by cannulating a peripheral vein or placing an intraosseous needle in the intraosseous space in the tibia.

12. Therapeutic hypothermia following perinatal asphyxia should be
    • Used only for babies ≥36 weeks' gestation who meet previously defined criteria for this therapy
    • Initiated before 6 hours after birth
    • Used only according to specific protocols coordinated by centers with specialized programs equipped to provide the therapy

## Lesson 7 Review

*(The answers follow.)*

1. Choanal atresia can be ruled out by what procedure? _____
   _____

2. Babies with Robin syndrome and airway obstruction may be helped by placing a _____ and positioning the babies _____.
   Endotracheal intubation of such babies is usually (easy) (difficult).

3. A pneumothorax or congenital diaphragmatic hernia should be considered if breath sounds are (equal) (unequal) on the 2 sides of the chest.

4. You should suspect a congenital diaphragmatic hernia if the abdomen is _____. Such babies should not be resuscitated with _____.

5. Persistent bradycardia and low SpO₂ during neonatal resuscitation most likely are caused by (heart problems) (inadequate ventilation).

6. Babies who do not have spontaneous respirations and whose mothers have been given narcotic drugs should first receive _____, and then, if spontaneous respirations do not begin, may be given _____ to confirm the cause of their respiratory depression.

## Lesson 7 Review—*continued*

7. After resuscitation of a term or near-term newborn, vascular resistance in the pulmonary circuit is more likely to be (high) (low). Adequate oxygenation is likely to cause the pulmonary blood flow to (increase) (decrease).

8. If a meconium-stained baby has been resuscitated and then develops acute respiratory deterioration, a _____ should be suspected.

9. A baby who required resuscitation still has low blood pressure and poor perfusion after having been given a blood transfusion for suspected perinatal blood loss. He may require an infusion of _____ to improve his cardiac output and vascular tone.

10. Babies who have been resuscitated may have kidney damage and are likely to need (more) (less) fluids after the resuscitation.

11. Because energy stores are consumed faster in the absence of oxygen, blood _____ levels may be low following resuscitation.

12. List 3 causes of seizures following resuscitation.

    1. _____

    2. _____

    3. _____

13. A baby has a seizure 10 hours after being resuscitated. A blood glucose screen and serum electrolytes are normal. What class of drug should be used to treat her seizure? _____

    _____

14. You are likely to have (more) (less) (about the same) difficulty controlling body temperature of babies requiring resuscitation beyond the immediate newborn period.

15. The priority for resuscitating babies beyond the immediate newborn period should be to

    A. Defibrillate the heart.
    B. Expand blood volume.
    C. Establish effective ventilation.
    D. Administer epinephrine.
    E. Deliver chest compressions.

16. If vacuum suction is not available to clear the airway, 2 alternative methods are _____ and _____.

17. If a 15-day-old baby requiring resuscitation had blood loss, vascular access routes include _____ and _____.

18. A baby was delivered at term by emergency cesarean section for persistent fetal bradycardia lasting 30 minutes. He required chest compressions and now is profoundly obtunded, with absent deep tendon reflexes. What procedure may decrease the subsequent severity of hypoxic-ischemic encephalopathy, if instituted before 6 hours following birth? _____ _____

## Answers to Questions

1. Choanal atresia can be ruled out by **passing a nasopharyngeal catheter through the nares.**

2. Babies with Robin syndrome who have upper airway obstruction may be helped by placing a **nasopharyngeal tube** and positioning them **on their abdomens (prone).** Endotracheal intubation of such babies is usually **difficult.**

3. A pneumothorax or congenital diaphragmatic hernia should be considered if breath sounds are **unequal** on different sides of the chest. If the trachea has been intubated, you also should check to be sure that the tube is not in too far.

4. You should suspect a congenital diaphragmatic hernia if the abdomen is **flat-appearing (scaphoid).** Such babies should not be resuscitated with **positive-pressure ventilation by mask.**

5. Persistent bradycardia and low $SpO_2$ during resuscitation most likely are caused by **inadequate ventilation.**

6. Babies who do not have spontaneous respirations and whose mothers have been given narcotic drugs should first receive **positive-pressure ventilation,** and then, if spontaneous respirations do not begin, may be given **naloxone.**

7. After resuscitation of a term or near-term newborn, vascular resistance in the pulmonary circuit is more likely to be **high.** Adequate oxygenation is likely to cause the pulmonary vascular resistance to fall, and thus blood flow to **increase.**

## Answers to Questions—*continued*

8.  If a meconium-stained baby has been resuscitated and then develops acute deterioration, a **pneumothorax** should be suspected. (An endotracheal tube plugged with meconium is also a consideration.)

9.  The baby may require an infusion of **dopamine (or other inotrope)** to improve his cardiac output and vascular tone.

10. Babies who have been resuscitated are more likely to need **less** fluids after the resuscitation.

11. Blood **glucose** levels may be low following resuscitation.

12. Seizures following resuscitation may be caused by (1) **hypoxic-ischemic encephalopathy,** (2) **metabolic disturbance, such as hypoglycemia,** or (3) **electrolyte abnormalities, such as hyponatremia or hypocalcemia.**

13. A baby with a seizure 10 hours after being resuscitated and with normal blood glucose levels should be treated with **an anticonvulsant (such as phenobarbital).**

14. You are likely to have **less** difficulty controlling body temperature of babies requiring resuscitation beyond the immediate newborn period, since they usually will not be wet.

15. The priority for resuscitating babies beyond the immediate newborn period should be to **establish effective ventilation.**

16. If vacuum suction is not available to clear the airway, 2 alternative methods are **bulb suction** and **wiping the airway with a clean cloth.**

17. If a 15-day-old baby requiring resuscitation had blood loss, vascular access routes include **cannulation of a peripheral vein** and **insertion of an intraosseous needle.**

18. A term baby who has required resuscitation and now shows early signs of hypoxic-ischemic encephalopathy may benefit from early administration of **therapeutic hypothermia.**

# Resuscitation of Babies Born Preterm

## In Lesson 8 you will learn

- The risk factors associated with preterm birth
- The additional resources needed to be prepared for a preterm delivery
- Additional strategies to maintain the preterm baby's body temperature
- Additional considerations for managing oxygen in a premature baby
- How to assist ventilation when a premature baby has difficulty breathing
- Ways to decrease the chances of brain injury in preterm babies
- Special precautions to take after resuscitating a premature baby

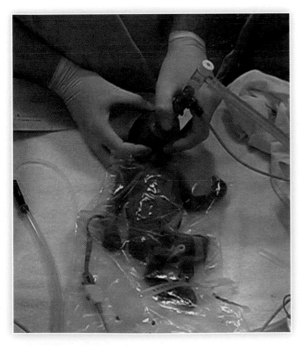

Photo kindly provided by Professor Colin Morley, University of Melbourne

The following case describes the delivery and resuscitation of an extremely preterm baby. As you read the case, imagine yourself as part of the team from the anticipation of the delivery through the resuscitation and stabilization and final transfer to an intensive care nursery.

## Case 8.
## Resuscitation and stabilization of a baby born extremely preterm

A 24-year-old woman is admitted to the hospital at 26 weeks' gestation. She reports that contractions began approximately 6 hours ago, that her membranes ruptured just before her arrival, and that the fluid was bloody. On examination, her cervix is 6-cm dilated and delivery is judged imminent.

A team with experience in neonatal resuscitation, including individuals with intubation and umbilical catheterization skills, is called to the delivery room. The equipment check is performed, which includes additional measures to prepare for a preterm birth. One member of the team checks that a blender is connected to oxygen and air sources, attaches a preterm-sized mask to the resuscitation bag, and prepares a laryngoscope with a size-0 blade and a 2.5-mm endotracheal tube. The blender is adjusted to the agreed-upon oxygen concentration of 40%. Another team member increases the temperature in the delivery room, activates a disposable warming pad, heats the radiant warmer, and places several layers of warming blankets under the radiant warmer. She then cuts the bottom from a reclosable food storage bag and places it in the resuscitation field. The team identifies a leader and reviews each team member's role, including who will be responsible for managing the airway and positive-pressure ventilation (PPV), monitoring the heart rate and pulse oximetry, preparing medications, inserting an emergency umbilical catheter if needed, and recording events. The leader identifies herself to the mother and father and explains the anticipated upcoming events.

The baby is delivered, and then handed to a member of the resuscitation team who places her up to her neck in the polyethylene bag and lays her gently on the pre-warmed towels under the radiant warmer (Figure 8.1). Bloody amniotic fluid is suctioned from her mouth and nose, her breathing is stimulated by gently rubbing her extremities, and another team member attaches an oximeter probe to the baby's right wrist, then connects the probe to the oximeter. The baby's tone is fairly good and there are labored respiratory efforts.

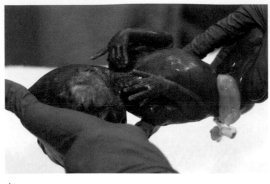

A

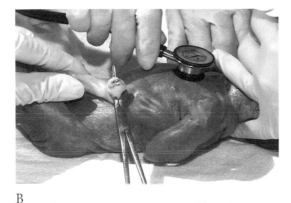

B

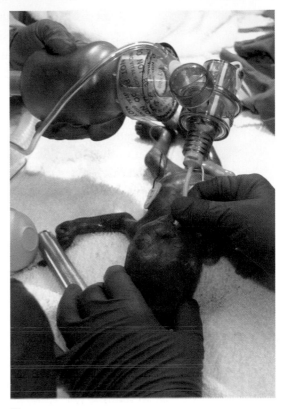

D

C

**Figure 8.1.** **A.** An extremely preterm baby is delivered and has poor muscle tone, has weak respiratory effort, and requires assisted ventilation. **B.** Heart rate is being determined by 2 methods: palpating the base of the cord and listening to the chest. **C.** Endotracheal intubation procedure is begun as assistant listens to the heart rate. **D.** Endotracheal tube is held in place as positive-pressure ventilation is provided. Thermoregulation could be improved by covering this newborn with polyethylene plastic wrap.

Continuous positive airway pressure (CPAP) is administered by mask, but, by 1 minute of age, she no longer has respiratory efforts, her heart rate is determined to be approximately 70 beats per minute (bpm), and her oxygen saturation as measured by pulse oximetry ($Spo_2$) is decreasing. Positive-pressure ventilation is administered with 40% supplemental oxygen, but, despite adjusting the mask and head position and suctioning the airway, it is difficult to hear breath sounds with a stethoscope, the chest is not moving, and the heart rate is not increasing. Successive pressure increases do not improve the situation, and the team leader elects to intubate the trachea. Intratracheal placement is verified with a carbon dioxide ($CO_2$) detector, breath sounds are noted to be equal bilaterally, and the tube is secured with the 7-cm mark noted to be at the baby's lip.

Intermittent PPV with 40% oxygen at approximately 20 cm $H_2O$ is gently administered. By 3 to 4 minutes after birth, the oximeter registers a heart rate greater than 100 bpm and an $Spo_2$ that is in the 70s and increasing. Breath sounds are audible and slight chest movement is present. As the saturation continues to rise, the oxygen concentration is gradually decreased. By 5 minutes of age, the heart rate is 150 bpm and the $Spo_2$ is approximately 85% as PPV with 30% oxygen is continued. At 10 minutes of age, surfactant is administered through the endotracheal tube and positive pressure is decreased while still maintaining a gentle chest rise with each breath. By 15 minutes, the oxygen concentration has been weaned to 25% to keep the baby's $Spo_2$ at 85% to 95%.

The baby is shown to her parents and transported to the nursery in a transport incubator while receiving PPV.

## What will this lesson cover?

In the first 7 lessons, you learned a systematic approach to resuscitating a baby after birth. When birth occurs before term, there are additional challenges that make the transition to extrauterine life more difficult. The likelihood that a preterm baby will need help making this transition increases as the degree of prematurity increases. Some of the complications of prematurity may be prevented by your management of these first transitional minutes. This lesson focuses on the additional problems associated with preterm birth and the actions that you can take to prevent or manage them.

## Why are premature babies at higher risk?

Babies who are born before term are at risk for a variety of complications following birth. Some of the complications of prematurity result from the factors that lead to preterm delivery; others are a reflection of the babies' relative anatomic and physiologic immaturity.

- Their thin skin, large surface area relative to body mass, and decreased fat allow them to lose heat easier.

- Their immature tissues may be damaged more easily by excessive oxygen.

- Their weak chest muscles may not allow them to take effective breaths, and their nervous system may not provide adequate stimulation to breathe.

- Their lungs may be immature and deficient in surfactant, making ventilation difficult and injury from positive-pressure ventilation (PPV) more likely.

- Their immune systems may be immature, increasing the risk of infection.

- Fragile capillaries within their developing brains may rupture.

- Their small blood volume makes them more susceptible to the hypovolemic effects of blood loss.

These and other aspects of prematurity should alert you to seek extra help when anticipating the birth of a baby born preterm.

## What additional resources do you need for resuscitating a preterm newborn?

- *Additional trained personnel*

The chance that a premature baby will require resuscitation is significantly higher than for a baby born at term. This is true even for late preterm babies (born at 34 to 36 weeks' gestation). You should have enough personnel present at the birth to perform a complex resuscitation, including someone skilled in endotracheal intubation and emergency umbilical venous catheterization.

- *Preparation of the environment and equipment*

Increase the temperature in the delivery room and preheat the radiant warmer to ensure a warm environment for the baby. If the baby is anticipated to be significantly preterm (eg, born at less than 29 weeks' gestation), you may want to have a reclosable, food-grade polyethylene bag and a chemically activated warming pad ready, as described in the next section. An oxygen blender and oximeter always should be available for preterm births. A transport incubator is important for maintaining the baby's temperature during the move to the nursery after resuscitation.

## How do you keep the baby warm?

Premature babies are particularly vulnerable to cold stress. Their larger surface-area-to-body-mass ratio, thin permeable skin, small amount of subcutaneous fat, and limited metabolic response to cold may lead to rapid heat loss and decrease in body temperature. Babies born prematurely should have all steps taken to reduce heat loss, even if they do not initially appear to require resuscitation. Therefore, when a preterm delivery is expected, anticipate that temperature regulation will be challenging and prepare for it.

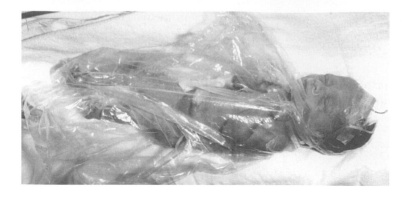

**Figure 8.2.** Use of a plastic bag for reducing evaporative heat loss. (From Vohra S, Frent G, et al. Effect of polyethylene occlusive skin wrapping on heat loss in very low birth weight infants at delivery: a randomized trial. *J Pediatr.* 1999;134:547-551)

- *Increase the temperature of the delivery room and the area where the baby will be resuscitated.*

  Frequently, delivery rooms and operating rooms are maintained relatively cool, but, when anticipating a preterm birth, you should try to increase the temperature of the room to approximately 25°C to 26°C (77°F-79°F).

- *Preheat the radiant warmer well before the birth.*

- *Place a portable warming pad under the layers of towels that are on the resuscitation table.*

  These pads are commercially available and are warmed only when needed, by activating a chemical reaction within the pad. Store the pads at room temperature, or they may overheat or under-heat when activated. Follow the manufacturer's recommendation for activation and place the correct side next to the baby.

- *Use polyethylene plastic wrap for babies delivered at less than 29 weeks' gestation (Figure 8.2).*

  Drying and placing the baby under a radiant warmer are not sufficient to prevent evaporative heat loss in a very premature newborn. Instead of drying the body with towels, these newborns should be wrapped up to their neck in polyethylene plastic immediately after birth. You may use a sheet of plastic food wrap, a food-grade 1-gallon plastic bag, or a commercially available sheet of polyethylene plastic *(Figure 8.2).*

- When the baby is transported to the nursery after resuscitation, *use a pre-warmed transport incubator* to maintain adequate temperature control *en route.*

Note: It is important to monitor the baby's temperature frequently after the initial resuscitation measures are completed because *overheating* has been described while using a plastic wrap with a chemical warming pad. Be sure to monitor the baby's temperature and avoid overheating as well as cooling. The goal should be an axillary temperature of approximately 36.5°C.

## Review

*(The answers are in the preceding section and at the end of the lesson.)*

1. List 5 factors that increase the likelihood of needing resuscitation with preterm deliveries.

   _____

   _____

   _____

   _____

   _____

2. A baby is about to be born at 30 weeks' gestation. What additional resources should you assemble?

   _____

   _____

3. You have turned on the radiant warmer in anticipation of the birth of a baby at 27 weeks' gestation. What else might you consider to help maintain this baby's temperature?

   _____

   _____

   _____

## How much oxygen should you use?

You have learned in previous lessons that injury during perinatal transition results from inadequate blood flow and limited oxygen delivery to body tissues, and that restoring these factors is an important goal in resuscitation. However, research at both the cellular and whole-body levels suggests that excessive oxygen delivered to tissues that have been deprived of perfusion and oxygen can result in even worse injury. The baby born preterm may be at higher risk for hyperoxic reperfusion injury because development of tissues during fetal life normally occurs in a relatively low oxygen environment, and the mechanisms that protect the body from oxidant injury have not yet fully developed.

As noted in earlier lessons, research studies so far have been unable to define precisely how quickly a baby who has been deprived of oxygen should be re-oxygenated. When resuscitating babies born at term, starting the resuscitation with no supplemental oxygen is reasonable until an oximeter can be attached to determine the oxygen need. However, when resuscitating a preterm baby with immature tissues, it is particularly important to balance the need to give sufficient oxygen to correct the baby's hypoxemic state against the need to avoid exposing the baby to excessive levels of oxygen. To accomplish both of these goals,

| Targeted Pre-ductal SpO$_2$ After Birth | |
|---|---|
| 1 min | 60%-65% |
| 2 min | 65%-70% |
| 3 min | 70%-75% |
| 4 min | 75%-80% |
| 5 min | 80%-85% |
| 10 min | 85%-95% |

 **If the heart rate does not respond by increasing rapidly to greater than 100 bpm, the baby likely is not being adequately ventilated. Correct the ventilation problem and adjust the oxygen concentration delivered to match the goals listed in the table. Increasing oxygen concentration without correcting inadequate ventilation will not result in improvement in heart rate and SpO$_2$.**

it is recommended that you begin resuscitation with a pulse oximeter and an oxygen blender to allow you to vary the amount of oxygen being given to achieve an appropriate level of oxygen in the baby's circulation as early as possible. This additional equipment is especially critical in preterm babies born at less than approximately 32 weeks' gestation.

## How do you adjust the oxygen?

As described in Lesson 2, observational studies conducted with full-term babies following uncomplicated birth and initiation of air breathing have shown that it normally may take up to 10 minutes for blood oxygen saturations to rise to 90%, and that occasional dips to the high 80% range are normal during the first few days of extrauterine life. Until more evidence becomes available about the optimum oxygen saturation as measured by pulse oximetry (SpO$_2$) for a preterm baby, it is recommended that you try to keep the preterm baby in the same saturation range as that shown for a term baby. That varying range is a function of the time from birth, as shown in the table on this page, which also appears in the resuscitation flow diagram discussed throughout this textbook. You should be able to titrate the baby's SpO$_2$ to the range shown in the table by adjusting the concentration of oxygen delivered from the blender.

## How do you assist ventilation?

Babies born significantly preterm have immature lungs that may be difficult to ventilate, but are also injured more easily with intermittent positive-pressure breaths. If the baby is breathing spontaneously and has a heart rate above 100 bpm, it may be preferable to let him continue to progress through the first few minutes of transition without assistance. However, use the same criteria for assisting ventilation with a preterm baby that you have learned for assisting ventilation with a term baby. (See flow diagram.) The following are special considerations for assisting ventilation of preterm babies:

*Consider giving continuous positive airway pressure (CPAP).* If the baby is breathing spontaneously and has a heart rate above 100 bpm, but has labored respirations, is cyanotic, or has low SpO$_2$, administration of CPAP may be helpful.

• **What is CPAP?**

CPAP is an acronym for continuous positive airway pressure, which is a technique for providing positive pressure to the airway of a spontaneously breathing baby throughout the respiratory cycle. (See Lesson 3.) When a baby exhales normally, he or she exhales by letting the pressure in the lungs passively flow into the neutral pressure in the atmosphere. To provide CPAP, a mask or special nasal prongs are connected to a resuscitation bag or T-piece resuscitator and held tightly to the baby's face or nose to provide continuous pressure in the baby's airway that is greater than the pressure in the surrounding atmosphere. CPAP keeps the lungs slightly inflated at all times and is most helpful for preterm babies whose lungs may be surfactant deficient and whose alveoli tend to collapse at the end of each exhalation. CPAP also may be beneficial for babies with infected or fluid-filled lungs that may not be fully expanded after transition. When CPAP is provided, the baby does not have to work as hard to reinflate the lungs with each inhalation.

• **How do you give CPAP during resuscitation, and how much do you give?**

CPAP is administered by placing the mask of a flow-inflating bag or T-piece resuscitator tightly on the baby's face and adjusting the flow-control valve (Figure 8.3) or positive end-expiratory pressure (PEEP) valve of a T-piece resuscitator (Figure 8.5) to the desired amount of CPAP. Generally, 4 to 6 cm $H_2O$ is an adequate amount of pressure. *CPAP cannot be delivered with a self-inflating bag.*

If CPAP will be administered for a prolonged period, it may be easier to use nasal prongs specially made for CPAP delivery rather than a mask, as the prongs are more easily kept in the proper position. CPAP also can be delivered via some mechanical ventilators.

Adjust the amount of CPAP by holding the mask tightly against your hand before applying it to the baby's face (Figures 8.4 and 8.5). Read

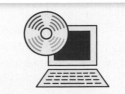

You are encouraged to view this video on the DVD that accompanies this textbook: *CPAP Administration*

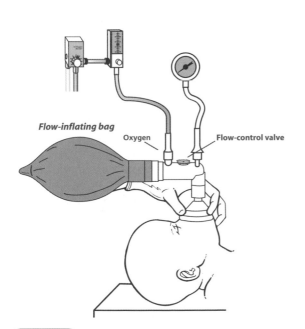

**Figure 8.3.** Administering continuous positive airway pressure (CPAP) to a baby with a face mask and flow-inflating bag. There must be a tight seal on the face and a pressure registering on the pressure gauge for CPAP to be delivered to the baby's airway.

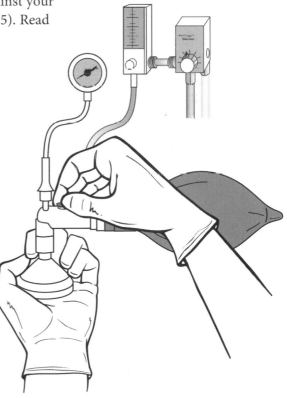

**Figure 8.4.** Adjustment of continuous positive airway pressure with a flow-inflating bag, before application of the mask to the baby's face

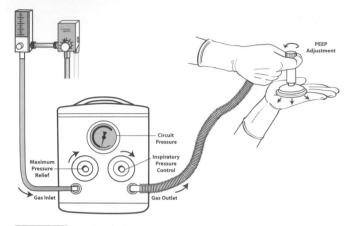

**Figure 8.5.** Adjustment of continuous positive airway pressure with a T-piece resuscitator, before application to the baby's face

the pressure gauge and adjust the valve or cap so that the gauge reads the desired starting pressure. Five to 6 cm $H_2O$ is a reasonable starting pressure.

After you have adjusted the CPAP to the desired pressure while holding the mask against your hand, place it firmly against the baby's face and check that the pressure is still at the selected level. If it is lower, you may not have a tight seal of the mask on the baby's face. During CPAP, the baby should breathe spontaneously without any additional breaths being provided via the ventilation bag or the T-piece resuscitator (ie, no PPV). Adjust the CPAP up or down depending on how hard the baby appears to be working to breathe. Usually, no more than 6 cm $H_2O$ is used. If the baby is not breathing sufficiently, you need to give PPV breaths instead of unassisted CPAP.

*If PPV is required, use the lowest inflation pressure necessary to achieve an adequate response.* An initial inflation pressure of 20 to 25 cm $H_2O$ is adequate for most preterm newborns. If there is not a prompt improvement in the heart rate, check if there is perceptible chest movement. If you cannot see any chest rise, check the mask seal and airway. If you still do not have any chest movement, you may need to increase the ventilating pressure cautiously, as described in Lesson 3 (the "P" in MR SOPA). However, avoid creating excessive chest rise while ventilating preterm newborns because their lungs are easily injured. Use the lowest inflation pressure necessary to maintain a heart rate greater than 100 bpm and a gradually improving oxygen saturation.

*If the baby has been intubated, use PEEP,* as described in Lesson 3. Generally, 2 to 5 cm $H_2O$ is sufficient. *(A special "PEEP valve" will be required with a self-inflating bag.)*

*Consider giving surfactant if the baby is significantly preterm.* Studies have shown that babies born at less than approximately 30 weeks' gestation benefit from early treatment with surfactant soon after resuscitation, even if they have not yet shown signs of respiratory distress. However, the indications for, and timing of, surfactant administration remain controversial. If the resuscitation team has not had expertise in surfactant administration and it is intended for the baby to be transported to another facility, it may be preferable to wait for arrival of the transport team. The use of prophylactic surfactant administration usually is determined by local care practices.

 **Babies should be fully resuscitated before surfactant is given.**

## What can you do to decrease the chances of neurologic injury in preterm newborns?

Before approximately 32 weeks' gestation, preterm babies have a fragile network of capillaries in an area of their brain called the germinal matrix. These capillaries are prone to rupture and bleeding. Rapid changes in blood carbon dioxide ($CO_2$) levels, blood pressure, or volume of blood in the brain blood vessels, as well as obstruction of the venous drainage from the head, may increase the risk of rupturing these capillaries. Bleeding in the germinal matrix may cause an intraventricular hemorrhage, hydrocephalus, and a lifelong disability. Inadequate blood flow and oxygen delivery may cause damage to the white matter of the brain, resulting in cerebral palsy, even in the absence of hemorrhage. Excessive oxygen administration may cause damage to the developing retina, resulting in retinopathy of prematurity and visual loss.

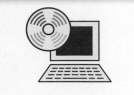

**You are encouraged to view this video on the DVD that accompanies this textbook:** *The ELBW Infant: Aspects of Delivery Room Management*

The following precautions apply to babies of all gestational ages, but are particularly important when resuscitating a preterm baby:

***Handle the baby gently.*** While this may seem obvious whenever treating any baby, this aspect of care may be forgotten during the stress of resuscitation when all members of the team are trying to act quickly and effectively.

***Avoid placing the baby in a head-down (Trendelenburg) position.*** The resuscitation table should be flat.

***Avoid delivering excessive positive pressure during PPV or CPAP.*** Sufficient pressure to achieve a rise in heart rate and adequate ventilation should be provided, but excessive inflation pressure or too much CPAP can restrict venous return from the head or create a pneumothorax, both of which have been associated with an increased risk of intraventricular hemorrhage.

***Use an oximeter and blood gases to adjust ventilation and oxygen concentration gradually and appropriately.*** Rapid changes in $CO_2$ levels result in corresponding changes in cerebral blood flow, which can increase the risk of bleeding. The $SpO_2$ should be monitored continuously during the resuscitation. An arterial or capillary blood gas should be obtained as soon as possible after resuscitation to ensure that the $CO_2$ level is neither too low nor too high.

***Do not give rapid infusions of fluid.*** If volume expansion becomes necessary (see Lesson 6), avoid giving the infusion too rapidly. Hypertonic intravenous solutions, such as sodium bicarbonate or hypertonic glucose, also should be avoided or given very slowly.

## What special precautions should be taken after a preterm baby has been resuscitated successfully?

Most of the physiologic preparation for a baby to become independent of his or her mother occurs during the last trimester. If a baby is born prematurely, many of these adaptations have not occurred and the preterm baby who has required resuscitation is even more susceptible to the stresses of independent survival. Consider the following precautions when initially managing a premature baby who required resuscitation at birth:

*Monitor blood glucose.* Babies born prematurely have lower glycogen stores than babies born at term. If resuscitation is required, it is more likely that these stores will be depleted quickly and the baby may become hypoglycemic.

*Monitor the baby for apnea and bradycardia.* Respiratory control is often unstable in preterm babies. Although premature babies can be expected to have breathing pauses, significant apnea and bradycardia during the stabilization period may be the first clinical sign of an abnormality in body temperature, oxygen, $CO_2$, electrolyte, blood glucose, or blood acid levels. Unexpected appearance of apnea and/or bradycardia also may be the first sign of an infection.

*Give an appropriate amount of oxygen and ventilation.* Following resuscitation, premature babies continue to be particularly vulnerable to both hypoxemia and hyperoxemia. Monitor $Spo_2$ until you are confident that the baby can maintain normal oxygenation while breathing room air. If the baby continues to require PPV or supplemental oxygen, measure blood gases at intervals to guide the amount of assistance required. If your hospital does not routinely care for preterm babies who require ongoing assisted ventilation, you will need to arrange transfer to an appropriate facility.

*Initiate feedings slowly and cautiously while you maintain nutrition intravenously.* Preterm babies who require resuscitation may have had bowel ischemia, and are at risk for early feeding intolerance and later problems with bowel function, such as necrotizing enterocolitis. Intravenous nutrition during the first few days and initiating feeds cautiously with expressed breast milk may be advisable.

*Increase suspicion for infection.* Chorioamnionitis is associated with premature onset of labor, and fetal infection may be the cause of perinatal asphyxia. Consider infection as a possible cause of premature delivery and draw blood cultures and administer antibiotic therapy promptly after birth if there is any chance that the baby could have an infection.

## Key Points

1. Preterm babies are at additional risk for requiring resuscitation because of their
   - Rapid heat loss
   - Vulnerability to hyperoxic injury
   - Immature lungs and diminished respiratory drive
   - Immature brains that are prone to bleeding
   - Vulnerability to infection
   - Small blood volume, increasing the implications of blood loss

2. Additional resources needed to prepare for an anticipated preterm birth include
   - Additional trained personnel, including someone with intubation and emergency umbilical venous catheterization expertise
   - Additional strategies for maintaining temperature
   - Compressed air source
   - Oxygen blender
   - Pulse oximeter

3. Premature babies are more vulnerable to hyperoxia; use an oximeter and blender to gradually achieve oxyhemoglobin saturations in the 85% to 95% range during and immediately following resuscitation.

4. Babies born very preterm are more susceptible to heat loss.
   - Increase temperature of room.
   - Preheat radiant warmer.
   - Consider using a chemically activated warming pad.
   - Use polyethylene wrap for babies less than approximately 29 weeks' gestation.
   - Use warmed transport incubator to transfer baby to nursery.

5. When assisting ventilation in preterm babies,
   - Follow the same criteria for initiating positive-pressure ventilation as with term babies.
   - Consider using continuous positive airway pressure (CPAP) if the baby is breathing spontaneously with a heart rate above 100 bpm, but has labored respirations or a low oxygen saturation. Use positive end-expiratory pressure if the baby has been intubated.
   - If positive-pressure ventilation is required, use the lowest inflation pressure necessary to achieve an adequate response.
   - Consider giving prophylactic surfactant.

6. Decrease the risk of brain injury by
   - Handling the baby gently
   - Avoiding the Trendelenburg position
   - Avoiding high airway pressures, when possible
   - Adjusting ventilation gradually, based on physical examination, oximetry, and blood gases
   - Avoiding rapid intravenous fluid boluses and hypertonic solutions

7. After resuscitation of a preterm baby,
   - Monitor and control blood glucose.
   - Monitor for apnea, bradycardia, or oxygen desaturations, and intervene promptly.
   - Monitor and control oxygenation and ventilation.
   - Consider delaying feeding or initiating feeds cautiously if perinatal compromise was significant.
   - Have a high level of suspicion for infection.

## Lesson 8 Review

*(The answers follow.)*

1. List 5 factors that increase the likelihood of needing resuscitation with preterm deliveries.

   _____
   _____
   _____
   _____
   _____

2. A baby is about to be born at 30 weeks' gestation. What additional resources should you assemble?

   _____
   _____
   _____
   _____
   _____

3. You have turned on the radiant warmer in anticipation of the birth of a baby at 27 weeks' gestation. What else might you consider to help maintain this baby's temperature?

   _____
   _____
   _____

## *Lesson 8 Review—continued*

4. A baby is delivered at 30 weeks' gestation. She requires positive-pressure ventilation for an initial heart rate of 80 beats per minute (bpm), despite tactile stimulation. She responds quickly with rising heart rate and spontaneous respirations. At 2 minutes of age, she is breathing, has a heart rate of 140 bpm, and is receiving continuous positive airway pressure (CPAP) with a flow-inflating mask and 50% oxygen. You have attached an oximeter that is now reading 95% and is increasing. You should (increase the oxygen concentration) (decrease the oxygen concentration) (leave the oxygen concentration the same).

5. CPAP may be given with a *(choose as many as are correct)*:
   A.  Self-inflating bag
   B.  Flow-inflating bag
   C.  T-piece resuscitator

6. To decrease the chance of brain hemorrhage, the best position is (table flat) (head down).

7. Intravenous fluids should be given (rapidly) (slowly) to preterm babies.

8. List 3 precautions that should be taken when managing a preterm baby who has required resuscitation.

   _____

   _____

   _____

# Answers to Questions

1. Risk factors include
   - **Lose heat easily**
   - **Tissues easily damaged from excess oxygen**
   - **Weak muscles, making it difficult to breathe**
   - **Lungs deficient in surfactant**
   - **Immature immune systems**
   - **Fragile capillaries in the brain**
   - **Small blood volume**

2. Additional resources include
   - **Additional personnel**
   - **Additional means to control temperature**
   - **Compressed air source**
   - **Oxygen blender**
   - **Oximeter**

3. Additional considerations include
   - **Increase temperature of delivery room.**
   - **Activate chemical heating pad.**
   - **Prepare plastic bag or wrap.**
   - **Prepare a transport incubator.**

4. **Decrease the oxygen concentration.**

5. CPAP may be given with a **flow-inflating bag** or a **T-piece resuscitator.**

6. The best position is **table flat.**

7. Intravenous fluids should be given **slowly.**

8. After resuscitation,
   - **Check blood glucose.**
   - **Monitor for apnea and bradycardia.**
   - **Control oxygenation.**
   - **Consider delaying feedings.**
   - **Increase suspicion for infection.**

# Ethics and Care at the End of Life

## In Lesson 9 you will learn

- The ethical principles associated with starting and stopping neonatal resuscitation
- How to communicate with parents and involve them in ethical decision making
- When it may be appropriate to withhold resuscitation
- What to do when the prognosis is uncertain
- How long to continue resuscitation attempts when the baby does not respond
- What to do when a baby dies
- How to help parents through the grieving process
- How to help staff through the grieving process

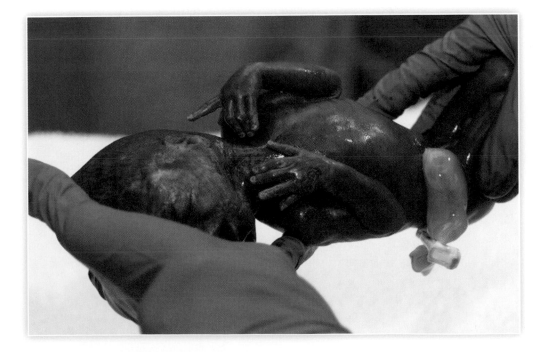

**Notes**

- Although this lesson is directed at the resuscitation team member who guides medical decision making, all members of the team should understand the reasoning behind the decisions. As much as possible, there should be unified support of the parents during their very personal period of crisis. This lesson refers to "parents," although it is recognized that sometimes the mother or father is alone during the crisis and, other times, support will be available through extended family or significant others. This lesson is applicable to health care professionals who participate in all aspects of care of pregnant women and newborns, from ambulatory antenatal care providers and pediatricians doing preconception and prenatal visits or consultations, to the inpatient perinatal care team, to professionals providing care to families who have experienced a neonatal death.

- Mortality and morbidity data by gestational age, compiled from data collected by perinatal centers in the United States and several other countries, may be found on the Neonatal Resuscitation Program™ (NRP™) Web site (http://www.aap.org/nrp).

- It is important to recognize that the recommendations made in this lesson are determined, to an extent, by the cultural context and available resources and may require adaptation before being applied to other cultures and countries. These recommendations were based on mortality and morbidity data available at the time of publication. Decisions regarding initiation or noninitiation of resuscitation are best made based on current local data and available therapies.

## *Case 9.*
## Care of a baby who could not be resuscitated

A gravida 3 woman at 23 weeks' gestation is admitted to the obstetrics floor of a rural community hospital with contractions, fever, and ruptured membranes. Gestation had been estimated by serial first- and second-trimester ultrasounds. The obstetrician asks you to join her in talking with the parents about the implications of a delivery at this early gestation. Before the meeting, the 2 of you discuss your regional mortality statistics over the past 5 years and consult the Web-based National Institute of Child Health & Human Development Outcomes Estimator about long-term morbidity of survivors following a birth at 23 weeks' gestation. The obstetrician advises against tocolysis because of suspected chorioamnionitis, and states that labor has progressed too far to try to transport the mother to a center that routinely cares for babies at this gestational age. You both enter the mother's room, introduce yourselves, and suggest that visitors may want to move to the waiting room while you talk with both parents, unless the parents prefer that they stay. The television is turned off and you both sit in chairs by the mother's bed. The obstetrician describes the obstetric care plan. You explain the implications of extremely preterm birth with the additional complication of probable chorioamnionitis, including available information on mortality and morbidity, and some of the expectations associated with neonatal intensive care. You describe the resuscitation team that will be available for the delivery, what procedures might be required to assist the baby's survival, and that some parents might elect not to attempt resuscitation in view of the risks involved for the likely outcome. The parents respond that they "want everything done if there is any chance that our baby can live."

Over the next hour, labor progresses, delivery becomes imminent, and the neonatal transport team at the regional medical center is alerted in case neonatal transport is needed. Appropriate preparations of equipment and staff are made for an extremely preterm delivery. When the baby is handed to the neonatal team, he has thin, gelatinous skin; no tone; and minimal respiratory efforts. The initial steps are performed and positive-pressure ventilation (PPV) by mask is administered. A pulse oximetry probe is placed and connected to the oximeter, and a heart rate of approximately 40 beats per minute is detected and confirmed by auscultation. The trachea is intubated and PPV via the endotracheal tube is continued. However, it is difficult to hear breath sounds despite using increased inflation pressures. Although further resuscitation measures are provided, the heart rate gradually falls. You explain to the parents that resuscitation has been unsuccessful. The endotracheal tube is removed, the baby is wrapped in a clean blanket, and the parents are asked if they would like to hold him. The parents do so and a member of the team remains with them to offer support. A picture is taken and given to the parents. The baby is pronounced dead when no signs of life remain.

Later that day, a member of the nursery team returns to the parents' room, expresses condolences, answers questions about the baby's failure to respond to initial resuscitation attempts and the team's assessment about his viability, and asks the parents about an autopsy. An anticipated follow-up visit is mentioned. The next day, a funeral home is identified. About 1 month later, a member of the nursery team contacts the parents, offering to schedule an office visit to discuss autopsy results and implications and problems the parents and siblings may be having adjusting to their loss, and to answer any questions that may remain about their son's death.

## What ethical principles apply to neonatal resuscitation?

The ethical principles of neonatal resuscitation are no different from those followed in resuscitating an older child or adult. Common ethical principles that apply to all medical care include respecting an individual's rights to make choices that affect his or her life (autonomy), acting so as to benefit others (beneficence), avoiding harm (nonmaleficence), and treating people truthfully and fairly (justice). These principles underlie why we ask patients for informed consent before proceeding with treatment. Exceptions to this rule include life-threatening medical emergencies and situations where patients are not competent to make their own decisions. Neonatal resuscitation is a medical treatment often complicated by both of these exceptions.

Unlike adults, newborns cannot make decisions for themselves and cannot express their desires. A surrogate decision maker must be identified to assume the responsibility of guarding the newborn's best interests. Generally, parents are considered to be the best surrogate decision makers for their own babies. For parents to fulfill this role responsibly, they need relevant, accurate, and honest information about the risks and benefits of each treatment option. In addition, they must have adequate time to thoughtfully consider each option, ask additional questions, and seek other opinions. Unfortunately, the need for resuscitation is often an unexpected emergency with little opportunity to achieve fully informed consent before proceeding. Even when you have the opportunity to meet with parents, uncertainty about the extent of congenital anomalies, the actual gestational age, the likelihood of survival, and the potential for severe disabilities may make it difficult for parents to decide before the delivery what is in their baby's best interest. In rare cases, the health care team may conclude that a decision made by a parent is not reasonable and is not in the baby's best interest.

The NRP endorses the following statement from the American Medical Association (AMA) Code of Medical Ethics*:

> The primary consideration for decisions regarding life-sustaining treatment for seriously ill newborns should be what is best for the newborn. Factors that should be weighed are as follows:
> 1. The chance that the therapy will succeed
> 2. The risks involved with treatment and nontreatment

---

*American Medical Association, Council on Ethical and Judicial Affairs. *Code of Medical Ethics: Current Opinions with Annotations*, 2010-2011 ed. Chicago, IL: American Medical Association (Opinion 2.215).

3. The degree to which the therapy, if successful, will extend life
4. The pain and discomfort associated with the therapy
5. The anticipated quality of life for the newborn with and without treatment

## What laws apply to neonatal resuscitation?

There is no federal law in the United States mandating delivery room resuscitation in all circumstances. There may be laws in your area that apply to the care of newborns in the delivery room. Health care professionals should be aware of the laws in the areas where they practice. If you are uncertain about the laws in your area, you should consult your hospital ethics committee or attorney. In most circumstances, it is ethically and legally acceptable to withhold or withdraw resuscitation efforts if the parents and health care professionals agree that further medical intervention would be futile, would merely prolong dying, or would not offer sufficient benefit to justify the burdens imposed. In many states, if the mother is a minor, she is considered "emancipated" and can legally make decisions about her fetus and newborn, but not necessarily for herself. Usually, the baby's father also has specific legal rights with regard to the baby, but only if he is married to the mother, or is listed as the father on the official birth certificate. Again, check the regulations for your specific state.

## What role should parents play in decisions about resuscitation?

Parents have a primary role in determining the goals of care delivered to their newborn. However, informed decisions should be based on complete and reliable information, and this may not be available until after delivery, and perhaps not until several hours after birth.

## Are there situations in which it is ethical not to initiate resuscitation?

The delivery of extremely immature babies and those with severe congenital anomalies frequently raises questions about the initiation of resuscitation. Although the survival rate for babies born between 22 and 25 weeks' gestation increases with each additional week of gestation, the incidence of moderate or severe neurodevelopmental disability among survivors is high. Where gestation, birth weight, and/or congenital anomalies are associated with almost certain early death, and unacceptably high morbidity is likely among the rare survivors, resuscitation is not indicated, although exceptions may be appropriate

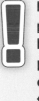

Both parents and providers should keep in mind that preliminary decisions regarding the level of care to be provided after delivery may need to be altered after initial assessment of the baby has been performed.

in specific cases to comply with parental request. Examples where noninitiation of resuscitation is appropriate may include the following*:

- Confirmed gestational age of less than 23 weeks or a birth weight of less than 400 g

- Anencephaly

- Confirmed lethal genetic disorder or malformation

- When available data support an unacceptably high likelihood of death or severe disability

In conditions associated with uncertain prognosis, where there is borderline survival and a relatively high rate of morbidity, and where the burden to the child is high, some parents will request that no attempt be made to resuscitate the baby. An example may include a baby born at 23 to 24 weeks' gestation. In such cases, the parents' views on either initiating or withholding resuscitation should be solicited and supported through well-coordinated communication by obstetric and pediatric team members. The provider should be proactively involved and exercise assessment and judgment leading to appropriate care. That care might be comfort care.

These recommendations must be interpreted according to current local outcomes and parental desires. Given the uncertainty of gestational age and birth-weight predictions, be cautious about making unalterable decisions about resuscitative efforts before the baby is born. When counseling parents, advise them that decisions made about neonatal management before birth may need to be modified in the delivery room, depending on the condition of the baby at birth and the postnatal gestational age assessment.

 Unless conception occurred via in vitro fertilization, techniques used for obstetric dating are accurate to 3 to 5 days if applied in the first trimester, and only to ± 1 to 2 weeks subsequently. Estimates of fetal weight are accurate only to ± 15% to 20%. Even small discrepancies of 1 or 2 weeks between estimated and actual gestational age or 100 to 200 g difference in birth weight may have implications for survival and long-term morbidity. Also, fetal weight can be misleading if there has been intrauterine growth restriction, and outcomes may be less predictable. These uncertainties underscore the importance of not making firm commitments about withholding or providing resuscitation until you have the opportunity to examine the baby after birth.

---

*These situations are examples based on currently available US outcomes data, and may vary depending on current local data and standards, available resources, and parental input.

### Are there times when you should resuscitate a baby against parental wishes?

Although parents generally are considered the best surrogate decision makers for their own children, health care professionals have a legal and an ethical obligation to provide appropriate care for the baby based on current medical information and their clinical assessment. In conditions associated with a high rate of survival and an acceptable risk of morbidity, resuscitation is nearly always indicated. In such cases, it may be helpful to solicit a second opinion from a colleague. When the health care team is unable to reach agreement with the parents on a reasonable treatment strategy, it may become necessary to consult the hospital ethics committee or legal counsel. If there is not enough time to consult additional resources, and the responsible physician concludes that the parents' decision is not in the best interest of the child, it is usually appropriate to resuscitate the baby over the parents' objection. Accurate documentation of the discussions with the parents, as well as documentation of the basis for the decision, is essential.

### What discussions should be held with parents prior to a very high-risk birth?

Meeting with parents prior to a very high-risk birth is important for both the parents and the neonatal care providers. Both the obstetric provider and the provider who will care for the baby after birth should talk with the parents. Studies have shown that obstetric and neonatal perspectives are often different. If possible, such differences should be discussed prior to meeting with the parents so that the information presented is consistent. Sometimes, such as when the woman is in active labor, it may seem as if there is inadequate time for such discussions. However, it is better to have some discussion of potential issues, even if brief, with the baby's family, than to wait until after the baby is born to initiate such conversations. Follow-up meetings can take place if the situation changes over subsequent hours and days.

### What should you say when you meet with parents for prenatal counseling before a high-risk birth?

Prenatal discussions provide an opportunity to begin establishing a trusting relationship, provide important information, establish realistic goals, and assist parents in making informed decisions for their baby. If it is impractical for you and a member of the obstetric team to meet the parents together, you should review the chart and, if possible, speak with the nurse caring for the mother before meeting with the parents, so that you can refer to the obstetric management plan during the meeting to provide consistent and coordinated communication. You should be prepared with accurate information about short- and long-term outcome data for the specific situation; ideally, you should be familiar with both national and local data. If necessary, consult with specialists at your regional referral center to obtain up-to-date information, or, if no one is available within the clinical time frame, check for pertinent information on the Internet (eg, the NRP or National Institute of Child Health & Human Development Web sites). If possible, meet with the parents before the mother has received medications that might make it difficult for her to understand or remember your conversation, and before the final stages of labor.

Before meeting with the parents, check with the mother's nurse to make sure it is a good time for a discussion. If possible, have the nurse attend the meeting. If a translator is necessary, use a hospital-trained and certified medical translator, not a friend or relative of the patient, and use simple and direct phrases to ensure accurate transmittal of information. It is best if you sit down during the meeting to make eye contact at the same level and to avoid the impression of being in a hurry. Use of clear, simple language, without medical abbreviations or jargon, is especially important. Stop talking when the mother is having a contraction or if a procedure, such as monitoring of vital signs, needs to be performed during the meeting. Resume the discussion when she is again able to concentrate on the information you are providing.

**The following issues might be covered:**

- Assessment of the baby's chances of survival and possible disability based on regional and national statistics. Be as accurate as possible, avoiding excessively negative or unrealistically positive prognoses (ie, present a balanced and objective picture of the possible outcomes).

- Consideration of palliative or "comfort-care-only" treatment as an acceptable option if the baby's viability is thought to be marginal. Do not avoid this issue. The discussion will be difficult for both you and the parents, but it is important that each of you understands the others' perspectives. If all options are discussed, most parents will quickly make clear what they want you to do. You can assure them that you will make every effort to support their wishes, but it is also important to advise them that decisions made about neonatal management before birth may need to be modified in the delivery room depending on the baby's condition at birth, the postnatal gestational age assessment, and the baby's response to resuscitative measures.

- How palliative or comfort care treatment will be provided, if agreed upon (subject to confirmation of the baby's status as described previously). Assure the parents that care would focus on preventing or relieving pain and suffering. Explain that, in this case, the baby is almost certain (or, in the case of malformations considered to be lethal, is likely) to die, but the timing could be minutes to hours, or even days, after birth. In a culturally sensitive manner, discuss ways in which the family might participate, and allow the family to make additional suggestions/requests.

- Where the resuscitation will occur, who will be in the delivery room, and what their roles will be. The events likely will be very different from the private birth the parents had originally imagined.

- Offer to give the mother and father (or support person) time alone to discuss what you have told them. Some parents may want to consult with other family members or clergy. Then make a return visit to confirm both their understanding of what may occur and your understanding of their wishes.

Review what you discussed with the obstetric care providers and the other members of your nursery's resuscitation team. *If it was decided that resuscitation would not be initiated, ensure that all members of your team, including on-call personnel and the obstetric care providers, are informed and in agreement with this decision.* If disagreements occur, discuss them in advance and consult additional professionals if necessary.

 **After you meet with the parents, document a summary of your conversation in the mother's chart.**

## What should you do if you are uncertain about the chances of survival or serious disability when you examine the baby immediately after birth?

If parents are uncertain how to proceed, or your examination suggests that the prenatal assessment of gestational age was incorrect, initial resuscitation and provision of life support allows you additional time to gather more complete clinical information and permits more time to review the situation with the parents. Once the parents and physicians have had an opportunity to evaluate additional clinical information, they may decide to discontinue critical care interventions and institute comfort care measures. In other situations, lack of response to initial resuscitative efforts may aid in decision making.

This approach also may be preferable for many parents, as they feel more comfortable that an effort was made. You should avoid a scenario where an initial decision is made not to resuscitate and then aggressive resuscitation is initiated many minutes after delivery due to a change of plan. If the newborn survives this delayed resuscitation, the risk of serious disability may increase.

**It should be noted that, although there is no ethical distinction between withholding and withdrawing support, many people find the latter more difficult. Nevertheless, resuscitation followed by withdrawal permits time for collecting more prognostic information.**

## You have followed the resuscitation recommendations, and the baby is not responding. For how long should you continue?

If you can confirm that no heart rate has been detectable for at least 10 minutes, discontinuation of resuscitation efforts may be appropriate. Current data indicate that, after 10 minutes of asystole, newborns are very unlikely to survive, and the rare survivors will have severe disability.

The decision to continue resuscitation efforts beyond 10 minutes with no heart rate should take into consideration factors such as the presumed etiology of the arrest, the gestational age of the baby, the presence or absence of complications, the potential role of therapeutic hypothermia, and the parents' previously expressed feelings about acceptable risk of morbidity.[*]

There may be other situations, such as in the case of prolonged bradycardia without improvement in the baby's condition, where, after complete and adequate resuscitation efforts, discontinuation of resuscitation may be appropriate. However, there is not enough information on outcomes in these situations to make specific recommendations, so decisions on how to proceed in these circumstances have to be made on a case-by-case basis.

## Once you have resuscitated a baby, are you obligated to continue life support?

In addition to the guideline of discontinuing resuscitation after 10 minutes of asystole, there is no obligation to continue life support if it is the judgment of experienced clinicians that such support would not be in the best interest of the baby or would serve no useful purpose (ie, would be futile). Although the parents' overall opinions regarding initiating or withdrawing therapy should be respected, the provider taking care of the baby must decide what specific treatments are medically indicated based on the baby's physical examination, physiologic status, and response to previous interventions. In the case of withdrawal of critical care interventions and institution of comfort care, the parents also should be in agreement with this judgment.

---

*Kattwinkel J, Perlman JM, Aziz K, et al. 2010 guidelines for cardiopulmonary resuscitation (CPR) and emergency cardiovascular care (ECC) of pediatric and neonatal patients: neonatal resuscitation guidelines. *Pediatrics* 2010;126;e1400–e1413.

## How do you tell the parents that their baby has died or is dying?

As soon as possible, sit down with the mother and the father (or another support person) to tell them that their baby has died (or is dying). There are no words that will make this conversation any less painful. Do not use euphemisms, such as, "Your baby has passed." Refer to the baby by name if the parents have already chosen one or by the correct gender if a name has not yet been chosen. Your role is to support the parents by giving clear and honest information in a supportive and caring manner. Express your sympathy, and reassure them that the outcome was not due to any actions or lack of actions on their part.

When interviewed, families have described comments made by some providers that were more upsetting than comforting. Be careful *not* to use phrases such as:

- "It was for the best" or "It was meant to be."

- "You can have more children."

- "At least it was only a baby and you didn't really have time to get to know her."

## How do you take care of a baby that is dying or has died?

The most important goal is to minimize suffering by providing humane and compassionate care. Offer to bring the baby to the mother and father to hold. Silence the alarms on monitors and medical equipment before removing them. Remove any unnecessary tubes, tape, monitors, or medical equipment and gently clean the baby's mouth and face. Wrap the baby in a clean blanket. Prepare the parents for what they may see, feel, and hear when they hold their baby, including the possibility of gasping, agonal respirations, color changes, persistent heart beat, and continuing movements. If the baby has obvious congenital anomalies, briefly explain to the parents what they will see. Help them look beyond any deformities by pointing out a good or memorable feature. Some institutions have specific protocols for these situations, including preparing "memory boxes" with the baby's handprints or footprints, a photo, and other items.

It is best to allow the parents private time with the baby in a comfortable environment, but a provider should check at intervals to see if anything is needed. The baby's chest should be auscultated intermittently for at least 60 seconds, as a very slow heart rate may persist for hours. Disturbing noises such as phone calls, pagers, monitor alarms, and staff conversations should be minimized. When the parents are ready for you to take the baby, the baby should be taken to a designated, private location until ready to be transported to the morgue.

It is very helpful to understand the cultural and religious expectations surrounding death in the community that you serve. Some families grieve quietly while others are more demonstrative; however, all modes are acceptable and should be accommodated. Some parents may prefer to be alone, while others may want their extended family, friends, community members, and/or clergy to be with them. Families may request to take their baby to a hospital chapel or a more peaceful setting outside, or may ask for help with arrangements for blessings or rites for their dead or dying baby. You should be as flexible as you can in responding to their wishes.

## What follow-up arrangements should be planned for the parents?

Before the parents leave the hospital, make sure you have contact information for them, and provide them with details about how to contact the attending physician, bereavement professionals, and, if available, a perinatal loss support group. If your institution does not provide these services, it may be helpful to contact your regional perinatal referral center to obtain contact information for the parents. It is important to involve the family's primary care physicians so they can provide additional support for the mother, father, and surviving siblings. The attending physician may want to schedule a follow-up appointment to answer any unresolved questions, review results of studies pending at the time of death or autopsy results, and assess the family's needs. Some hospitals sponsor parent-to-parent support groups and plan an annual memorial service, bringing together families who have suffered a perinatal loss. Recognize that some families may not want any additional contact from the hospital staff. This desire must be respected. Unexpected communications, such as a quality assurance survey from the hospital, or newsletters about baby care, may be an unwanted reminder of the family's loss. Parents should be urged to direct questions to the obstetric provider regarding concerns they may have about events and care before birth; providers responsible for pediatric care should be careful not to make comments that might be considered judgmental about obstetric care.

## How do you support the staff in the nursery after a perinatal death?

Staff members who participated in the care of the baby and family also need support. They will have feelings of sadness and also may be feeling anger and guilt. Consider holding a debriefing session shortly after the baby's death so you can openly discuss questions and feelings in a professional, supportive, and nonjudgmental forum. However, speculation based on secondhand information should be avoided in such meetings, and questions and issues regarding care decisions and actions should be discussed only in a qualified peer review session and should follow hospital policy for such sessions.

## Key Points

1. The ethical principles regarding the resuscitation of a newborn should be no different from those followed in resuscitating an older child or adult.

2. Ethical and current national legal principles do not mandate attempted resuscitation in all circumstances, and withdrawal of critical care interventions and institution of comfort care are considered acceptable if there is agreement by health care professionals and the parents that further resuscitation efforts would be futile, would merely prolong dying, or would not offer sufficient benefit to justify the burdens imposed.

3. Parents are considered to be the appropriate surrogate decision makers for their own babies. For parents to fulfill this role responsibly, they must be given relevant and accurate information about the risks and benefits of each treatment option.

4. Where gestation, birth weight, and/or congenital anomalies are associated with almost certain early death, or unacceptably high morbidity is likely among the rare survivors, resuscitation is not indicated, although exceptions may be reasonable to comply with parental wishes.

5. In conditions associated with uncertain prognosis, where there is borderline survival and a high rate of morbidity, and where the burden to the child is high, parental desires regarding initiation of resuscitation should be supported.

6. Unless conception occurred via in vitro fertilization, techniques used for obstetrics dating are accurate to 3 to 5 days if applied in the first trimester, and only to ± 1 to 2 weeks subsequently. Estimates of fetal weight are accurate only to ± 15% to 20%. When counseling parents about the births of babies born at the extremes of prematurity, advise them that decisions made about neonatal management before birth may need to be modified in the delivery room, depending on the condition of the baby at birth and the postnatal gestational age assessment.

7. Discontinuation of resuscitation efforts should be considered after 10 minutes of absent heart rate. The decision to continue resuscitation efforts beyond this point should take into consideration factors such as the presumed etiology of the arrest, the gestational age of the baby, the presence or absence of complications, the potential role of therapeutic hypothermia, and the parents' previously expressed feelings about acceptable risk of morbidity.

## Lesson 9 Review

*(The answers follow.)*

1. The 4 common principles of medical ethics are
   * _____
   * _____
   * _____
   * _____

2. Generally, parents are considered to be the best "surrogate" decision makers for their own newborns. (True/False)

3. The parents of a baby about to be born at 23 weeks' gestation have requested that, if there is any possibility of brain damage, they do not want any attempt made to resuscitate their baby. Which of the following is most appropriate?
   A. Support their wishes and promise to give "comfort care only" to the baby after birth.
   B. Tell them that you will try to support their decision, but must wait until you examine the baby after birth to determine what you will do.
   C. Tell them that all medical decisions regarding resuscitation are made by the medical team and the physician-in-charge.
   D. Try to convince them to change their mind.

## Lesson 9 Review—*continued*

4. You have been asked to be present for the impending birth of a baby known from prenatal ultrasound and laboratory assessments to have major congenital malformations. List 4 issues that should be covered when you meet the parents.

   • _____
   • _____
   • _____
   • _____

5. A mother enters the delivery suite in active labor at 34 weeks' gestation after having had no prenatal care. She proceeds to deliver a live-born baby with major malformations that appear to be consistent with trisomy 18 syndrome. An attempt to resuscitate the baby in an adjacent room is unsuccessful. Which of the following is the most appropriate action?
   A. Explain the situation to the parents and ask them if they would like to hold the baby.
   B. Take the baby away from the area, tell the parents that she was stillborn, and tell them that it would be best if they did not see her.
   C. Tell the parents that she had a major malformation and it "was for the best" that she died because she would have been "disabled anyway."

6. Which of the following is (are) appropriate to say to parents whose baby just died after an unsuccessful resuscitation? (Select all that apply):
   A. "I'm sorry, we tried to resuscitate your baby, but the resuscitation was unsuccessful and your baby died."
   B. "This is a terrible tragedy, but, in view of the malformations, it was meant to be."
   C. "I'm so sorry that your baby died. She is a beautiful baby."
   D. "Fortunately, you are both young and can have another baby."

# Lesson 9 Answers to Questions

1. The 4 principles are
   - Respect individual's rights of freedom and liberty to make choices that affect his or her life *(autonomy)*.
   - Act so as to benefit others *(beneficence)*.
   - Avoid harming people unjustifiably *(nonmaleficence)*.
   - Treat people truthfully and fairly *(justice)*.

2. True.

3. B. Tell them that you will try to support their decision, but must wait until you examine the baby after birth to determine what you will do.

4. Any of the following:
   - Review the current obstetric plans and expectations.
   - Explain who will be present, and their respective roles.
   - Explain the statistics and your assessment of the baby's chances for survival and possible disability.
   - Determine the parents' wishes and expectations.
   - Inform the parents that decisions may need to be modified after you examine the baby.

5. A. Explain the situation to the parents and ask them if they would like to hold the baby.

6. Either or both of the following are appropriate:
   A. "I'm sorry, we tried to resuscitate your baby, but the resuscitation was unsuccessful and your baby died."
   C. "I'm so sorry that your baby died. She is a beautiful baby."

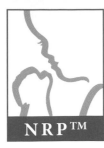

# Integrated Skills Station Performance Checklist (Basic)

**The Integrated Skills Station is a required course component used for learner evaluation.**

The instructor may use several scenarios to allow the learner to demonstrate all steps of the Neonatal Resuscitation Program™ (NRP™) Flow Diagram (Lessons 1 through 4) in correct order, using proper technique, without coaching from the instructor. If the learner makes significant errors in timing, sequence, or technique, the learner returns to the appropriate Performance Skills Station for additional help and practice.

If the instructor wants more detail and sample vital signs, Performance Checklist 4 may be used.

**Participant Name:** _____

| Critical Performance Steps | Details |
|---|---|
| ☐ Obtains relevant perinatal history | Gestational age, fluid, expected number of babies, additional risk factors? |
| ☐ Performs Equipment Check | Warm, Clear airway, Auscultate, Oxygenate, Ventilate, Intubate, Medicate, Thermoregulate. |
| ☐ Discusses plan and assigns team member roles | Use NRP Key Behavioral Skills throughout resuscitation to improve teamwork and communication. |
| ☐ Completes initial assessment | Term, tone, crying, or breathing? |
| ☐ *(option) Meconium management* | *If NOT vigorous, indicate need for endotracheal intubation and suction.* |
| ☐ Performs initial steps | Warm, clear airway if necessary, dry, remove wet linen, stimulate. |
| ☐ Evaluates respirations and heart rate (HR) | Auscultate apical pulse or palpate umbilicus. **Heart rate less than 60 beats per minute (bpm), apneic or gasping.** |
| ☐ Initiates positive-pressure ventilation (PPV) with 21% oxygen | Apply mask correctly, rate 40-60/minute. |
| ☐ Calls for additional help, if necessary | A minimum of 2 resuscitators necessary if PPV required. |
| ☐ Requests pulse oximetry | Place probe on right hand before plugging into monitor. |
| ☐ Assesses for rising heart rate and oxygen saturation within first 5-10 breaths. | **HR remains below 60 bpm.** Heart rate not rising. Pulse oximetry might not be functioning. |
| ☐ Assesses chest movement and bilateral breath sounds. | Initially respond that **bilateral breath sounds are absent and chest is NOT moving with PPV.** |
| ☐ Takes ventilation corrective steps (MR SOPA) | Instructor decides how many corrective steps are necessary. **M**ask adjustment and **R**eposition head. **S**uction mouth and nose and **O**pen mouth. Increase **P**ressure (do not exceed 40 cm H$_2$O). *Indicate need to* Use **A**lternative airway (endotracheal [ET] tube or laryngeal mask airway). |
| ☐ Requests assessment of bilateral breath sounds and chest movement<br>☐ Performs 30 seconds of effective PPV | **Bilateral breath sounds and chest movement are present.** |
| ☐ Evaluates HR, breathing, and oxygen saturation | **Heart rate remains below 60 bpm.** **Apneic.** **Pulse oximetry might not be functioning.** |

| | |
|---|---|
| ☐ Increases oxygen to 100% in preparation for chest compressions | **Increase oxygen concentration to 100% when chest compressions begin.** |
| ☐ Initiates chest compressions coordinated with PPV | 2 thumbs (preferred) on lower third of sternum,<br>3 compressions: 1 ventilation.<br>Compress one-third of the anterior-posterior diameter of the chest. |
| ☐ Calls for additional help | **Indicates need for help with intubation, line placement, and medication.** |
| ☐ After at least 45-60 seconds of chest compressions, evaluates HR, breathing, and oxygen saturation | **Heart rate above 60 bpm.**<br>**Occasional spontaneous breath.**<br>**Pulse oximetry functioning.** |
| ☐ Discontinues compressions, continues ventilation for 30 seconds | **Discontinue compressions if heart rate above 60 bpm.**<br>**Reassess every 30 seconds.** |
| ☐ Evaluates HR, breathing, and oxygen saturation. Continues/discontinues PPV appropriately. May provide free-flow oxygen and adjust oxygen concentration per oximetry. | **Adjust oxygen concentration based on oximetry and newborn's age. Continue PPV until HR above 100 bpm with adequate breathing.** |
| ☐ Directs post-resuscitation care | Ongoing evaluation and monitoring.<br>Communicate effectively with parent(s). |

**Reflective Questions:**

1. What did you think you would need to do when this baby was placed on the radiant warmer?
2. What went well during this resuscitation? What would you do differently next time?
3. What NRP Key Behavioral Skills were used? Give examples.

### Neonatal Resuscitation Program Key Behavioral Skills

| | | |
|---|---|---|
| Know your environment. | Delegate workload optimally. | Use all available resources. |
| Anticipate and plan. | Allocate attention wisely. | Call for help when needed. |
| Assume the leadership role. | Use all available information. | Maintain professional behavior. |
| Communicate effectively. | | |

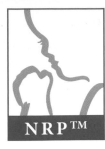

# Integrated Skills Station Performance Checklist (Advanced)

**The Integrated Skills Station is a required course component used for learner evaluation.**

The instructor may use several scenarios to allow the learner to demonstrate all steps of the Neonatal Resuscitation Program™ (NRP™) Flow Diagram (Lessons 1 through 4 and additional lessons relevant to course objectives) in correct order, using proper technique, without coaching from the instructor. If the learner makes significant errors in timing, sequence, or technique, the learner returns to the appropriate Performance Skills Station for additional help and practice.

If the instructor wants more detail and sample vital signs, Performance Checklist 6 may be used.

**Participant Name:** _____

| Critical Performance Steps | Details |
|---|---|
| ☐ Obtains relevant perinatal history | Gestational age, fluid, expected number of babies, additional risk factors? |
| ☐ Performs Equipment Check | Warm, Clear airway, Auscultate, Oxygenate, Ventilate, Intubate, Medicate, Thermoregulate. |
| ☐ Discusses plan and assigns team member roles | Use NRP Key Behavioral Skills throughout resuscitation to improve teamwork and communication. |
| ☐ Completes initial assessment | Term, tone, crying or breathing? |
| ☐ *(option) Meconium management* | *If NOT vigorous, assist with/performs tracheal suction.* |
| ☐ Performs initial steps | Warm, clear airway if necessary, dry, remove wet linen, stimulate. |
| ☐ Evaluates respirations and heart rate (HR) | Auscultate apical pulse or palpate umbilicus. **Heart rate less than 60 beats per minute (bpm), apneic or gasping.** |
| ☐ Initiates positive-pressure ventilation (PPV) with 21% oxygen | Apply mask correctly, rate 40-60/minute. |
| ☐ Calls for additional help, if needed | A minimum of 2 resuscitators necessary if PPV required. |
| ☐ Requests pulse oximetry | Place probe on right hand before plugging into monitor. |
| ☐ Assesses for rising heart rate and oxygen saturation within first 5-10 breaths. | **HR remains below 60 bpm.** Heart rate not rising. Pulse oximetry might not be functioning. |
| ☐ Assesses chest movement and bilateral breath sounds. | Initially respond that **bilateral breath sounds are absent and chest is NOT moving with PPV.** |
| ☐ Takes ventilation corrective steps (MR SOPA) | Instructor decides how many corrective steps are necessary. **M**ask adjustment and **R**eposition head. **S**uction mouth and nose and **O**pen mouth. Increase **P**ressure (do not exceed 40 cm H$_2$O). Use **A**lternative airway (endotracheal [ET] tube or laryngeal mask airway). |
| ☐ Requests assessment of bilateral breath sounds and chest movement<br>☐ Performs 30 seconds of effective PPV | **Bilateral breath sounds and chest movement are present.** |
| ☐ Evaluates HR, breathing, and oxygen saturation | **Heart rate remains below 60 bpm.** **Apneic.** **Pulse oximetry might not be functioning.** |

| | |
|---|---|
| ☐ Intubates or directs intubation and assesses ET tube placement | Intubation is recommended prior to beginning chest compressions. |
| ☐ Increases oxygen to 100% in preparation for chest compressions (CC) | **Increase oxygen concentration to 100% when chest compressions begin.** |
| ☐ Initiates chest compressions coordinated with PPV | 2 thumbs (preferred) on lower third of sternum, 3 compressions: 1 ventilation. Compress one-third of the anterior-posterior diameter of the chest. |
| ☐ Calls for additional help | Complex scenario may require more help. |
| ☐ After at least 45-60 seconds of chest compressions, evaluates HR, breathing, and oxygen saturation | **HR remains below 60 bpm.** **Apneic.** **Pulse oximetry might not be functioning.** |
| ☐ May consider intratracheal epinephrine while umbilical venous catheter (UVC) is being placed. | Epinephrine dose: 1:10,000 (0.1-0.3 mL/kg). *Intratracheal dose:* 0.5 to 1 mL/kg. No response expected from intratracheal epinephrine for at least 1 minute and perhaps longer. |
| ☐ Places or directs placement of UVC | CC may be performed from head of infant after intubation. Insert UVC 2-4 cm. Hold or tape catheter to avoid dislodgement. |
| ☐ After at least 45-60 seconds of chest compressions, evaluates HR, breathing, and oxygen saturation | **Heart rate remains below 60 bpm.** **Apneic.** **Pulse oximeter might not be functioning.** |
| ☐ Administers or directs administration of IV epinephrine | Epinephrine dose: 1:10,000 (0.1-0.3 mL/kg). *IV dose:* 0.1 to 0.3 mL/kg. Flush UVC with 0.5-1 mL normal saline. |
| ☐ After at least 45-60 seconds of chest compressions, evaluates HR, breathing, and oxygen saturation. | **Heart rate above 60 bpm.** **Occasional gasp.** **Pulse oximetry functioning.** |
| ☐ Discontinues compressions, continues ventilation at 40-60 breaths/minute | Discontinue compressions if HR above 60 bpm. Reassess every 30 seconds. |
| ☐ (Option) Based on scenario, identifies need for volume replacement (states solution, dose, route, rate) | *Risk factors:* Placenta previa, abruption, blood loss from umbilical cord. *Solutions:* Normal saline, Ringer's lactate or O Rh-negative packed cells. *Dose:* 10 mL/kg over 5-10 minutes. *Route:* Umbilical vein. *Rate:* Over 5-10 minutes. |
| ☐ Continues to monitor HR, breathing, and oxygen saturation every 30 seconds during resuscitation | Adjust oxygen based on oximetry and newborn's age. Continue PPV until HR above 100 bpm with adequate respiratory effort (newborn may remain intubated). |
| ☐ Directs post-resuscitation care | Ongoing evaluation and monitoring. Communicate effectively with parent(s). |

**Reflective Questions:**

1. What did you think you would need to do when this baby was placed on the radiant warmer?
2. What went well during this resuscitation? What would you do differently next time?
3. What NRP Key Behavioral Skills were used? Give examples.

### Neonatal Resuscitation Program Key Behavioral Skills

| | | |
|---|---|---|
| Know your environment. | Delegate workload optimally. | Use all available resources. |
| Anticipate and plan. | Allocate attention wisely. | Call for help when needed. |
| Assume the leadership role. | Use all available information. | Maintain professional behavior. |
| Communicate effectively. | | |

# Appendix

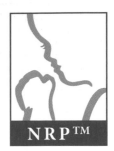

# PEDIATRICS®

OFFICIAL JOURNAL OF THE AMERICAN ACADEMY OF PEDIATRICS

**Neonatal Resuscitation: 2010 American Heart Association Guidelines for Cardiopulmonary Resuscitation and Emergency Cardiovascular Care**

John Kattwinkel, Jeffrey M. Perlman, Khalid Aziz, Christopher Colby, Karen Fairchild, John Gallagher, Mary Fran Hazinski, Louis P. Halamek, Praveen Kumar, George Little, Jane E. McGowan, Barbara Nightengale, Mildred M. Ramirez, Steven Ringer, Wendy M. Simon, Gary M. Weiner, Myra Wyckoff and Jeanette Zaichkin
*Pediatrics* 2010;126;e1400-e1413; originally published online Oct 18, 2010;
DOI: 10.1542/peds.2010-2972E

The online version of this article, along with updated information and services, is located on the World Wide Web at:
http://www.pediatrics.org/cgi/content/full/126/5/e1400

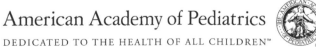

American Academy of Pediatrics
DEDICATED TO THE HEALTH OF ALL CHILDREN™

# Special Report—Neonatal Resuscitation: 2010 American Heart Association Guidelines for Cardiopulmonary Resuscitation and Emergency Cardiovascular Care

The following guidelines are an interpretation of the evidence presented in the *2010 International Consensus on Cardiopulmonary Resuscitation and Emergency Cardiovascular Care Science With Treatment Recommendations[1]*). They apply primarily to newly born infants undergoing transition from intrauterine to extrauterine life, but the recommendations are also applicable to neonates who have completed perinatal transition and require resuscitation during the first few weeks to months following birth. Practitioners who resuscitate infants at birth or at any time during the initial hospital admission should consider following these guidelines. For the purposes of these guidelines, the terms *newborn* and *neonate* are intended to apply to any infant during the initial hospitalization. The term *newly born* is intended to apply specifically to an infant at the time of birth.

Approximately 10% of newborns require some assistance to begin breathing at birth. Less than 1% require extensive resuscitative measures.[2,3] Although the vast majority of newly born infants do not require intervention to make the transition from intrauterine to extrauterine life, because of the large total number of births, a sizable number will require some degree of resuscitation.

Those newly born infants who do not require resuscitation can generally be identified by a rapid assessment of the following 3 characteristics:

- Term gestation?
- Crying or breathing?
- Good muscle tone?

If the answer to all 3 of these questions is "yes," the baby does not need resuscitation and should not be separated from the mother. The baby should be dried, placed skin-to-skin with the mother, and covered with dry linen to maintain temperature. Observation of breathing, activity, and color should be ongoing.

If the answer to any of these assessment questions is "no," the infant should receive one or more of the following 4 categories of action in sequence:

A. Initial steps in stabilization (provide warmth, clear airway if necessary, dry, stimulate)

B. Ventilation

John Kattwinkel, Co-Chair*, Jeffrey M. Perlman, Co-Chair*, Khalid Aziz, Christopher Colby, Karen Fairchild, John Gallagher, Mary Fran Hazinski, Louis P. Halamek, Praveen Kumar, George Little, Jane E. McGowan, Barbara Nightengale, Mildred M. Ramirez, Steven Ringer, Wendy M. Simon, Gary M. Weiner, Myra Wyckoff, Jeanette Zaichkin

**KEY WORDS**
cardiopulmonary resuscitation

The American Heart Association requests that this document be cited as follows: Kattwinkel J, Perlman JM, Aziz K, Colby C, Fairchild K, Gallagher J, Hazinski MF, Halamek LP, Kumar P, Little G, McGowan JE, Nightengale B, Ramirez MM, Ringer S, Simon WM, Weiner GM, Wyckoff M, Zaichkin J. Part 15: neonatal resuscitation: 2010 American Heart Association Guidelines for Cardiopulmonary Resuscitation and Emergency Cardiovascular Care. *Circulation.* 2010;122:S909–S919.

*Co-chairs and equal first co-authors.

(Circulation. 2010;122:S909–S919.)
© 2010 American Heart Association, Inc.

Circulation is available at http://circ.ahajournals.org.

doi:10.1542/peds.2010-2972E

## Newborn Resuscitation

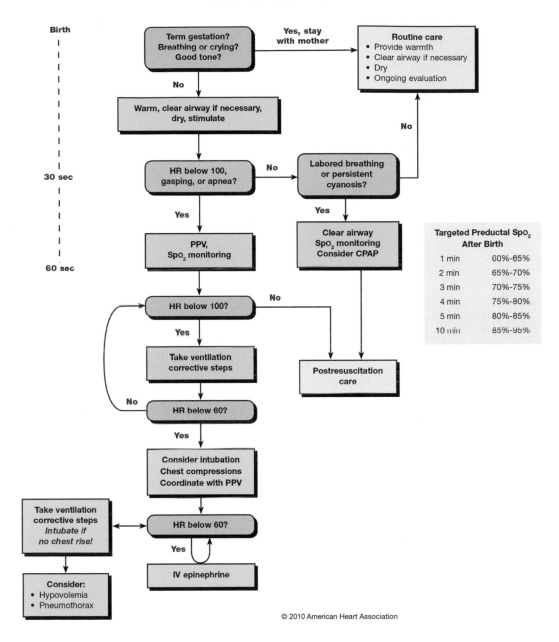

© 2010 American Heart Association

C. Chest compressions

D. Administration of epinephrine and/ or volume expansion

Approximately 60 seconds ("the Golden Minute") are allotted for completing the initial steps, reevaluating, and beginning ventilation if required (see Figure). The decision to progress beyond the initial steps is determined by simultaneous assessment of 2 vital characteristics: respirations (apnea, gasping, or labored or unlabored breathing) and heart rate (whether greater than or less than 100 beats per minute). Assessment of heart rate should be done by intermittently auscultating the precordial pulse. When a pulse is detectable, palpation of the umbilical pulse can also provide a rapid estimate of the pulse and is more accurate than palpation at other sites.[4,5]

A pulse oximeter can provide a continuous assessment of the pulse without interruption of other resuscitation measures, but the device takes 1 to 2 minutes to apply, and it may not function during states of very poor cardiac output or perfusion. Once positive pressure ventilation or supplementary oxygen administration is begun, assessment should consist of simultaneous evaluation of 3 vital characteristics: heart rate, respirations, and the state of oxygenation, the latter optimally determined by a pulse oximeter as discussed under "Assessment of Oxygen Need and Administration of Oxygen" below. The most sensitive indicator of a successful response to each step is an increase in heart rate.

## ANTICIPATION OF RESUSCITATION NEED

Anticipation, adequate preparation, accurate evaluation, and prompt initiation of support are critical for successful neonatal resuscitation. At every delivery there should be at least 1 person whose primary responsibility is the newly born. This person must be capable of initiating resuscitation, including administration of positive-pressure ventilation and chest compressions. Either that person or someone else who is promptly available should have the skills required to perform a complete resuscitation, including endotracheal intubation and administration of medications.[6] Several studies have demonstrated that a cesarean section performed under regional anesthesia at 37 to 39 weeks, without antenatally identified risk factors, versus a similar vaginal delivery performed at term, does not increase the risk of the baby requiring endotracheal intubation.[7–10]

With careful consideration of risk factors, the majority of newborns who will need resuscitation can be identified before birth. If the possible need for resuscitation is anticipated, additional skilled personnel should be recruited and the necessary equipment prepared. Identifiable risk factors and the necessary equipment for resuscitation are listed in the *Textbook of Neonatal Resuscitation, 6th Edition*

(American Academy of Pediatrics, *in press*).[11] If a preterm delivery (<37 weeks of gestation) is expected, special preparations will be required. Preterm babies have immature lungs that may be more difficult to ventilate and are also more vulnerable to injury by positive-pressure ventilation. Preterm babies also have immature blood vessels in the brain that are prone to hemorrhage; thin skin and a large surface area, which contribute to rapid heat loss; increased susceptibility to infection; and increased risk of hypovolemic shock related to small blood volume.

## INITIAL STEPS

The initial steps of resuscitation are to provide warmth by placing the baby under a radiant heat source, positioning the head in a "sniffing" position to open the airway, clearing the airway if necessary with a bulb syringe or suction catheter, drying the baby, and stimulating breathing. Recent studies have examined several aspects of these initial steps. These studies are summarized below.

### Temperature Control

Very low-birth weight (<1500 g) preterm babies are likely to become hypothermic despite the use of traditional techniques for decreasing heat loss.[12] For this reason additional warming techniques are recommended (eg, prewarming the delivery room to 26°C,[13] covering the baby in plastic wrapping (food or medical grade, heat-resistant plastic) (Class I, LOE A[14,15]), placing the baby on an exothermic mattress (Class IIb, LOE B[16]), and placing the baby under radiant heat (Class IIb, LOE C[17]). The infant's temperature must be monitored closely because of the slight, but described risk of hyperthermia when these techniques are used in combination (Class IIb, LOE B[16]). Other techniques for maintaining temperature during stabilization of the baby in the delivery room have been used (eg,

prewarming the linen, drying and swaddling, placing the baby skin-to-skin with the mother and covering both with a blanket) and are recommended, but they have not been studied specifically (Class IIb, LOE C). All resuscitation procedures, including endotracheal intubation, chest compression, and insertion of intravenous lines, can be performed with these temperature-controlling interventions in place (Class IIb, LOE C).

Infants born to febrile mothers have been reported to have a higher incidence of perinatal respiratory depression, neonatal seizures, and cerebral palsy and an increased risk of mortality.[18,19] Animal studies indicate that hyperthermia during or after ischemia is associated with progression of cerebral injury. Lowering the temperature reduces neuronal damage.[20] Hyperthermia should be avoided (Class IIb, LOE C). The goal is to achieve normothermia and avoid iatrogenic hyperthermia.

### Clearing the Airway

#### When Amniotic Fluid Is Clear

There is evidence that suctioning of the nasopharynx can create bradycardia during resuscitation[21,22] and that suctioning of the trachea in intubated babies receiving mechanical ventilation in the neonatal intensive care unit (NICU) can be associated with deterioration of pulmonary compliance and oxygenation and reduction in cerebral blood flow velocity when performed routinely (ie, in the absence of obvious nasal or oral secretions).[23,24] However, there is also evidence that suctioning in the presence of secretions can decrease respiratory resistance.[25] Therefore it is recommended that suctioning immediately following birth (including suctioning with a bulb syringe) should be reserved for babies who have obvious obstruction to spontaneous breathing or who require positive-pressure ventilation (PPV) (Class IIb, LOE C).

### When Meconium is Present

Aspiration of meconium before delivery, during birth, or during resuscitation can cause severe meconium aspiration syndrome (MAS). Historically a variety of techniques have been recommended to reduce the incidence of MAS. Suctioning of the oropharynx before delivery of the shoulders was considered routine until a randomized controlled trial demonstrated it to be of no value.[26] Elective and routine endotracheal intubation and direct suctioning of the trachea were initially recommended for all meconium-stained newborns until a randomized controlled trial demonstrated that there was no value in performing this procedure in babies who were vigorous at birth.[27] Although depressed infants born to mothers with meconium-stained amniotic fluid (MSAF) are at increased risk to develop MAS,[28,29] tracheal suctioning has not been associated with reduction in the incidence of MAS or mortality in these infants.[30,31] The only evidence that direct tracheal suctioning of meconium may be of value was based on comparison of suctioned babies with historic controls, and there was apparent selection bias in the group of intubated babies included in those studies.[32–34]

In the absence of randomized, controlled trials, there is insufficient evidence to recommend a change in the current practice of performing endotracheal suctioning of nonvigorous babies with meconium-stained amniotic fluid (Class IIb, LOE C). However, if attempted intubation is prolonged and unsuccessful, bag-mask ventilation should be considered, particularly if there is persistent bradycardia.

### Assessment of Oxygen Need and Administration of Oxygen

There is a large body of evidence that blood oxygen levels in uncompromised babies generally do not reach extrauterine values until approximately 10 minutes following birth. Oxyhemoglo-bin saturation may normally remain in the 70% to 80% range for several minutes following birth, thus resulting in the appearance of cyanosis during that time. Other studies have shown that clinical assessment of skin color is a very poor indicator of oxyhemoglobin saturation during the immediate neonatal period and that lack of cyanosis appears to be a very poor indicator of the state of oxygenation of an uncompromised baby following birth.

Optimal management of oxygen during neonatal resuscitation becomes particularly important because of the evidence that either insufficient or excessive oxygenation can be harmful to the newborn infant. Hypoxia and ischemia are known to result in injury to multiple organs. Conversely there is growing experimental evidence, as well as evidence from studies of babies receiving resuscitation, that adverse outcomes may result from even brief exposure to excessive oxygen during and following resuscitation.

### Pulse Oximetry

Numerous studies have defined the percentiles of oxygen saturation as a function of time from birth in uncompromised babies born at term (see table in Figure). This includes saturations measured from both preductal and postductal sites, following both operative and vaginal deliveries, and those occurring at sea level and at altitude.[35–40]

Newer pulse oximeters, which employ probes designed specifically for neonates, have been shown to provide reliable readings within 1 to 2 minutes following birth.[41–43] These oximeters are reliable in the large majority of newborns, both term and preterm, and requiring resuscitation or not, as long as there is sufficient cardiac output and skin blood flow for the oximeter to detect a pulse. It is recommended that oximetry be used when resuscitation can be anticipated,[2] when positive pressure is administered for more than a few breaths, when cyanosis is persistent, or when supplementary oxygen is administered (Class I, LOE B).

To appropriately compare oxygen saturations to similar published data, the probe should be attached to a preductal location (ie, the right upper extremity, usually the wrist or medial surface of the palm).[43] There is some evidence that attaching the probe to the baby before connecting the probe to the instrument facilitates the most rapid acquisition of signal (Class IIb, LOE C).[42]

### Administration of Supplementary Oxygen

Two meta-analyses of several randomized controlled trials comparing neonatal resuscitation initiated with room air versus 100% oxygen showed increased survival when resuscitation was initiated with air.[44,45] There are no studies in term infants comparing outcomes when resuscitations are initiated with different concentrations of oxygen other than 100% or room air. One study in preterm infants showed that initiation of resuscitation with a blend of oxygen and air resulted in less hypoxemia or hyperoxemia, as defined by the investigators, than when resuscitation was initiated with either air or 100% oxygen followed by titration with an adjustable blend of air and oxygen.[46]

In the absence of studies comparing outcomes of neonatal resuscitation initiated with other oxygen concentrations or targeted at various oxyhemoglobin saturations, it is recommended that the goal in babies being resuscitated at birth, whether born at term or preterm, should be an oxygen saturation value in the interquartile range of preductal saturations (see table in Figure) measured in healthy term babies following vaginal birth at sea level (Class IIb, LOE B). These targets may be achieved by initiating resuscitation with air or a blended oxygen and titrating the oxygen concentration to achieve an $Spo_2$ in the target range as described above using pulse oximetry (Class IIb, LOE C). If blended oxygen is not available, resuscitation should be initiated with air (Class IIb, LOE B). If the baby is bradycardic (HR <60 per minute) after 90 seconds of resuscitation with a lower concentration of oxygen, oxygen concentration should be increased to 100% until recovery of a normal heart rate (Class IIb, LOE B).

### Positive-Pressure Ventilation (PPV)

If the infant remains apneic or gasping, or if the heart rate remains <100 per minute after administering the initial steps, start PPV.

### Initial Breaths and Assisted Ventilation

Initial inflations following birth, either spontaneous or assisted, create a functional residual capacity (FRC).[47–50] The optimal pressure, inflation time, and flow rate required to establish an effective FRC when PPV is administered during resuscitation have not been determined. Evidence from animal studies indicates that preterm lungs are easily injured by large-volume inflations immediately after birth.[51,52] Assisted ventilation rates of 40 to 60 breaths per minute are commonly used, but the relative efficacy of various rates has not been investigated.

The primary measure of adequate initial ventilation is prompt improvement in heart rate.[53] Chest wall movement should be assessed if heart rate does not improve. The initial peak inflating pressures needed are variable and unpredictable and should be individualized to achieve an increase in heart rate or movement of the chest with each breath. Inflation pressure should be monitored; an initial inflation pressure of 20 cm $H_2O$ may be effective, but ≥30 to 40 cm $H_2O$ may be required in some term babies without spontaneous ventilation (Class IIb, LOE C).[48,50,54] If circumstances preclude the use of pressure monitoring, the minimal inflation required to achieve an increase in heart rate should be used. There is insufficient evidence to recommend an optimum inflation time. In summary, assisted ventilation should be delivered at a rate of 40 to 60 breaths per minute to promptly achieve or maintain a heart rate >100 per minute (Class IIb, LOE C).

The use of colorimetric $CO_2$ detectors during mask ventilation of small numbers of preterm infants in the intensive care unit and in the delivery room has been reported, and such detectors may help to identify airway obstruction.[55,56] However, it is unclear whether the use of $CO_2$ detectors during mask ventilation confers additional benefit above clinical assessment alone (Class IIb, LOE C).

### End-Expiratory Pressure

Many experts recommend administration of continuous positive airway pressure (CPAP) to infants who are breathing spontaneously, but with difficulty, following birth, although its use has been studied only in infants born preterm. A multicenter randomized clinical trial of newborns at 25 to 28 weeks gestation with signs of respiratory distress showed no significant difference in the outcomes of death or oxygen requirement at 36 weeks postmenstrual age between infants started on CPAP versus those intubated and placed on mechanical ventilation in the delivery room. Starting infants on CPAP reduced the rates of intubation and mechanical ventilation, surfactant use, and duration of ventilation, but increased the rate of pneumothorax.[57] Spontaneously breathing preterm infants who have respiratory distress may be supported with CPAP or with intubation and mechanical ventilation (Class IIb, LOE B). The most appropriate choice may be guided by local expertise and preferences. There is no evidence to support or refute the use of CPAP in the delivery room in the term baby with respiratory distress.

Although positive end–expiratory pressure (PEEP) has been shown to be beneficial and its use is routine during mechanical ventilation of neonates in intensive care units, there have been no studies specifically examining PEEP versus no PEEP when PPV is used during establishment of an FRC following birth. Nevertheless, PEEP is likely to be beneficial and should be used if suitable equipment is available (Class IIb, LOE C). PEEP can easily be given with a flow-inflating bag or T-piece resuscitator, but it cannot be given with a self-inflating bag unless an optional PEEP valve is used. There is, however, some evidence that such valves often deliver inconsistent end-expiratory pressures.[58,59]

### ASSISTED-VENTILATION DEVICES

Effective ventilation can be achieved with either a flow-inflating or self-inflating bag or with a T-piece mechanical device designed to regulate pressure.[60–63] The pop-off valves of self-inflating bags are dependent on the flow rate of incoming gas, and pressures generated may exceed the value specified by the manufacturer. Target inflation pressures and long inspiratory times are more consistently achieved in mechanical models when T-piece devices are used rather than bags,[60,61] although the clinical implications of these findings are not clear (Class IIb, LOE C). It is likely that inflation pressures will need to change as compliance improves following birth, but the relationship of pressures to delivered volume and the optimal volume to deliver with each breath as FRC is being established have not been studied. Resuscitators are insensitive to changes in lung compliance, regardless of the device being used (Class IIb, LOE C).[64]

## Laryngeal Mask Airways

Laryngeal mask airways that fit over the laryngeal inlet have been shown to be effective for ventilating newborns weighing more than 2000 g or delivered $\geq$34 weeks gestation (Class IIb, LOE B[65–67]). There are limited data on the use of these devices in small preterm infants, ie, < 2000 g or <34 weeks (Class IIb, LOE C[65–67]). A laryngeal mask should be considered during resuscitation if facemask ventilation is unsuccessful and tracheal intubation is unsuccessful or not feasible (Class IIa, LOE B). The laryngeal mask has not been evaluated in cases of meconium-stained fluid, during chest compressions, or for administration of emergency intratracheal medications.

## Endotracheal Tube Placement

Endotracheal intubation may be indicated at several points during neonatal resuscitation:

- Initial endotracheal suctioning of non-vigorous meconium-stained newborns
- If bag-mask ventilation is ineffective or prolonged
- When chest compressions are performed
- For special resuscitation circumstances, such as congenital diaphragmatic hernia or extremely low birth weight

The timing of endotracheal intubation may also depend on the skill and experience of the available providers.

After endotracheal intubation and administration of intermittent positive pressure, a prompt increase in heart rate is the best indicator that the tube is in the tracheobronchial tree and providing effective ventilation.[53] Exhaled $CO_2$ detection is effective for confirmation of endotracheal tube placement in infants, including very low-birth-weight infants (Class IIa, LOE B[68–71]). A positive test result (detection of exhaled $CO_2$) in patients with adequate cardiac output confirms placement of the endotracheal tube within the trachea, whereas a negative test result (ie, no $CO_2$ detected) strongly suggests esophageal intubation.[68–72] Exhaled $CO_2$ detection is the recommended method of confirmation of endotracheal tube placement (Class IIa, LOE B). However, it should be noted that poor or absent pulmonary blood flow may give false-negative results (ie, no $CO_2$ detected despite tube placement in the trachea). A false-negative result may thus lead to unnecessary extubation and re-intubation of critically ill infants with poor cardiac output.

Other clinical indicators of correct endotracheal tube placement are condensation in the endotracheal tube, chest movement, and presence of equal breath sounds bilaterally, but these indicators have not been systematically evaluated in neonates (Class 11b, LOE C).

## Chest Compressions

Chest compressions are indicated for a heart rate that is <60 per minute despite adequate ventilation with supplementary oxygen for 30 seconds. Because ventilation is the most effective action in neonatal resuscitation and because chest compressions are likely to compete with effective ventilation, rescuers should ensure that assisted ventilation is being delivered optimally before starting chest compressions.

Compressions should be delivered on the lower third of the sternum to a depth of approximately one third of the anterior-posterior diameter of the chest (Class IIb, LOE C[73–75]). Two techniques have been described: compression with 2 thumbs with fingers encircling the chest and supporting the back (the 2 thumb–encircling hands technique) or compression with 2 fingers with a second hand supporting the back. Because the 2 thumb–encircling hands technique may generate higher peak systolic and coronary perfusion pressure than the 2-finger technique,[76–80] the 2 thumb–encircling hands technique is recommended for performing chest compressions in newly born infants (Class IIb, LOE C). The 2-finger technique may be preferable when access to the umbilicus is required during insertion of an umbilical catheter, although it is possible to administer the 2 thumb–encircling hands technique in intubated infants with the rescuer standing at the baby's head, thus permitting adequate access to the umbilicus (Class IIb, LOE C).

Compressions and ventilations should be coordinated to avoid simultaneous delivery.[81] The chest should be permitted to reexpand fully during relaxation, but the rescuer's thumbs should not leave the chest (Class IIb, LOE C). There should be a 3:1 ratio of compressions to ventilations with 90 compressions and 30 breaths to achieve approximately 120 events per minute to maximize ventilation at an achievable rate. Thus each event will be allotted approximately 1/2 second, with exhalation occurring during the first compression after each ventilation (Class IIb, LOE C).

There is evidence from animals and non-neonatal studies that sustained compressions or a compression ratio of 15:2 or even 30:2 may be more effective when the arrest is of primary cardiac etiology. One study in children suggests that CPR with rescue breathing is preferable to chest compressions alone when the arrest is of noncardiac etiology.[82] It is recommended that a 3:1 compression to ventilation ratio be used for neonatal resuscitation where compromise of ventilation is nearly always the primary cause, but rescuers should consider using higher ratios (eg, 15:2) if the arrest is believed to be of cardiac origin (Class IIb, LOE C).

Respirations, heart rate, and oxygenation should be reassessed periodically, and coordinated chest compressions and ventilations should continue until the spontaneous heart rate is ≥60 per minute (Class IIb, LOE C). However, frequent interruptions of compressions should be avoided, as they will compromise artificial maintenance of systemic perfusion and maintenance of coronary blood flow (Class IIb, LOE C).

## MEDICATIONS

Drugs are rarely indicated in resuscitation of the newly born infant. Bradycardia in the newborn infant is usually the result of inadequate lung inflation or profound hypoxemia, and establishing adequate ventilation is the most important step toward correcting it. However, if the heart rate remains <60 per minute despite adequate ventilation (usually with endotracheal intubation) with 100% oxygen and chest compressions, administration of epinephrine or volume expansion, or both, may be indicated. Rarely, buffers, a narcotic antagonist, or vasopressors may be useful after resuscitation, but these are not recommended in the delivery room.

### Rate and Dose of Epinephrine Administration

Epinephrine is recommended to be administered intravenously (Class IIb, LOE C). Past guidelines recommended that initial doses of epinephrine be given through an endotracheal tube because the dose can be administered more quickly than when an intravenous route must be established. However, animal studies that showed a positive effect of endotracheal epinephrine used considerably higher doses than are currently recommended,[83,84] and the one animal study that used currently recommended doses via endotracheal tube showed no effect.[85] Given the lack of supportive data for endotracheal epinephrine, the IV route should be used as soon as

venous access is established (Class IIb, LOE C).

The recommended IV dose is 0.01 to 0.03 mg/kg per dose. Higher IV doses are not recommended because animal[86,87] and pediatric[88,89] studies show exaggerated hypertension, decreased myocardial function, and worse neurological function after administration of IV doses in the range of 0.1 mg/kg. If the endotracheal route is used, doses of 0.01 or 0.03 mg/kg will likely be ineffective. Therefore, IV administration of 0.01 to 0.03 mg/kg per dose is the preferred route. While access is being obtained, administration of a higher dose (0.05 to 0.1 mg/kg) through the endotracheal tube may be considered, but the safety and efficacy of this practice have not been evaluated (Class IIb, LOE C). The concentration of epinephrine for either route should be 1:10,000 (0.1 mg/mL).

## VOLUME EXPANSION

Volume expansion should be considered when blood loss is known or suspected (pale skin, poor perfusion, weak pulse) and the baby's heart rate has not responded adequately to other resuscitative measures (Class IIb, LOE C).[90] An isotonic crystalloid solution or blood is recommended for volume expansion in the delivery room (Class IIb, LOE C). The recommended dose is 10 mL/kg, which may need to be repeated. When resuscitating premature infants, care should be taken to avoid giving volume expanders rapidly, because rapid infusions of large volumes have been associated with intraventricular hemorrhage (Class IIb, LOE C).

## POSTRESUSCITATION CARE

Babies who require resuscitation are at risk for deterioration after their vital signs have returned to normal. Once adequate ventilation and circulation have been established, the infant should be maintained in, or transferred to an environment where close

monitoring and anticipatory care can be provided.

### Naloxone

Administration of naloxone is not recommended as part of initial resuscitative efforts in the delivery room for newborns with respiratory depression. Heart rate and oxygenation should be restored by supporting ventilation.

### Glucose

Newborns with lower blood glucose levels are at increased risk for brain injury and adverse outcomes after a hypoxic-ischemic insult, although no specific glucose level associated with worse outcome has been identified.[91,92] Increased glucose levels after hypoxia or ischemia were not associated with adverse effects in a recent pediatric series[93] or in animal studies,[94] and they may be protective.[95] However, there are no randomized controlled trials that examine this question. Due to the paucity of data, no specific target glucose concentration range can be identified at present. Intravenous glucose infusion should be considered as soon as practical after resuscitation, with the goal of avoiding hypoglycemia (Class IIb, LOE C).

### Induced Therapeutic Hypothermia

Several randomized controlled multicenter trials of induced hypothermia (33.5°C to 34.5°C) of newborns ≥36 weeks gestational age, with moderate to severe hypoxic-ischemic encephalopathy as defined by strict criteria, showed that those babies who were cooled had significantly lower mortality and less neurodevelopmental disability at 18-month follow-up than babies who were not cooled.[96–98] The randomized trials produced similar results using different methods of cooling (selective head versus systemic).[96–100] It is recommended that infants born at ≥36 weeks gestation with evolving moderate to severe hypoxic-ischemic encephalopathy should be offered therapeutic hypothermia. The treatment should be implemented according to the studied protocols, which currently include commencement within 6 hours following birth, continuation for 72 hours, and slow rewarming over at least 4 hours. Therapeutic hypothermia should be administered under clearly defined protocols similar to those used in published clinical trials and in facilities with the capabilities for multidisciplinary care and longitudinal follow-up (Class IIa, LOE A). Studies suggest that there may be some associated adverse effects, such as thrombocytopenia and increased need for inotropic support.

## GUIDELINES FOR WITHHOLDING AND DISCONTINUING RESUSCITATION

For neonates at the margins of viability or those with conditions which predict a high risk of mortality or morbidity, attitudes and practice vary according to region and availability of resources. Studies indicate that parents desire a larger role in decisions to initiate resuscitation and continue life support of severely compromised newborns. Opinions among neonatal providers vary widely regarding the benefits and disadvantages of aggressive therapies in such newborns.

### Withholding Resuscitation

It is possible to identify conditions associated with high mortality and poor outcome in which withholding resuscitative efforts may be considered reasonable, particularly when there has been the opportunity for parental agreement (Class IIb, LOE C[101,102]).

A consistent and coordinated approach to individual cases by the obstetric and neonatal teams and the parents is an important goal. Noninitiation of resuscitation and discontinuation of life-sustaining treatment during or after resuscitation are ethically equivalent, and clinicians should not hesitate to withdraw support when

functional survival is highly unlikely.[103] The following guidelines must be interpreted according to current regional outcomes:

- When gestation, birth weight, or congenital anomalies are associated with almost certain early death and when unacceptably high morbidity is likely among the rare survivors, resuscitation is not indicated. Examples include extreme prematurity (gestational age <23 weeks or birth weight <400 g), anencephaly, and some major chromosomal abnormalities, such as trisomy 13 (Class IIb, LOE C).

- In conditions associated with a high rate of survival and acceptable morbidity, resuscitation is nearly always indicated. This will generally include babies with gestational age ≥25 weeks and those with most congenital malformations (Class IIb, LOE C).

- In conditions associated with uncertain prognosis in which survival is borderline, the morbidity rate is relatively high, and the anticipated burden to the child is high, parental desires concerning initiation of resuscitation should be supported (Class IIb, LOE C).

Assessment of morbidity and mortality risks should take into consideration available data, and may be augmented by use of published tools based on data from specific populations. Decisions should also take into account changes in medical practice that may occur over time.

Mortality and morbidity data by gestational age compiled from data collected by perinatal centers in the US and several other countries may be found on the Neonatal Resuscitation Program (NRP) website (www.aap.org/nrp). A link to a computerized tool to estimate mortality and morbidity from a population of extremely low-

birth-weight babies born in a network of regional perinatal centers may be found at that site. However, unless conception occurred via in vitro fertilization, techniques used for obstetric dating are accurate to only ±3 to 4 days if applied in the first trimester and to only ±1 to 2 weeks subsequently. Estimates of fetal weight are accurate to only ±15% to 20%. Even small discrepancies of 1 or 2 weeks between estimated and actual gestational age or a 100- to 200-g difference in birth weight may have implications for survival and long-term morbidity. Also, fetal weight can be misleading if there has been intrauterine growth restriction, and outcomes may be less predictable. These uncertainties underscore the importance of not making firm commitments about withholding or providing resuscitation until you have the opportunity to examine the baby after birth.

### Discontinuing Resuscitative Efforts

In a newly born baby with no detectable heart rate, it is appropriate to consider stopping resuscitation if the heart rate remains undetectable for 10 minutes (Class IIb, LOE C[104–106]). The decision to continue resuscitation efforts beyond 10 minutes with no heart rate should take into consideration factors such as the presumed etiology of the arrest, the gestation of the baby, the presence or absence of complications, the potential role of therapeutic hypothermia, and the parents' previously expressed feelings about acceptable risk of morbidity.

## STRUCTURE OF EDUCATIONAL PROGRAMS TO TEACH NEONATAL RESUSCITATION

Studies have demonstrated that use of simulation-based learning methodologies enhances performance in both real-life clinical situations and simulated resuscitations,[107–110] although a few studies have found no differences when compared to standard or other nonsimulated training.[111,112] Also, studies examining briefings or debriefings of resuscitation team performance have generally shown improved knowledge or skills.[113–118] Interpretation of data is complicated by the heterogeneity and limitations of the studies, including a paucity of data about clinical outcomes. Based on available evidence, it is recommended that the AAP/AHA Neonatal Resuscitation Program adopt simulation, briefing, and debriefing techniques in designing an education program for the acquisition and maintenance of the skills necessary for effective neonatal resuscitation (Class IIb, LOE C).

## REFERENCES

1. 2010 International Consensus on Cardiopulmonary Resuscitation and Emergency Cardiovascular Care Science with Treatment Recommendations. *Circulation.* In Press

2. Perlman JM, Risser R. Cardiopulmonary resuscitation in the delivery room: associated clinical events. *Arch Pediatr Adolesc Med.* 1995;149:20–25

3. Barber CA, Wyckoff MH. Use and efficacy of endotracheal versus intravenous epinephrine during neonatal cardiopulmonary resuscitation in the delivery room. *Pediatrics.* 2006;118:1028–1034

4. Owen CJ, Wyllie JP. Determination of heart rate in the baby at birth. *Resuscitation.* 2004;60:213–217

5. Kamlin CO, Dawson JA, O'Donnell CP, Morley CJ, Donath SM, Sekhon J, Davis PG. Accuracy of pulse oximetry measurement of heart rate of newborn infants in the delivery room. *J Pediatr.* 2008;152:756–760

6. Am Academy of Pediatrics, Am College of Obstetricians and Gynecologists. In: Lockwood C, Lemons J, eds. *Guidelines for Perinatal Care.* 6th ed. Elk Grove Village, IL: Am Academy of Pediatrics;2007:205

7. Annibale DJ, Hulsey TC, Wagner CL, Southgate WM. Comparative neonatal morbidity of abdominal and vaginal deliveries after uncomplicated pregnancies. *Arch Pediatr Adolesc Med.* 1995;149:862–867

8. Atherton N, Parsons SJ, Mansfield P. Attendance of paediatricians at elective Caesarean sections performed under regional anaesthesia: is it warranted? *J Paediatr Child Health.* 2006;42:332–336

9. Gordon A, McKechnie EJ, Jeffery H. Pediatric presence at cesarean section: justified or not? *Am J Obstet Gynecol.* 2005;193(3 Pt 1):599–605

10. Parsons SJ, Sonneveld S, Nolan T. Is a paediatrician needed at all Caesarean sections? *J Paediatr Child Health.* 1998;34: 241–244

11. Kattwinkel J, ed. *Textbook of Neonatal Resuscitation.* 6th ed. Elk Grove Village: Am Academy of Pediatrics; In Press

12. Cramer K, Wiebe N, Hartling L, Crumley E, Vohra S. Heat loss prevention: a systematic review of occlusive skin wrap for premature neonates. *J Perinatol.* 2005;25: 763–769

13. Kent AL, Williams J. Increasing ambient operating theatre temperature and wrapping in polyethylene improves admission temperature in premature infants. *J Paediatr Child Health.* 2008;44:325–331

14. Vohra S, Frent G, Campbell V, Abbott M, Whyte R. Effect of polyethylene occlusive skin wrapping on heat loss in very low birth weight infants at delivery: a randomized trial. *J Pediatr.* 1999;134:547–551

15. Vohra S, Roberts RS, Zhang B, Janes M, Schmidt B. Heat Loss Prevention (HeLP) in the delivery room: A randomized controlled trial of polyethylene occlusive skin wrapping in very preterm infants. *J Pediatr.* 2004;145:750–753

16. Singh A, Duckett J, Newton T, Watkinson M. Improving neonatal unit admission temperatures in preterm babies: exothermic mattresses, polythene bags or a traditional approach? *J Perinatol.* 2010;30: 45–49

17. Meyer MP, Bold GT. Admission temperatures following radiant warmer or incubator transport for preterm infants <28 weeks: a randomised study. *Arch Dis Child Fetal Neonatal Ed.* 2007;92:F295–F297

18. Petrova A, Demissie K, Rhoads GG, Smulian JC, Marcella S, Ananth CV. Association of maternal fever during labor with neonatal and infant morbidity and mortality. *Obstet Gynecol.* 2001;98:20–27

19. Lieberman E, Lang J, Richardson DK, Frigoletto FD, Heffner LJ, Cohen A. Intrapartum maternal fever and neonatal outcome. *Pediatrics.* 2000;105(1 Pt 1):8–13

20. Coimbra C, Boris-Moller F, Drake M, Wieloch T. Diminished neuronal damage in the rat brain by late treatment with the antipyretic drug dipyrone or cooling following cerebral ischemia. *Acta Neuropathol.* 1996;92:447–453

21. Gungor S, Kurt E, Teksoz E, Goktolga U, Ceyhan T, Baser I. Oronasopharyngeal suction versus no suction in normal and term infants delivered by elective cesarean section: a prospective randomized controlled trial. *Gynecol Obstet Invest.* 2006; 61:9–14

22. Waltman PA, Brewer JM, Rogers BP, May WL. Building evidence for practice: a pilot study of newborn bulb suctioning at birth. *J Midwifery Womens Health.* 2004;49: 32–38

23. Perlman JM, Volpe JJ. Suctioning in the preterm infant: effects on cerebral blood flow velocity, intracranial pressure, and arterial blood pressure. *Pediatrics.* 1983; 72:329–334

24. Simbruner G, Coradello H, Fodor M, Havelec L, Lubec G, Pollak A. Effect of tracheal suction on oxygenation, circulation, and lung mechanics in newborn infants. *Arch Dis Child.* 1981;56:326–330

25. Prendiville A, Thomson A, Silverman M. Effect of tracheobronchial suction on respiratory resistance in intubated preterm babies. *Arch Dis Child.* 1986;61:1178–1183

26. Vain NE, Szyld EG, Prudent LM, Wiswell TE, Aguilar AM, Vivas NI. Oropharyngeal and nasopharyngeal suctioning of meconium-stained neonates before delivery of their shoulders: multicentre, randomised controlled trial. *Lancet.* 2004;364:597–602

27. Wiswell TE, Gannon CM, Jacob J, Goldsmith L, Szyld E, Weiss K, Schutzman D, Cleary GM, Filipov P, Kurlat I, Caballero CL, Abassi S, Sprague D, Oltorf C, Padula M. Delivery room management of the apparently vigorous meconium-stained neonate: results of the multicenter, international collaborative trial. *Pediatrics.* 2000;105(1 Pt 1): 1–7

28. Rossi EM, Philipson EH, Williams TG, Kalhan SC. Meconium aspiration syndrome: intrapartum and neonatal attributes. *Am J Obstet Gynecol.* 1989;161:1106–1110

29. Usta IM, Mercer BM, Sibai BM. Risk factors for meconium aspiration syndrome. *Obstet Gynecol.* 1995;86:230–234

30. Gupta V, Bhatia BD, Mishra OP. Meconium stained amniotic fluid: antenatal, intrapartum and neonatal attributes. *Indian Pediatr.* 1996;33:293–297

31. Al Takroni AM, Parvathi CK, Mendis KB, Hassan S, Reddy I, Kudair HA. Selective tracheal suctioning to prevent meconium aspiration syndrome. *Int J Gynaecol Obstet.* 1998;63:259–263

32. Carson BS, Losey RW, Bowes WA, Jr, Sim-

mons MA. Combined obstetric and pediatric approach to prevent meconium aspiration syndrome. *Am J Obstet Gynecol.* 1976; 126:712–715

33. Ting P, Brady JP. Tracheal suction in meconium aspiration. *Am J Obstet Gynecol.* 1975;122:767–771

34. Gregory GA, Gooding CA, Phibbs RH, Tooley WH. Meconium aspiration in infants—a prospective study. *J Pediatr.* 1974;85: 848–852

35. Toth B, Becker A, Seelbach-Gobel B. Oxygen saturation in healthy newborn infants immediately after birth measured by pulse oximetry. *Arch Gynecol Obstet.* 2002;266: 105–107

36. Gonzales GF, Salirrosas A. Arterial oxygen saturation in healthy newborns delivered at term in Cerro de Pasco (4340 m) and Lima (150 m). *Reprod Biol Endocrinol.* 2005;3:46

37. Altuncu E, Ozek E, Bilgen H, Topuzoglu A, Kavuncuoglu S. Percentiles of oxygen saturations in healthy term newborns in the first minutes of life. *Eur J Pediatr.* 2008; 167:687–688

38. Kamlin CO, O'Donnell CP, Davis PG, Morley CJ. Oxygen saturation in healthy infants immediately after birth. *J Pediatr.* 2006; 148:585–589

39. Mariani G, Dik PB, Ezquer A, Aguirre A, Esteban ML, Perez C, Fernandez Jonusas S, Fustinana C. Pre-ductal and post-ductal O2 saturation in healthy term neonates after birth. *J Pediatr.* 2007;150:418–421

40. Rabi Y, Yee W, Chen SY, Singhal N. Oxygen saturation trends immediately after birth. *J Pediatr.* 2006;148:590–594

41. Hay WW, Jr, Rodden DJ, Collins SM, Melara DL, Hale KA, Fashaw LM. Reliability of conventional and new pulse oximetry in neonatal patients. *J Perinatol.* 2002;22: 360–366

42. O'Donnell CP, Kamlin CO, Davis PG, Morley CJ. Feasibility of and delay in obtaining pulse oximetry during neonatal resuscitation. *J Pediatr.* 2005;147:698–699

43. Dawson JA, Kamlin CO, Wong C, te Pas AB, O'Donnell CP, Donath SM, Davis PG, Morley CJ. Oxygen saturation and heart rate during delivery room resuscitation of infants <30 weeks' gestation with air or 100% oxygen. *Arch Dis Child Fetal Neonatal Ed.* 2009;94:F87–F91

44. Davis PG, Tan A, O'Donnell CP, Schulze A. Resuscitation of newborn infants with 100% oxygen or air: a systematic review and meta-analysis. *Lancet.* 2004;364: 1329–1333

45. Rabi Y, Rabi D, Yee W. Room air resuscitation of the depressed newborn: a systematic review and meta-analysis. *Resuscitation.* 2007;72:353–363

46. Escrig R, Arruza L, Izquierdo I, Villar G, Saenz P, Gimeno A, Moro M, Vento M. Achievement of targeted saturation values in extremely low gestational age neonates resuscitated with low or high oxygen concentrations: a prospective, randomized trial. *Pediatrics.* 2008;121:875–881

47. Karlberg P, Koch G. Respiratory studies in newborn infants. III. Development of mechanics of breathing during the first week of life. A longitudinal study. *Acta Paediatr.* 1962;(Suppl 135):121–129

48. Vyas H, Milner AD, Hopkin IE, Boon AW. Physiologic responses to prolonged and slow-rise inflation in the resuscitation of the asphyxiated newborn infant. *J Pediatr.* 1981;99:635–639

49. Vyas H, Field D, Milner AD, Hopkin IE. Determinants of the first inspiratory volume and functional residual capacity at birth. *Pediatr Pulmonol.* 1986;2:189–193

50. Boon AW, Milner AD, Hopkin IE. Lung expansion, tidal exchange, and formation of the functional residual capacity during resuscitation of asphyxiated neonates. *J Pediatr.* 1979;95:1031–1036

51. Hillman NH, Moss TJ, Kallapur SG, Bachurski C, Pillow JJ, Polglase GR, Nitsos I, Kramer BW, Jobe AH. Brief, large tidal volume ventilation initiates lung injury and a systemic response in fetal sheep. *Am J Respir Crit Care Med.* 2007;176:575–581

52. Polglase GR, Hooper SB, Gill AW, Allison BJ, McLean CJ, Nitsos I, Pillow JJ, Kluckow M. Cardiovascular and pulmonary consequences of airway recruitment in preterm lambs. *J Appl Physiol.* 2009;106:1347–1355

53. Dawes GS. Foetal and Neonatal Physiology. A Comparative Study of the Changes at Birth. Chicago: Year Book Medical Publishers, Inc; 1968

54. Lindner W, Vossbeck S, Hummler H, Pohlandt F. Delivery room management of extremely low birth weight infants: spontaneous breathing or intubation? *Pediatrics.* 1999;103(5 Pt 1):961–967

55. Leone TA, Lange A, Rich W, Finer NN. Disposable colorimetric carbon dioxide detector use as an indicator of a patent airway during noninvasive mask ventilation. *Pediatrics.* 2006;118:e202–204

56. Finer NN, Rich W, Wang C, Leone T. Airway obstruction during mask ventilation of very low birth weight infants during neonatal resuscitation. *Pediatrics.* 2009;123: 865–869

57. Morley CJ, Davis PG, Doyle LW, Brion LP, Hascoet JM, Carlin JB. Nasal CPAP or intubation at birth for very preterm infants. *N Engl J Med.* 2008;358:700–708

58. Kelm M, Proquitte H, Schmalisch G, Roehr CC. Reliability of two common PEEP-generating devices used in neonatal resuscitation. *Klin Padiatr.* 2009;221: 415–418

59. Morley CJ, Dawson JA, Stewart MJ, Hussain F, Davis PG. The effect of a PEEP valve on a Laerdal neonatal self-inflating resuscitation bag. *J Paediatr Child Health.* 46(1–2):51–56, 2010

60. Oddie S, Wyllie J, Scally A. Use of self-inflating bags for neonatal resuscitation. *Resuscitation.* 2005;67:109–112

61. Hussey SG, Ryan CA, Murphy BP. Comparison of three manual ventilation devices using an intubated mannequin. *Arch Dis Child Fetal Neonatal Ed.* 2004;89:F490–493

62. Finer NN, Rich W, Craft A, Henderson C. Comparison of methods of bag and mask ventilation for neonatal resuscitation. *Resuscitation.* 2001;49:299–305

63. Bennett S, Finer NN, Rich W, Vaucher Y. A comparison of three neonatal resuscitation devices. *Resuscitation.* 2005;67.113–118

64. Kattwinkel J, Stewart C, Walsh B, Gurka M, Paget-Brown A. Responding to compliance changes in a lung model during manual ventilation: perhaps volume, rather than pressure, should be displayed. *Pediatrics.* 2009;123:e465–470

65. Trevisanuto D, Micaglio M, Pitton M, Magarotto M, Piva D, Zanardo V. Laryngeal mask airway: is the management of neonates requiring positive pressure ventilation at birth changing? *Resuscitation.* 2004;62: 151–157

66. Gandini D, Brimacombe JR. Neonatal resuscitation with the laryngeal mask airway in normal and low birth weight infants. *Anesth Analg.* 1999;89:642–643

67. Esmail N, Saleh M, et al. Laryngeal mask airway versus endotracheal intubation for Apgar score improvement in neonatal resuscitation. *Egyptian Journal of Anesthesiology.* 2002;18:115–121

68. Hosono S, Inami I, Fujita H, Minato M, Takahashi S, Mugishima H. A role of end-tidal CO monitoring for assessment of tracheal intubations in very low birth weight infants during neonatal resuscitation at birth. *J Perinat Med.* 2009;37:79–84

69. Repetto JE, Donohue P-CP, Baker SF, Kelly L, Nogee LM. Use of capnography in the delivery room for assessment of endotracheal tube placement. *J Perinatol.* 2001;21: 284–287

70. Roberts WA, Maniscalco WM, Cohen AR,

Litman RS, Chhibber A. The use of capnography for recognition of esophageal intubation in the neonatal intensive care unit. *Pediatr Pulmonol.* 1995;19:262–268

71. Aziz HF, Martin JB, Moore JJ. The pediatric disposable end-tidal carbon dioxide detector role in endotracheal intubation in newborns. *J Perinatol.* 1999;19:110–113

72. Garey DM, Ward R, Rich W, Heldt G, Leone T, Finer NN. Tidal volume threshold for colorimetric carbon dioxide detectors available for use in neonates. *Pediatrics.* 2008;121: e1524–1527

73. Orlowski JP. Optimum position for external cardiac compression in infants and young children. *Ann Emerg Med.* 1986;15: 667–673

74. Phillips GW, Zideman DA. Relation of infant heart to sternum: its significance in cardiopulmonary resuscitation. *Lancet.* 1986; 1:1024–1025

75. Braga MS, Dominguez TE, Pollock AN, Niles D, Meyer A, Myklebust H, Nysaether J, Nadkarni V. Estimation of optimal CPR chest compression depth in children by using computer tomography. *Pediatrics.* 2009; 124:e69–e74

76. Menegazzi JJ, Auble TE, Nicklas KA, Hosack GM, Rack L, Goode JS. Two-thumb versus two-finger chest compression during CRP in a swine infant model of cardiac arrest. *Ann Emerg Med.* 1993;22:240–243

77. Houri PK, Frank LR, Menegazzi JJ, Taylor R. A randomized, controlled trial of two-thumb vs two-finger chest compression in a swine infant model of cardiac arrest. *Prehosp Emerg Care.* 1997;1:65–67

78. Udassi JP, Udassi S, Theriaque DW, Shuster JJ, Zaritsky AL, Haque IU. Effect of alternative chest compression techniques in infant and child on rescuer performance. *Pediatr Crit Care Med.* 2009;10:328–333

79. David R. Closed chest cardiac massage in the newborn infant. *Pediatrics.* 1988;81: 552–554

80. Thaler MM, Stobie GH. An improved technique of external caridac compression in infants and young children. *N Engl J Med.* 1963;269:606–610

81. Berkowitz ID, Chantarojanasiri T, Koehler RC, Schleien CL, Dean JM, Michael JR, Rogers MC, Traystman RJ. Blood flow during cardiopulmonary resuscitation with simultaneous compression and ventilation in infant pigs. *Pediatr Res.* 1989;26:558–564

82. Kitamura T, Iwami T, Kawamura T, Nagao K, Tanaka H, Nadkarni VM, Berg RA, Hiraide A. Conventional and chest-compression-only cardiopulmonary resuscitation by bystanders for children who have out-of-hospital cardiac arrests: a prospective, nationwide, population-based cohort study. *Lancet.* 2010;375:1347–1354

83. Mielke LL, Frank C, Lanzinger MJ, Wilhelm MG, Entholzner EK, Hargasser SR, Hipp RF. Plasma catecholamine levels following tracheal and intravenous epinephrine administration in swine. *Resuscitation.* 1998; 36:187–192

84. Roberts JR, Greenberg MI, Knaub MA, Kendrick ZV, Baskin SI. Blood levels following intravenous and endotracheal epinephrine administration. *JACEP.* 1979;8: 53–56

85. Hornchen U, Schuttler J, Stoeckel H, Eichelkraut W, Hahn N. Endobronchial instillation of epinephrine during cardiopulmonary resuscitation. *Crit Care Med.* 1987;15: 1037–1039

86. Berg RA, Otto CW, Kern KB, Hilwig RW, Sanders AB, Henry CP, Ewy GA. A randomized, blinded trial of high-dose epinephrine versus standard-dose epinephrine in a swine model of pediatric asphyxial cardiac arrest. *Crit Care Med.* 1996;24:1695–1700

87. Burchfield DJ, Preziosi MP, Lucas VW, Fan J. Effects of graded doses of epinephrine during asphyxia-induced bradycardia in newborn lambs. *Resuscitation.* 1993;25: 235–244

88. Perondi MB, Reis AG, Paiva EF, Nadkarni VM, Berg RA. A comparison of high-dose and standard-dose epinephrine in children with cardiac arrest. *N Engl J Med.* 2004;350:1722–1730

89. Patterson MD, Boenning DA, Klein BL, Fuchs S, Smith KM, Hegenbarth MA, Carlson DW, Krug SE, Harris EM. The use of high-dose epinephrine for patients with out-of-hospital cardiopulmonary arrest refractory to prehospital interventions. *Pediatr Emerg Care.* 2005;21:227–237

90. Wyckoff MH, Perlman JM, Laptook AR. Use of volume expansion during delivery room resuscitation in near-term and term infants. *Pediatrics.* 2005;115:950–955

91. Salhab WA, Wyckoff MH, Laptook AR, Perlman JM. Initial hypoglycemia and neonatal brain injury in term infants with severe fetal acidemia. *Pediatrics.* 2004;114:361–366

92. Ondoa-Onama C, Tumwine JK. Immediate outcome of babies with low Apgar score in Mulago Hospital, Uganda. *East Afr Med J.* 2003;80:22–29

93. Klein GW, Hojsak JM, Schmeidler J, Rapaport R. Hyperglycemia and outcome in the pediatric intensive care unit. *J Pediatr.* 2008;153:379–384

94. LeBlanc MH, Huang M, Patel D, Smith EE, Devidas M. Glucose given after hypoxic ischemia does not affect brain injury in piglets. *Stroke.* 25:1443–1447, 1994; discussion 1448

95. Hattori H, Wasterlain CG. Posthypoxic glucose supplement reduces hypoxic-ischemic brain damage in the neonatal rat. *Ann Neurol.* 1990;28:122–128

96. Gluckman PD, Wyatt JS, Azzopardi D, Ballard R, Edwards AD, Ferriero DM, Polin RA, Robertson CM, Thoresen M, Whitelaw A, Gunn AJ. Selective head cooling with mild systemic hypothermia after neonatal encephalopathy: multicentre randomised trial. *Lancet.* 2005;365:663–670

97. Shankaran S, Laptook AR, Ehrenkranz RA, Tyson JE, McDonald SA, Donovan EF, Fanaroff AA, Poole WK, Wright LL, Higgins RD, Finer NN, Carlo WA, Duara S, Oh W, Cotten CM, Stevenson DK, Stoll BJ, Lemons JA, Guillet R, Jobe AH. Whole-body hypothermia for neonates with hypoxic-ischemic encephalopathy. *N Engl J Med.* 2005;353: 1574–1584

98. Azzopardi DV, Strohm B, Edwards AD, Dyet L, Halliday HL, Juszczak E, Kapellou O, Levene M, Marlow N, Porter E, Thoresen M, Whitelaw A, Brocklehurst P. Moderate hypothermia to treat perinatal asphyxial encephalopathy. *N Engl J Med.* 2009;361: 1349–1358

99. Eicher DJ, Wagner CL, Katikaneni LP, Hulsey TC, Bass WT, Kaufman DA, Horgan MJ, Languani S, Bhatia JJ, Givelichian LM, Sankaran K, Yager JY. Moderate hypothermia in neonatal encephalopathy: safety outcomes. *Pediatr Neurol.* 2005;32:18–24

100. Lin ZL, Yu HM, Lin J, Chen SQ, Liang ZQ, Zhang ZY. Mild hypothermia via selective head cooling as neuroprotective therapy in term neonates with perinatal asphyxia: an experience from a single neonatal intensive care unit. *J Perinatol.* 2006;26: 180–184

101. Field DJ, Dorling JS, Manktelow BN, Draper ES. Survival of extremely premature babies in a geographically defined population: prospective cohort study of 1994–9 compared with 2000–5. *BMJ.* 2008;336: 1221–1223

102. Tyson JE, Parikh NA, Langer J, Green C, Higgins RD. Intensive care for extreme prematurity—moving beyond gestational age. *N Engl J Med.* 2008;358:1672–1681

103. Paris JJ. What standards apply to resuscitation at the borderline of gestational age? *J Perinatol.* 2005;25:683–684

104. Jain L, Ferre C, Vidyasagar D, Nath S, Sheftel D. Cardiopulmonary resuscitation of apparently stillborn infants: survival and long-term outcome. *J Pediatr.* 1991;118: 778–782

105. Casalaz DM, Marlow N, Speidel BD. Outcome of resuscitation following unexpected apparent stillbirth. *Arch Dis Child Fetal Neonatal Ed.* 1998;78:F112–F115

106. Laptook AR, Shankaran S, Ambalavanan N, Carlo WA, McDonald SA, Higgins RD, Das A. Outcome of term infants using apgar scores at 10 minutes following hypoxic-ischemic encephalopathy. *Pediatrics.* 2009; 124:1619–1626

107. Knudson MM, Khaw L, Bullard MK, Dicker R, Cohen MJ, Staudenmayer K, Sadjadi J, Howard S, Gaba D, Krummel T. Trauma training in simulation: translating skills from SIM time to real time. *J Trauma.* 64: 255–263, 2008; discussion 263–254

108. Wayne DB, Didwania A, Feinglass J, Fudala MJ, Barsuk JH, McGaghie WC. Simulation-based education improves quality of care during cardiac arrest team responses at an academic teaching hospital: a case-control study. *Chest.* 2008;133:56–61

100. Kory PD, Eisen LA, Adachi M, Ribaudo VA, Rosenthal ME, Mayo PH. Initial airway management skills of senior residents: simulation training compared with traditional training. *Chest.* 2007;132:1927–1931

110. Schwid HA, Rooke GA, Michalowski P, Ross BK. Screen-based anesthesia simulation with debriefing improves performance in a mannequin-based anesthesia simulator. *Teach Learn Med.* 2001;13:92–96

111. Shapiro MJ, Morey JC, Small SD, Langford V, Kaylor CJ, Jagminas L, Suner S, Salisbury ML, Simon R, Jay GD. Simulation based teamwork training for emergency department staff: does it improve clinical team performance when added to an existing didactic teamwork curriculum? *Qual Saf Health Care.* 2004;13:417–421

112. Cherry RA, Williams J, George J, Ali J. The effectiveness of a human patient simulator in the ATLS shock skills station. *J Surg Res.* 2007;139:229–235

113. Savoldelli GL, Naik VN, Park J, Joo HS, Chow R, Hamstra SJ. Value of debriefing during simulated crisis management: oral versus video-assisted oral feedback. *Anesthesiology.* 2006;105:279–285

114. Edelson DP, Litzinger B, Arora V, Walsh D, Kim S, Lauderdale DS, Vanden Hoek TL, Becker LB, Abella BS. Improving in-hospital cardiac arrest process and outcomes with performance debriefing. *Arch Intern Med.* 2008;168:1063–1069

115. DeVita MA, Schaefer J, Lutz J, Wang H, Dongilli T. Improving medical emergency team (MET) performance using a novel curriculum and a computerized human patient simulator. *Qual Saf Health Care.* 2005;14:326–331

116. Wayne DB, Butter J, Siddall VJ, Fudala MJ, Linquist LA, Feinglass J, Wade LD, McGaghie WC. Simulation-based training of internal medicine residents in advanced cardiac life support protocols: a randomized trial. *Teach Learn Med.* 2005;17: 210–216

117. Clay AS, Que L, Petrusa ER, Sebastian M, Govert J. Debriefing in the intensive care unit: a feedback tool to facilitate bedside teaching. *Crit Care Med.* 2007;35:738–754

118. Blum RH, Raemer DB, Carroll JS, Dufresne RL, Cooper JB. A method for measuring the effectiveness of simulation-based team training for improving communication skills. *Anesth Analg.* 2005;100:1375–1380

# DISCLOSURES

**GUIDELINES PART 15:** Neonatal Resuscitation Writing Group Disclosures

| Writing Group Member | Employment | Research Grant | Other Research Support | Speakers' Bureau/ Honoraria | Ownership Interest | Consultant/ Advisory Board | Other |
|---|---|---|---|---|---|---|---|
| John Kattwinkel | University of Virginia—Professor of Pediatrics | None | None | None | None | None | None |
| Jeffrey M. Perlman | Weill Cornell-Professor of Pediatrics | †NIH-NIH- Improving antimicrobial prescribing practices in the NICU | None | None | None | None | None |
| Khalid Aziz | University of Alberta— Associate Professor of Pediatrics | None | None | None | None | None | None |
| Christopher Colby | Mayo Clinic–physician | None | None | None | None | None | None |
| Karen Fairchild | University of Virginia Health System—Associate Professor of Pediatrics | None | None | None | None | None | None |
| John Gallagher | Univ. Hosp of Cleveland-Crit Care Coordinator of Ped.Resp Care | None | None | None | None | None | None |
| Mary Fran Hazinski | Vanderbilt University School of Nursing—Professor; AHA ECC Product Development-Senior Science Editor †Significant AHA compensation to write, edit and review documents such as the 2010 AHA Guidelines for CPR and ECC. | None | None | None | None | None | None |
| Louis P. Halamek | Stanford University—Associate Professor | †Laerdal Foundation: The Laerdal Foundation (not company) provided a grant to the Center for Advanced Pediatric and Perinatal Education at Packard Children's Hospital at Stanford during the academic years 2006–07, 2007–08, 2008–09; I develop simulation-based training programs and conduct research at CAPE. This support was provided directly to my institution. | None | *I have received < 10 honoraria in amounts of $500 or less from speaking at various academic meetings in the past 24 months; none of these meetings were conducted by for-profit entities. | None | *Laerdal Medical Advanced Medical Simulation Both of these companies reimburse me directly. | *I provide medical consultation to the legal profession for which I am reimbursed directly. |
| Praveen Kumar | PEDIATRIC FACULTY FOUNDATION- ATTENDING NEONATOLOGIST | None | None | None | None | None | None |
| George Little | Dartmouth College- Ped. Professor; Dartmouth Hitchcock Medfont. Center Neonatologist | None | None | None | None | None | None |
| Jane E. McGowan | St Christopher's Pediatric Associate/ Tenet Healthcare—Attending neonatologist; medical director, NICU | None | None | None | None | None | * reviewed records of cases involving neonatal resuscitation on one or two occasions over the past 5 years. *As co-editor for Textbook of Neonatal Resuscitation 6th edition, to be published by the AAP, being paid a total of $4000 over 3 years by the AAP. |
| Barbara Nightengale | Univ.Health Assoc,Nurse Practitioner | None | None | None | None | None | None |
| Mildred M. Ramirez | Univ of Texas Med School Houston-Physician | None | None | *Signed as consultant for Cyto-kine Pharmasciences, Inc., for a lecture in Mexico City. Product Propress for cervical rippening. $2,000 Money to Univ. | None | None | *Expert for Current expert case of triplets and preterm delivery. Money to the university '09 |
| Steven Ringer | Brigham and Women's Hospital–Chief, Newborn Medicine | None | None | *Vermont Oxford Neonatal Network, $1000, comes to me | None | *Alere $2000, consultation Dey Pharamaceutical $1000 Consultation Forrest Pharmaceuticals $1500 Grant Review Committee | †Several Attorneys, serving as expert witness in Medical malpractice cases |
| Wendy M. Simon | American Academy of Pediatrics–Director, Life Support Programs | None | None | None | None | None | None |
| Gary M. Weiner | St. Joseph Mercy Hospital-Ann Arbor Michigan—Attending Neonatologist | None | †Received equipment on-loan (3 resuscitation mannequins, 2 sets of video recording equipment) from Laerdal Medical Corporation to be used to complete a research project evaluating educational methods for teaching neonatal resuscitation. The value of the on-loan equipment is approximately $35,000. | None | None | None | None |

*(Continued)*

**GUIDELINES PART 15:** Neonatal Resuscitation Writing Group Disclosures, *Continued*

| Writing Group Member | Employment | Research Grant | Other Research Support | Speakers' Bureau/ Honoraria | Ownership Interest | Consultant/ Advisory Board | Other |
|---|---|---|---|---|---|---|---|
| Myra Wyckoff | UT Southwestern Medical Center–Associate Professor of Pediatrics | †American Academy of Pediatrics Neonatal Research Grant-Ergonomics of Neonatal CPR 2008–2009 | †Received a SimNewB neonatal simulator for help in Beta testing prior to final production | *Speaker at Symposia on Neonatal Care from University of Miami-honoraria paid to me Speaker at Symposia on Neonatal Care from Columbia/ Cornell-honoraria paid directly to me Speaker for Grand Rounds from University of Oklahoma-honoraria paid directly to me | None | None | None |
| Jeanette Zaichkin | Seattle Children's Hospital–Neonatal Outreach Coordinator | None | None | *I receive honoraria directly to me from the AAP as compensation for editorial activities for NRP instructor ms. | None | None | None |

This table represents the relationships of writing group members that may be perceived as actual or reasonably perceived conflicts of interest as reported on the Disclosure Questionnaire, which all members of the writing group are required to complete and submit. A relationship is considered to be "significant" if (a) the person receives $10 000 or more during any 12-month period, or 5% or more of the person's gross income; or (b) the person owns 5% or more of the voting stock or share of the entity, or owns $10 000 or more of the fair market value of the entity. A relationship is considered to be "modest" if it is less than "significant" under the preceding definition.

*Modest.

†Significant.

**Neonatal Resuscitation: 2010 American Heart Association Guidelines for Cardiopulmonary Resuscitation and Emergency Cardiovascular Care**

John Kattwinkel, Jeffrey M. Perlman, Khalid Aziz, Christopher Colby, Karen Fairchild, John Gallagher, Mary Fran Hazinski, Louis P. Halamek, Praveen Kumar, George Little, Jane E. McGowan, Barbara Nightengale, Mildred M. Ramirez, Steven Ringer, Wendy M. Simon, Gary M. Weiner, Myra Wyckoff and Jeanette Zaichkin

*Pediatrics* 2010;126;e1400-e1413; originally published online Oct 18, 2010;
DOI: 10.1542/peds.2010-2972E

| | |
|---|---|
| **Updated Information & Services** | including high-resolution figures, can be found at: http://www.pediatrics.org/cgi/content/full/126/5/e1400 |
| **References** | This article cites 113 articles, 33 of which you can access for free at: http://www.pediatrics.org/cgi/content/full/126/5/e1400#BIBL |
| **Permissions & Licensing** | Information about reproducing this article in parts (figures, tables) or in its entirety can be found online at: http://www.pediatrics.org/misc/Permissions.shtml |
| **Reprints** | Information about ordering reprints can be found online: http://www.pediatrics.org/misc/reprints.shtml |

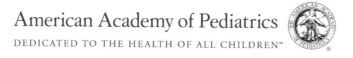

American Academy of Pediatrics
DEDICATED TO THE HEALTH OF ALL CHILDREN™

# Index

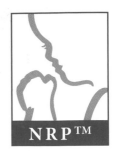

# Index

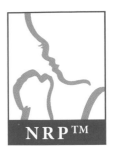

expansion of blood volume, 223–224
infusion of dopamine, 251
lack of improvement, 226
magnesium sulfate, 248
naloxone, 214, 247, 248
for neonatal resuscitation, 32
nitric oxide, 250
performance checklist and, 230–236
resuscitation with positive-pressure ventilation, chest compressions, and, 212–214
shock and, 223
via umbilical vein, performance checklist and, 230–236
Metabolic acidosis, 250–251
Methadone maintenance, 248
Mortality, 284
Mouth
anomalies of, and need for laryngeal mask airway, 191
suctioning of, 46
"MR SOPA," 95, 98, 238, 239, 276
Multiple births, personnel present at, 18
Muscle tone, 15, 40
Myocardial function
compromised, 223
deterioration of, 7, 9, 136
epinephrine for, 136

## N

Naloxone, 214, 247, 248
Narcotics, 8, 247, 248
Neck, anomalies of, and need for laryngeal mask airway, 191
Necrosis, tubular, 251
Necrotizing enterocolitis, 252, 278
Neonatal deaths, 2
Neonatal pneumonia, 250
Neonatal resuscitation. *See also* Resuscitation
actions after successful, 249
advantages and disadvantages of ventilation devices, 77–78
Apgar score and, 15
application of ethical principles to, 286–287
for babies born outside of hospital, 255–256
characteristics of devices used in, 79–81
characteristics of face masks and effectiveness of, 88
clearing airway and, 42, 46
concentration of oxygen used in positive-pressure ventilation, 85–86
determining need for, 40
endotracheal intubation, discontinuation of, 168
equipment/supplies needed for, 19, 162–164
establishing intravenous access during, 215–217
ethics in not initiating, 287–288
giving free-flow oxygen using device, 87
initial steps in, 41–42
laryngeal mask airway in, 160
legal applications, 287
life support following, 292
against parental wishes, 289
performance checklist for, 65–69
position of baby, 41–42
post-resuscitation care following, 20
preparing for, 15
preparing resuscitation device for anticipated, 88–89
presence of meconium, 42–44
prevention of heat loss, 47
prioritizing actions in, 14
provision of warmth, 41
reasons for learning, 2
risk factors associated with need for, 16
role of parents in decisions on, 287
routine care following, 20
safety feature of devices, 82–83
stimulating breathing, 47–49
supplies and equipment, 32–33
types of devices in, 75–77
Neurologic injuries
brain injury. *See* Brain injury
decreasing chances of, 277
Neuromuscular disorder, congenital, 247
Newborns
assisting ventilation in compromised, 50–51
birth at term, 40
breech presentation of, 16
care of, who could not be resuscitated, 284–285
caring for dead or dying, 293–294
characteristics of face masks and effectiveness of, for, 88
heart rate in evaluating, 50
need for resuscitation, 2
nonimprovement of, and chest compressions, 146
perinatal compromise in, 8–9
positioning of, in endotracheal intubation, 170
positioning of head, 90
respirations in evaluating, 50
response of, to interruption in normal transition, 7–8
resuscitation of apparently healthy, 256–258
uncertainty about chances of survival, 291
Nitric oxide, 250
Nutrition, 278

## O

Obstetric care plan, 285
Obstetrical dating, 288
Oligohydramnios, 16, 246
Oral airway in endotracheal intubation, 162
Orogastric tube
bag-and-mask ventilation and, 72, 73
equipment in inserting, 100
laryngeal mask airway placement and, 192
need for, 98, 99, 116, 208
removal of, 73, 192
steps in inserting, 100–101
in venting stomach, 146
Oropharynx
blocked airway and, 94
cleaning meconium from, 39
PPV mask ventilation, 99, 240
Overheating, 252, 272
Oximeter/oximetry, 57, 58. *See also* Pulse oximeter
how oximeters work, 53–54
use of oximeter, 52, 53–54
Oxygen, 55–56. *See also* Free-flow oxygen; Supplemental oxygen
adjusting, 274
concentration of, in T-piece resuscitator, 130
flow of concentration and pressure in flow-inflating bags, 125–126
if oxygen saturation not rising, 93–95
amount to be used, 273–274
appropriate amount of, 278
capability to deliver variable concentration, 80
checking for adequate, 98
compressed air and oxygen source, 80
excessive, 13
in positive-pressure ventilation, 85–86
receipt of
before birth, 4–5
from lungs, 5–6
Oxygen blender, 32, 54, 55, 56, 72, 80, 88, 89, 125, 130, 271, 274
Oxygen (gas) inlet
in flow-inflating resuscitation bags, 122
in self-inflating resuscitation bags, 117
in T-piece resuscitator, 128
Oxygen mask, 55
Oxygen reservoir, need for self-inflating bags, 118–119
Oxygen tubing, 56
Oxyhemoglobin saturation, 85, 274, 279

## P

Palliative treatment, 290, 291
Parents
    follow-up arrangements with, 294
    role of, in decisions about neonatal
        resuscitation, 9–5
    telling, newborn is dead or dying, 293
Partial pressure of oxygen ($Po_2$) in fetus, 4
Patient (gas) outlet
    in flow-inflating resuscitation
        bags, 122
    in self-inflating resuscitation bags, 117
    in T-piece resuscitator, 128
Patient T-piece in T-piece resuscitator, 128
Peak inspiratory pressure (PIP), 74, 75, 76,
        77, 78, 82, 83, 128, 129, 130
Peak pressure, capability to control, 81
Pediatric Advanced Life Support (PALS),
        256, 277
Pediatric Education for Prehospital
        Professionals (PEPP) program of
        American Academy of
        Pediatrics, 256
Performance checklists
    chest compressions and, 153–157
    endotracheal intubation and, 202–210
    epinephrine via endotracheal tube and,
        230–236
    medications and, 230–236
    medications via umbilical vein and,
        230–236
    for positive-pressure ventilation,
        112–116
Perinatal compromise, 8–9, 20
Perinatal death, support for staff in nursing
        after, 295
Perinatal loss support group, 294
Peripheral vasoconstriction, 219
Persistent pulmonary hypertension of
        newborn, 7, 58
Pharyngeal airway malformation, 241–242
Pharynx anomalies, and need for laryngeal
        mask airway, 191
Phenobarbital, 252
Placenta previa, 223
Placental membrane, 4
Plastic-bag technique, 272
Pleural effusions, 243
Pneumonia, 250, 254
    congenital, 246
    neonatal, 250
Pneumothorax, 82, 93, 99, 117, 126, 226,
        242–243, 250, 277
    complication of, in endotracheal
        intubation, 187
    evacuation of, 243–246
Pop-off valve, 30, 78, 82, 83, 117

Positive end-expiratory pressure (PEEP),
        74, 75, 76, 77, 78, 79, 81, 82, 87,
        104, 124, 128, 129, 130
    assisting ventilation, 274–276
Positive end-expiratory pressure (PEEP)
    cap in T-piece resuscitator,
        95, 128
Positive-pressure device
    in endotracheal intubation, 162
    preparing, for administering, 167
Positive-pressure ventilation, 9, 18, 48, 51,
        72, 73, 160, 258
    advantages and disadvantages of
        assisted-ventilation devices,
        77–78
    characteristics of face masks in, 88
    characteristics of resuscitation devices
        in, 79–81
    checks before beginning, 90
    components of, 74
    concentration of oxygen used, 85–86
    controls of respiratory limits during,
        with resuscitation devices, 83
    effectiveness, assessment of, 85–86
    failure to result in adequate ventilation,
        238–240
    giving free-flow oxygen using
        resuscitation devices, 87
    indications for, 74
    insertion of orogastric tube, 100–101
    lack of improvement with, 98–99
    medication and, 212–214
    need for orogastric tube, 99
    people needed to perform, 17, 18
    performance checklist, 112–116
    preparing resuscitation devices for,
        88–89
    proper ventilation rate in, 95
    resuscitation with chest compressions
        and, 134–135, 212–214
    safety features of resuscitation devices,
        82–83
    types of resuscitation devices for, 75–77
    use of resuscitation devices for, 71–132
Post-resuscitation care, 249, 254
    following neonatal resuscitation, 20
Premature babies
    risk factors for, 17
    vulnerability of, to injury from excess
        oxygen, 57
Premature newborn, length of trachea
        in, 164
Pressure, controlling in self-inflating
        bag, 121
Pressure gauge in self-inflating
        resuscitation bags, 117
Pressure-gauge attachment site in flow-
        inflating resuscitation bags, 122

Pressure-release valve, 78
    in self-inflating resuscitation bags, 117
Preterm babies
    evaluation of, 40
    lungs of, 40
Primary apnea, 8, 9, 48
Prophylactic administration of
        surfactant, 276
Pulmonary arterioles, sustained
        constriction of, 7
Pulmonary hypertension, 16, 245,
        249–250, 254
    persistent, in newborn, 7, 58
Pulmonary hypoplasia, 246
Pulse oximeter, 258, 274
    in endotracheal intubation, 162

## R

Radiant warmer, 19, 40, 41, 268
    for preterm newborns, 271, 272
    resuscitation using, 10, 39, 72, 134
    supplies and equipment at, 34
    therapeutic hypothermia, 253
Reflex irritability, 15
Respirations
    actions on abnormal, 50–51
    in evaluating newborn, 50
    failure to begin spontaneous, 247–248
Respiratory distress, 242, 243
    after resuscitation, 249, 250
    choanal atresia and, 240
    cyanosis and, 54
    diaphragmatic hernia, baby with, 245
    PPV upon persistency or worsening of,
        11, 55
Resuscitation. *See also* Neonatal
        resuscitation
    of apparently healthy newborn,
        256–258
    with bag and mask and oxygen, 72–73
    complications after initial attempts
        at, 238
    discontinuation of, 292
    endotracheal intubation during, 168
    flow diagram, 10–13
    initial steps in, 65–69
    involving meconium, 39
    maintaining body temperature
        during, 2
    with positive-pressure ventilation, chest
        compressions and, 134–135
    preparing for, 47
    of preterm babies, 267–282
        assisting ventilation, 274–276
        decreasing chances of brain injury,
        277
        keeping baby warm, 272

# Textbook of Neonatal Resuscitation, 6th Edition
## Evaluation

1. In which Neonatal Resuscitation Program™ (NRP™) course did you use the *Textbook of Neonatal Resuscitation, 6th Edition*?
   ☐ Standard Provider Course      ☐ Instructor Course With a Provider Component

2. Please indicate your medical credentials.
   MD   DO   RN   NNP   RT   PA   EMT-P   EMT      Other (please indicate): _____

3. Have you previously taken an NRP course?      ☐ Yes      ☐ No

4. Please use the scale below to rate the *Textbook of Neonatal Resuscitation, 6th Edition*, on the qualities listed.
   **1** = Strongly Disagree      **2** = Disagree      **3** = Agree      **4** = Strongly Agree

| | 1 | 2 | 3 | 4 |
|---|---|---|---|---|
| The textbook was well written. | 1 | 2 | 3 | 4 |
| The textbook effectively communicates the principles of the Neonatal Resuscitation Program. | 1 | 2 | 3 | 4 |
| The resuscitation flow diagram is easy to use. | 1 | 2 | 3 | 4 |
| Information follows a logical sequence from lesson to lesson. | 1 | 2 | 3 | 4 |
| The textbook adequately prepares a health care worker to participate in a neonatal resuscitation. | 1 | 2 | 3 | 4 |
| The case scenarios are useful. | 1 | 2 | 3 | 4 |
| The illustrations are useful. | 1 | 2 | 3 | 4 |
| The Performance Checklists match the course content. | 1 | 2 | 3 | 4 |
| The textbook is attractive and well designed. | 1 | 2 | 3 | 4 |
| The color photos throughout the text are useful. | 1 | 2 | 3 | 4 |
| The overall design of the textbook supports independent learning. | 1 | 2 | 3 | 4 |
| The practice activities aid in the learning process. | 1 | 2 | 3 | 4 |

5. Have you used the *Textbook of Neonatal Resuscitation, 6th Edition, Multimedia DVD-ROM*?      ☐ Yes      ☐ No
   5a. Were the boxes within the text directing you to view segments of the DVD-ROM helpful?      ☐ Yes      ☐ No
   5b. If you answered yes to the above question, feel free to include any comments about the DVD-ROM below.

   _____
   _____
   _____

6. What aspects or features of the textbook enhanced your learning?

   _____
   _____
   _____

7. How could the textbook be improved?

   _____
   _____
   _____

This evaluation also may be completed online at *http://www.aap.org/nrp/survey,* or you may turn in this completed evaluation to your course instructor. Fax completed evaluations to 847/228-1350, or mail to American Academy of Pediatrics, Division of Life Support Programs, 141 Northwest Point Blvd, Elk Grove Village, IL 60007-1098.